Status epilepticus, *the maximum expression of epilepsy*, is a distinctive condition, much more than simply a severe version of ordinary epilepsy. This is the definitive reference book on the subject, taking a modern look at the clinical features, pathophysiology and treatment of status, in both adults and in children.

All forms of status are considered, including the classical convulsive (grand mal) type, the less well-understood yet common and fascinating nonconvulsive variants, boundary syndromes and also pseudostatus epilepticus. The history, clinical aspects, treatment and outcome of each form are explored in their scientific context. Research findings in the fields of epidemiology, neurophysiology, neuroanatomy, neuropathology, neurochemistry and neuropharmacology are reviewed. Received ideas are examined critically, the existing schemes of classification revised, and current practice is challenged where it seems inadequate.

Treatment is dealt with in depth, and schemes of management outlined for both convulsive and nonconvulsive forms. For each drug used in status, a systematic review is given of the pharmacology, clinical and toxic effects in status, administration and dosage. Summary tables outline key clinical information.

The text is based on extensive clinical experience of the author, and a practical and theoretical perspective is taken throughout. The world literature is marshalled to provide a comprehensive review of the topic in all its aspects. The book is therefore both a reference work and a practical guide, useful for a wide range of clinicians, including neurologists, psychiatrists, paediatricians, including other specialists and generalists, and all those dealing with emergency and intensive care medicine.

Status epilepticus
its clinical features and treatment in children and adults

Frontispiece Poriomania (ambulatory fugue) in nonconvulsive status epilepticus: a famous case. A map of Paris showing the routes of three episodes of long fugue in a patient described by Charcot during his Tuesday lectures on 31 January 1888. These remarkable ambulatory fugues were attributed by Charcot to epilepsy in a long and interesting discourse. The patient was a 37 year old delivery man.

Fugue 1: This started in the Avenue de Villiers (1) where the patient was on an errand. He then vaguely remembers being near Mont Valerien (2), and then crossing Pont de St Cloud (3). He then regained consciousness finding himself in Place de la Concorde (4), 14 hours after the onset of the fugue.

Fugue 2: The patient delivered in a parcel in rue de Passy (5), then the amnestic period began. He remembers walking to the bottom of Trocadero (6), seeing the foundations of the Eiffel Tower (7), and then nothing more for 42 hours. He awakened to find himself swimming in the River Seine, having jumped into the water near the Pont National in Bercy (8).

Fugue 3: He visited a house on rue du Chemin Vert (9), where this long fugue began. He left Paris (10) and his next memory is awakening in the town of Claye (about 29 km to the northwest). Here he visited a restaurant, and remembers nothing more again until consciousness was regained on the banks of the Seine near the Asnières bridge (11), two days later.

The patient experienced amnesia for the attacks, except for these fragments of memory, yet witnesses apparently noticed nothing amiss. He was treated successfully with potassium bromide for 1 year, the drug was then withdrawn and a further fugure occurred, lasting 8 days, in which the patient found himself inexplicably in Brest on the French southwest coast (where he was promptly arrested, in spite of the evidence of a prescription from Charcot, who was famed throughout France). Although there were no other positive features of nonconvulsive status (either of the absence or complex partial type), Charcot was convinced that the attacks had an epileptic origin, although some features are more suggestive of psychogenic fugue. The term poriomania, to describe unconscious wandering, was coined by Kraepelin. (The details are taken from the excerpts of Charcot's (1889) case presentations prepared and translated by Goetz (1987), whose idea of mapping the fugues was the model for this illustration. The exact perambulations of the patient between the numbered positions is speculative, and the map illustrates commonly used routes.)

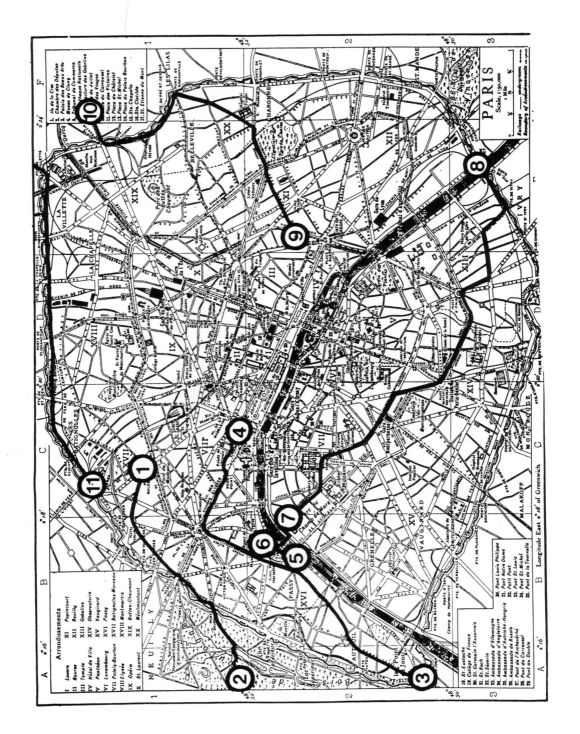

Status Epilepticus

its clinical features and treatment in children and adults

SIMON SHORVON

*Reader in Neurology, Institute of Neurology, University of London;
Consultant Neurologist, National Hospital for Neurology and Neurosurgery,
Queen Square, London; Medical Director, National Society for Epilepsy,
Chalfont St Peter, Buckinghamshire*

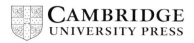
CAMBRIDGE
UNIVERSITY PRESS

Published by the Press Syndicate of the University of Cambridge
The Pitt Building, Trumpington Street, Cambridge CB2 1RP
40 West 20th Street, New York, NY 10011-4211, USA
10 Stamford Road, Oakleigh, Melbourne 3166, Australia

© Cambridge University Press 1994

First published 1994

Set in 10 on 12pt Ehrhardt, headings in Ehrhardt and Univers.

Printed in Great Britain at the University Press, Cambridge

A catalogue record for this book is available from the British Library

Library of Congress cataloguing in publication data

Shorvon, S. D. (Simon D.)

Status epilepticus : its clinical features and treatment in children and adults /
Simon Shorvon.
    p.   cm.
Includes bibliographical references and index.
ISBN 0-521-42065-2 (hardback)
1. Epilepsy.   I. Title.
[DNLM: 1. Status Epilepticus.   WL 385 S559s 1994]
RC372.S53   1994
616.8′53—dc20   93-24228 CIP

ISBN 0 521 42065 2 hardback

Contents

Frontispiece   iii–iv

Preface   xv

1   The concept of status epilepticus and its history   1

Pre-history of status epilepticus   1
Origins of status epilepticus   2
Classical descriptions of status epilepticus   4
Era of electroencephalography   13
Les Colloques de Marseille, and the definition and classification
    of status epilepticus   14
        Notes   17

**2   Definition, classification and frequency of status
epilepticus**   21

Definition of status epilepticus   21
Classification of status epilepticus   23
A new classification of status epilepticus   25
Frequency of status epilepticus   27
    Status epilepticus as a proportion of hospital admissions   28
    Status epilepticus as a proportion of all epileptic cases   28
    The timing of status epilepticus   28
    Factors influencing the frequency of tonic–clonic status epilepticus   29
Population estimates of the frequency of status epilepticus   30

3   Clinical forms of status epilepticus   34

Status epilepticus confined to the neonatal period   34
Neonatal status epilepticus   34
    Frequency   34
    Definition   35

Contents

Clinical forms 35
Electroencephalography 37
Causes 39
Status epilepticus in neonatal epilepsy syndromes 40
Early infantile epileptic encephalopathy 40
Neonatal myoclonic encephalopathy 40
Benign familial neonatal seizures 41
Benign neonatal convulsions 41
Status epilepticus confined largely to infancy and childhood 41
Infantile spasm (West syndrome) 42
Frequency and clinical form 43
Electroencephalography 43
Causes 44
Febrile status epilepticus 45
Status in childhood myoclonic epilepsies 46
Cryptogenic and symptomatic childhood myoclonic epilepsies 46
Syndrome of severe myoclonic epilepsy in infants 46
Syndrome of myoclonic status epilepticus in nonprogressive encephalopathy 47
Syndrome of myoclonic–astatic epilepsy 47
Status epilepticus in the benign childhood epilepsy syndromes 48
Benign rolandic epilepsy (benign epilepsy of childhood with
   rolandic spikes) 48
Benign occipital epilepsy 48
Electrical status epilepticus during slow wave sleep 49
Syndrome of acquired epileptic aphasia (Landau–Kleffner or
   Worster–Drought syndrome) 51
Status epilepticus occurring in late childhood and adult life 53
Tonic–clonic status epilepticus 53
Clinical features 53
Electroencephalography 61
Causes 66
Absence status epilepticus 76
Distinction between typical and atypical absence status
   epilepticus and other nosological problems 76
Frequency and clinical features 79
Electroencephalography 82
Cause 83
Epilepsia partialis continua 84
Russian descriptions (Russian spring–summer encephalitis) 85
Canadian descriptions (Rasmussen's chronic encephalitis) 85
Evidence for a cortical or subcortical origin, and the
   differentiation from myoclonus 86
EPC as focal motor epilepsy 91
Clinical and electroencephalographic features of EPC 94
Causes 95
Myoclonic status epilepticus in coma 98
Specific forms of status epilepticus in mental retardation 100
Lennox–Gastaut syndrome 101

Forms of status epilepticus in the Lennox–Gastaut syndrome
and other types of mental retardation — 103
Other syndromes of myoclonic status epilepticus — 109
Myoclonic status epilepticus in primary generalised epilepsy — 109
Status epilepticus in the progressive myoclonic epilepsies — 109
Nonconvulsive simple partial status epilepticus — 110
Complex partial status epilepticus — 116
Definition and subclassification of complex partial status epilepticus — 116
Clinical features — 118
Electroencephalography — 127
Anatomical site — 128
Causes — 129
Boundary conditions — 130
Electrographic status epilepticus with subtle clinical signs — 130
Prolonged postictal confusional states — 131
Epileptic behavioural disturbances and psychosis — 131
Status epilepticus confined to adult life — 135
De novo absence status epilepticus of late onset — 135
Pseudostatus epilepticus — 137

**4   Neurophysiology, neuropathology and neurochemistry
of status epilepticus** — 139

Experimental neurophysiology of status epilepticus — 140
Initiation of seizure activity in status epilepticus — 140
Spread and maintenance of seizure activity in status epilepticus — 141
Termination of status epilepticus — 149
Cerebral energy in status epilepticus — 150
Neuropathology of status epilepticus — 151
Neuropathological changes in status epilepticus: cause or effect? — 152
Human pathological studies — 152
Animal pathological studies — 158
Neurochemistry of status epilepticus — 165
Inhibitory mechanisms — 167
Excitatory mechanisms — 168

5   Emergency treatment of status epilepticus — 175

General measures — 175
Cardiorespiratory function and resuscitation — 176
Patient monitoring — 177
Intravenous lines — 177
Emergency investigations — 177
Intravenous glucose and thiamine — 177
Acidosis — 178

Contents

Aetiology	178
Pressor therapy	178
Other physiological changes and medical complications	179
Seizure and electroencephalographic monitoring	180
Intracranial pressure monitoring and cerebral oedema	182
Antiepileptic drug pharmacokinetics in status epilepticus	183
Drug absorption	183
Route of administration	183
Drug distribution, metabolism and excretion	185
Blood–brain barrier, lipid solubility and ionisation	185
Distribution of drugs and half-lives	186
Apparent volume of distribution	190
Clearance	192
Loading dose	192
Hepatic metabolism	192
Active metabolites	193
Excretion	193
Blood levels and interactions	194
Relation of blood level to activity	194
Drug interactions	194
Ideal antiepileptic drug in tonic–clonic status epilepticus	195
Physical characteristics	195
Side-effects and selectivity of pharmacological action	195
Pharmacokinetics	196
Antiepileptic action	197
Stages of drug treatment in tonic–clonic status epilepticus,	
and drug treatment regimens	198
Premonitory stage	198
Stage of early status epilepticus (0–30 minutes)	198
Stage of established status epilepticus (30–60 or 90 minutes)	201
Stage of refractory status epilepticus (after 60 or 90 minutes)	201
Long-term maintenance antiepileptic therapy	202
Failure of antiepileptic drug treatment	202
Antiepileptic drugs used in status epilepticus	203
Premonitory status epilepticus	203
Diazepam	203
Absorption	204
Distribution	205
Biotransformation and excretion	207
Clinical effect in status epilepticus	207
Toxic effects in status epilepticus	209
Administration and dosage in status epilepticus	211
Summary of use in status epilepticus	212
Midazolam	213
Absorption	214
Distribution	214
Biotransformation and excretion	214
Clinical effect in status epilepticus	214

Toxic effects in status epilepticus   215
Administration and dosage in status epilepticus   217
Summary of use in status epilepticus   217
Paraldehyde   218
   Absorption   218
   Distribution   219
   Biotransformation and excretion   219
   Clinical effect in status epilepticus   219
   Toxic effects in status epilepticus   220
   Administration and dosage in status epilepticus   221
   Summary of use in status epilepticus   223
Early and established status epilepticus   223
Chlormethiazole (chlomethiazole)   224
   Absorption   224
   Distribution   224
   Biotransformation and excretion   225
   Clinical effect in status epilepticus   226
   Toxic effects in status epilepticus   228
   Administration and dosage in status epilepticus   229
   Summary of use in status epilepticus   230
Clonazepam   230
   Absorption   231
   Distribution   231
   Biotransformation and excretion   232
   Clinical effect in status epilepticus   232
   Toxic effects in status epilepticus   233
   Administration and dosage in status epilepticus   234
   Summary of use in status epilepticus   234
Lignocaine (lidocaine)   235
   Pharmacokinetics   235
   Clinical effect in status epilepticus   236
   Toxic effects in status epilepticus   237
   Administration and dosage in status epilepticus   237
   Summary of use in status epilepticus   237
Lorazepam   238
   Absorption   239
   Distribution   239
   Biotransformation and excretion   241
   Clinical effect in status epilepticus   241
   Toxic effects in status epilepticus   243
   Administration and dosage in status epilepticus   243
   Summary of use in status epilepticus   243
Phenytoin   244
   Absorption   245
   Distribution   245
   Biotransformation and excretion   249
   Clinical effect in status epilepticus   250
   Toxic effects in status epilepticus   251

Contents

Administration and dosage in status epilepticus	252
Summary of use in status epilepticus	253
Phenobarbitone (phenobarbital)	254
Absorption	255
Distribution	255
Biotransformation and excretion	257
Clinical effect in status epilepticus	258
Toxic effects in status epilepticus	260
Administration and dosage in status epilepticus	260
Summary of use in status epilepticus	261
Stage of refractory status epilepticus: general anaesthesia	262
Thiopentone sodium (thiopental sodium)	262
Absorption	263
Distribution	263
Biotransformation and excretion	264
Clinical effect in status epilepticus	265
Toxic effects in status epilepticus	266
Administration and dosage in status epilepticus	267
Summary of use in status epilepticus	267
Pentobarbitone sodium (pentobarbital sodium)	269
Pharmacokinetics	269
Clinical and toxic effects in status epilepticus	270
Administration and dosage in status epilepticus	273
Summary of use in status epilepticus	274
Isoflurane	274
Pharmacokinetics	275
Clinical effect in status epilepticus	275
Toxic effects in status epilepticus	276
Administration and dosage in status epilepticus	277
Summary of use in status epilepticus	277
Etomidate	279
Pharmacokinetics	279
Clinical effect in status epilepticus	279
Toxic effects in status epilepticus	280
Administration and dosage in status epilepticus	281
Summary of use in status epilepticus	282
Propofol	282
Pharmacokinetics	282
Clinical effect in status epilepticus	283
Toxic effects in status epilepticus	283
Administration and dosage in status epilepticus	284
Summary of use in status epilepticus	285
Other drugs used in status epilepticus	285
Emergency treatment of other forms of status epilepticus	287
Neonatal status epilepticus	288
Status epilepticus in neonatal epilepsy syndromes	288
Infantile spasm (West syndrome)	288
Febrile status epilepticus	288

Status epilepticus in childhood myoclonic syndromes   289

Status epilepticus in benign childhood epilepsy syndromes   289

Electrical status epilepticus during slow wave sleep and
the syndrome of acquired epileptic aphasia   289

Absence status epilepticus and de novo *absence status*
epilepticus of late onset   290

Epilepsia partialis continua   290

Myoclonic status epilepticus in coma   290

Specific forms of status epilepticus in mental retardation   291

Other forms of myoclonic status epilepticus   291

Nonconvulsive simple partial status epilepticus   291

Complex partial status epilepticus and boundary syndromes   291

Prologue to therapy in status epilepticus   292

6   **Prognosis and outcome of status epilepticus**   293

Outcome of tonic–clonic status epilepticus (including generic
studies of status epilepticus)   293

Mortality and morbidity statistics from early series   293

Recent studies of mortality   294

Recent studies of morbidity   298

Factors influencing outcome   300

Outcome of other syndromes of status epilepticus   301

Neonatal status epilepticus   301

Status epilepticus in neonatal epilepsy syndromes   303

Infantile spasm (West syndrome)   303

Febrile status epilepticus   304

Status epilepticus in the childhood myoclonic epilepsies   306

Status epilepticus in benign childhood epilepsy syndromes   306

Electrical status epilepticus during slow wave sleep   307

Syndrome of acquired epileptic aphasia   307

Absence status epilepticus   308

Epilepsia partialis continua   308

Myoclonic status epilepticus in coma   309

Specific forms of status epilepticus in mental retardation   309

Other syndromes of myoclonic status epilepticus   310

Nonconvulsive simple partial status epilepticus   310

Complex partial status epilepticus   311

De novo *absence status epilepticus of late onset*   311

References   313

Index   365

Preface

Status epilepticus, the *maximum expression of epilepsy*, has been unrightfully ignored. Amongst the 35 000 published papers in the *Epilepsy Indexes*, which contain almost all the scientific citations to epilepsy between 1945 and 1978, only 370 were primary or secondary references to status. The first monograph devoted to the subject (*Les états de mal épileptique*; Gastaut *et al.* 1967) was the collected proceedings of the Xth Marseilles Colloquium of 1962, a providential meeting which was a landmark in status history. The only widely known English language monograph is the proceedings of the next international conference held in 1981 (*Advances in Neurology*, 34: *Status epilepticus: mechanisms of brain damage and treatment*; Delgado-Escueta *et al.* 1983). In the past three decades, interest in the condition has greatly intensified, stimulated particularly by improvements in its therapy. Status has now come to be seen, correctly, not simply as an iterative version of ordinary epilepsy, but as a condition in its own right with specific clinical and experimental features. The conceptual basis of status today is very different from that defined in Marseilles in the 1960s, and substantial advances have been made in the understanding of its clinical aspects, its treatment and its scientific basis. Contemporary status epilepticus encompasses more than just the grand mal condition, although this is still its most hazardous type. There are other less well-known forms, some much commoner than the tonic–clonic variant yet fascinating and ill understood.

The book aims to be a definitive text on status and to provide a thorough reappraisal of the subject, in the light of this modern research. I have attempted to examine current practice rigorously and critically, and in doing so to challenge existing tenets where these seem flawed. The conventional classification of status, designed as it is to parallel the seizure type classification scheme, is quite inadequate to describe the plurality of the clinical forms of status. A new scheme is proposed, encompassing the various nonconvulsive and myoclonic forms of status that fit uneasily into a seizure type approach. In this book, the clinical forms of status are grouped by age, and are categorised according to this revised classification scheme. Although electroencephalography is central to any understanding of epilepsy, the overreliance on electrographic form in defining and classifying seizure type and syndrome has tended in my view to inhibit clinical research in status, and this is given less weight here. Where possible, the clinical aspects of status are considered in the context of their scientific base, whether this be epidemiology, neurophysiology, neurochemistry, neuropathology or neuropharmacology. Similarly, I have endeavoured to relate experimental physiological, pathological and chemical research in status to a clinical context. A large space has been devoted to treatment, to provide a critical review of the published evidence of efficacy and toxicity of the individual drugs used in status (some of which, even for widely used drugs, is remarkably sparse), in relation to their pharmacokinetics and pharmacology. I have emphasised the currently fasionable drugs, even where these are relatively new and untried in status. Finally, in considering therapy, I have tried to maintain a practical bias, to give clear advice on anticonvulsant drug treatment and other points of management, and to provide a useful scheme for emergency therapy.

This book provides a comprehensive discourse on these aspects of status, embedded where possible in my own clinical experience. At the same time, I have striven to review rigorously the whole of the anglophone and most of the European literature, much of which is in relatively unknown and not easily accessible specialist journals. Our current clinical perspectives are best understood in terms of the evolution of the concept of status. I therefore make no apology for having, at times, adopted a deliberately historical approach to the basic scientific and clinical features, in a book otherwise intended as a reference work for neurologists, psychiatrists, paediatricians and other physicians with duties in emergency medicine and an interest in epilepsy.

I thank many colleagues at the Institute of Neurology, the National Hospital for Neurology and Neurosurgery and the National Society for Epilepsy for their advice and help in writing this book. I am particularly grateful to Drs Ley Sander and Mark Cook for their clinical comments, Drs David Fish and John Jefferys for their authoritative remarks on neurophysiological issues, Dr Martin Smith for an intensive-care physician's view on chapter 5, Dr Philip Thompson for helping me to come to grips with myoclonus and EPC, Dr Philip Patsalos for guidance on pharmacokinetic equations, Dr Brian Harding for his comments on neuropathology, Ms Bailey for help with historical detail from the magnificent library at Queen Square, and Dr Mohammed Sharief for his unstinting help in researching and preparing case material, and for his pharmacological perspective on chapter 5. I am grateful to Drs David Fish, Shelagh Smith and Brian Harding for providing material for illustrations, to Dr Sveinbjornsdottir for her beautiful drawing of the hippocampus for figure 4.4, to Ms Sue Gerrard and her team for expert pharmacy advice and to Mr George Kaim for his skill in preparing illustrations. Professor Jean Aicardi has also most kindly helped to clarify many issues particularly of childhood status. I also thank Dr Elizabeth Whitcombe for her skilful translations, discussions and help in chapter 1. I am enormously indebted to Mrs Anne Prasad of the Pharmaceutical Society of Great Britain for her very careful scrutiny of and comments concerning chapter 5, and to Professor George Mawer for his authoritative and detailed comments on the same chapter (there is no-one else in Britain with his depth of pharmacological knowledge of status). I am very grateful to Ms Carolyn Cowey for ordering and checking the reference section, and helpful comments on the text, and to my wife, Penelope Farmer, for civilising the text. The book would be much the poorer without all of this assistance, which was so kindly and freely given. Finally, I thank Dr Richard Barling, at Cambridge University Press, for his original suggestion that such a book be written, and along with his colleague, Dr Jocelyn Foster, for kindness and forbearance during the execution (a word, carefully chosen) of the task; Mrs Sandi Irvine for her excellent editing; and Peter Ducker, who designed the book. At the National Hospital for Neurology and Neurosurgery and the National Society for Epilepsy, there is a large epilepsy practice which forms the basis of my clinical experience and from which the case histories cited in the text are drawn. I am indebted to and thank both institutions and their patients.

Simon Shorvon

CHAPTER 1

The concept of status epilepticus and its history

If the possessing demon possesses him many times during the middle
watch of the night, and at the time of his possession his hands
and feet are cold, he is much darkened, keeps opening and shutting
his mouth, is brown and yellow as to the eyes... It may go on for
some time, but he will die.

(XXV–XXVIth tablet (obverse) of the Sakikku cuneiform[1],
718/612 BC)

Pre-history of status epilepticus

Epilepsy, that unrivalled hierophant of neurology, has an ancient pedigree. The
Sakikku cuneiform is the earliest known record, and there, with due foreboding,
is the first allusion to status (fig. 1.1). Surprisingly, though, in the long line of
historical reference to epilepsy which followed, status received scant attention.
No condition resembling status was recorded by Hippocrates in the fourth century
BC in his great work on epilepsy, nor by Galen in the second century. The
fifth-century Numidian, Caelius Aurelianus, gave a grave prognosis to protracted
epileptic attacks 'which extended into a second day', but there was little other
mention of prolonged seizures in the classical literature. Mediaeval medicine left
status undisturbed, although epilepsy was extensively described because of its
demoniacal associations. In renaissance times there were sporadic reports:

> the illustrious cardinal Commendoni suffered sixty epileptic paroxysms in
> the space of 24 hours, under which nature being debilitated and oppress'd
> he at leangth sank, and died. His skull being immediately taken off, I found
> his brain affected with a disorder of the hydrocephalous kind.
>
> (Gavassetti 1586)

> . . . whenas fits are often repeated, and every time grow more cruell, the
> animal function is quickly debilitated; and from thence, but the taint, by degrees
> brought on the spirits, and the Nerves serving the Praecordia, the vital
> function is by little and little enervated, till at length, the whole body
> languishing, and the pulse loosened, and at length ceasing, at last the vital
> flame is extinguished.
>
> (Thomas Willis 1667)[2]

1

After the mid-eighteenth century, more clinical observations were made of status, cases which were generally considered to be isolated curiosities (see Lysons 1772, Heberden 1802, and Good 1822 cited by Hunter 1959/60). It was only in the nineteenth century that status was clearly differentiated from the ordinary condition. The expression *état de mal* is first found in the University Dissertation of Louis Calmeil (1824)[3], where the term, coined by the patients themselves, was said to be common currency in the Bicêtre and Salpêtrière (see also Bouchet & Cazauvieilh 1825/6; Beau 1836) and how strangely appropriate it is that status should be christened in that 'museum of living pathology', so important to the history of epilepsy. The first appearance of the latinised English expression *status epilepticus* was in Bazire's translation of Trousseau's lectures on clinical medicine in 1867 (Trousseau 1868*a,b*).

Why, in contrast to epilepsy, was status so infrequently recorded, and so long in its recognition? Hunter (1959/60)[4] speculates that the condition was actually rare before powerful anticonvulsant drugs became available (bromides were introduced into clinical practice in 1857), and that the condition had become common due largely to the risks of sudden anticonvulsant drug withdrawal; a view that can be only partly substantiated, as many drug-naive patients presenting with status are encountered today. Status may have increased in frequency from the mid-nineteenth century, however, and it would be an irony indeed if this 'maximum expression' of epilepsy was in fact caused by its treatment.

Origins of status epilepticus

When Calmeil defined the term, status epilepticus was a condition barely recognised, probably rare, and not differentiated from the greater subject of epilepsy. Within a few years, however, began a growth in conceptual thought which has continued to the present day. This evolution can be divided conveniently, albeit artificially, into three phases, the first of which is that of classical description. Research was concentrated upon accurate clinical and pathological description; to this period we owe meticulous observations of individual cases, and the establishment of classical histology and morbid anatomy. The underlying assumption that status was simply a severe form of repetitive epilepsy was rejected, and the condition was viewed rather as a separate entity, 'a maximum expression of epilepsy', with clinical features distinct from ordinary seizures. The term was confined to grand mal status, and although other forms of continuing epilepsy had also been recognised these were not categorically linked. Rudimentary drug treatment was now possible – as always, a potent stimulus to research. The second phase was ushered in by the discovery of electroencephalography (EEG) in 1924 by Berger[5]. That single invention changed profoundly the theoretical basis of epilepsy and of status. EEG dominated research on status for the next four decades. During this time, the electrographic correlates of status were described and the basic neurophysiological principles of epilepsy established. Other clinical and experimental research was carried out, but was mainly subservient to EEG. Treatment was also advanced. The Marseilles Colloquia of 1962 and 1964 (of which

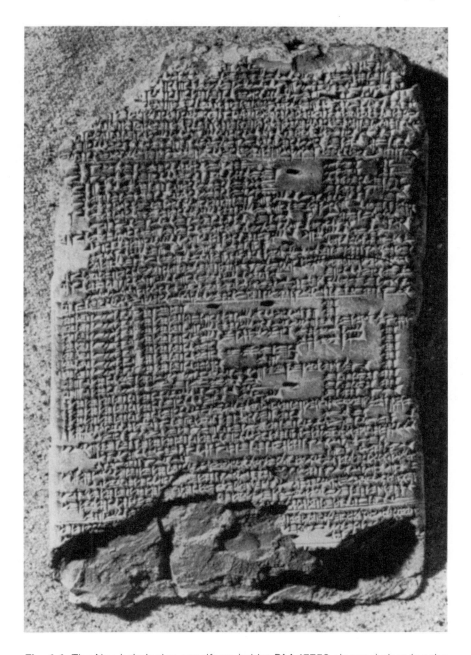

Fig. 1.1. The Neo-babylonian cuneiform (tablet BM 47753 obverse) showing the text of the XXV/XXVIth tablet of Sakikku (all diseases), which contains the first known reference to epilepsy and to status epilepticus. (From Kinnier Wilson & Reynolds 1990, with kind permission.)

3

more later) were landmarks in this evolution, and at these conferences definitions and classifications of seizures and of status were proposed, heavily influenced by EEG. Here was made implicit the concept that status was simply iterative seizures, rather than a specific entity (a return to pre-nineteenth century thought). The definition of status was also widened to include iterative versions of other seizure types (a logical step given the nosological basis), and the view was established that there are *as many types of status as there are types of seizure*. There was a relative neglect of other aspects of status, particularly study of its basic mechanisms, aetiology and anatomy. In the succeeding years, a third phase of activity has begun in which pharmacology, neurochemistry and experimental physiology have increasingly replaced human EEG as the focus of status research, and great advances in treatment have also been made. The clinical concepts of status have again expanded to include conditions crossing seizure type boundaries, and the utility of underpinning classification on the basis of seizure type is being challenged. New imaging methods have revived interest in the structural and anatomical basis of status, and in developmental aspects. Status is now again increasingly seen as an entity distinct from other seizure types. These topics form the substance of this book.

Before proceeding to these modern developments, though, in the rest of this chapter, the two earlier phases are discussed, some classical descriptions given, and the history of definition and classification traced from the Marseilles Colloquia; the current conceptual basis of status can best be understood in the context of such an historical approach.

Classical descriptions of status epilepticus

Modern neurology can be said to have emerged in the mid-nineteenth century, in London and Paris, with epilepsy its mystagogue. This was the age of meticulous scientific observation, made possible in epilepsy by the establishment of asylums and hospitals in which great numbers of epileptics were confined (Temkin 1971). In England, asylums for the mentally ill had existed at least since 1547 (when the hospital of St Mary of Bethlehem was incorporated as a royal foundation for the reception of lunatics; the famed 'Bedlam'), but such institutions specifically excluded sufferers from epilepsy. In the nineteenth century, attitudes changed, and epileptic cases were admitted first to county asylums, and then to the metropolitan institutions. It was the newly opened *National Hospital for the Paralysed and the Epileptic* that proved the most fertile ground in this golden age for epilepsy research. Here physicians such as Jackson, Ferrier, Gowers, Horsley, Sieveking, Turner and Colman saw and described cases of status[6]. In Paris, the Salpêtrière, the biggest asylum in Europe (housing up to 8000 persons in the eighteenth century when the total population of Paris was only 500 000, and 5000 persons in Charcot's time), and its sister institution the Bicêtre admitted epileptics from the early nineteenth century. In 1813, there were 389 epileptic women at the Salpêtrière and 162 epileptic men at the Bicêtre, but by the middle of the century these numbers had grown enormously. Esquirol, Calmeil, Pinel, Charcot and

Bourneville all cut their epileptic teeth at these institutions, and throughout Europe alienist physicians led this developing field.[7]

To Paris went the privilege of bringing status into the modern world, for it was here that Bourneville[8] at the Bicêtre, and Trousseau [9] at the Hôtel Dieu recorded the first clinical descriptions of status. Desiré Bourneville, favoured pupil of Charcot, published his celebrated paper in 1876. *Etat de mal* was defined as a 'serious complication' of epilepsy, distinguished by five characteristic features: (1) the repetition, more or less incessant, of seizures that in consequence often became subintrant; (2) collapsus, which varied in degree of severity from transitory loss of consciousness to complete and irreversible coma; (3) hemiplegia, more or less complete, but transitory; (4) characteristic rates of pulse and respiration; and (5) marked rise in temperature, persisting in intervals between seizures and intensifying after the seizures ceased. From personal observation, he recognised convulsive status to be an entity with 'progressive clinical stages', a concept only recently rediscovered (see pp. 53–4 and pp. 61–6), and his observations on temperature (his primary interest), pulse and the systemic effects of status have not been bettered.

He detailed the status in the case of Marie Lamb . . ., an epileptic hemiplegic and retarded girl of 19 years, in the Salpêtrière, starting on 8 June 1874 (Bourneville 1876). This is worth quoting at length as a masterful depiction of secondarily generalised tonic–clonic status, and a classic instance of meticulous observation. On the previous day Marie had had her habitual seizures at increasing frequency (17 in all). On the morning of 8 June, the seizures began to occur in series of three initially with consciousness intervening, but by 10.45 a.m. consciousness was lost, there were 17 seizures in 1¼ hours, her pulse rate was 128/ minute and vaginal temperature 39.3 °C; status had occurred. Bourneville identified three phases in each seizure:

> In the first phase – initiation – the legs, more so the left, were flexed slowly
> over the thighs and the patient uttered a kind of grunt, then several
> raucous cries in succession. In the second phase, her eyelids were closed;
> when opened, her eyes were seen to be strongly deviated to the left, and
> her face turned less sharply in the same direction; within four or five seconds,
> her eyes and face turned to the right; her left arm lay flexed and rigid
> across her body, the fingers tightly flexed across the thumb; her right arm
> was also stiff, but extended and raised 20 or 30 cm above her body, the fingers
> flexed but alongside the thumb; the lower limbs remained flexed and rigid.
> The third phase was marked by very strong and rapid convulsions of the
> right facial muscles, followed in several seconds by convulsions of the eyelids
> and the left frontalis; the mouth was deviated to the extreme right, the right
> nasolabial furrow strongly accentuated, the left obliterated; at the same time,
> clonic jerks of moderate intensity were observed in the lower limbs, more so
> the right; breathing was stertorous and there was much frothing at the mouth.

Bourneville noted certain modifications of this pattern in subsequent seizures:

> at the onset, flushing of the face; in the second phase, an asymmetry of the
> eyelids, the right closed, the left half-open; in the third phase, more

5

violent clonic jerks, the face purple and covered with sweat, more marked on one side than the other, with urinary incontinence.

Treatment was given with 'sinapismes, lavement purgatif' and quinine sulphate – to no effect. Between midday and 6.00 p.m., a further 122 seizures were recorded and another 7 between 6.00 and 6.30. Leeches were applied behind each ear and ammoniac inhalations administered. The patient moved her head, opened her eyes and moaned several times, as though waking. At 7.00, the pulse rate slowed from 124 to 100 and the temperature had fallen to 39.8. Treatment with quinine sulphate and ammoniac inhalations was continued. In the next two hours, two further seizures were recorded, bringing the total number over the 24 hours to 9.00 p.m. on June 8 to 168. Another 20 were recorded overnight, to 6.00 a.m. At intervals around midnight, the patient had become semi-conscious; she had seemed to recognise the nurse and had swallowed two spoonfuls of soup. At 9.00 a.m., the patient shook her head when an attempt was made at ophthalmoscopic examination and she moved her left arm; she opened her eyes from time to time; her gaze was dulled, and eyes and face turned mostly to the left, the pupils equal and constricted; a very fine nystagmus could sometimes be detected; her lips, gums and tongue were dry. The left arm was held above the bed, while the right arm was now completely flaccid, as were both lower limbs, more so the right. Pinprick repeated rapidly over all four limbs produced grimaces and sometimes little moans; when the face was pricked, the grimaces intensified. The pulse rate had now risen to 146, small, regular and readily palpable at the wrist; respirations were 60 per minute and (vaginal) temperature 40.6. By 11.00 a.m. no further seizures had been recorded but slight convulsive movements were noted from time to time in the limbs. Three hours later, the coma deepened; the skin had now taken on a yellowish pallor and breathing had become stertorous. At 4.00 the following morning, the patient died.

At autopsy on 10 June, the brain was found to be grossly abnormal, showing marked asymmetries, softening, swelling, atrophy of Ammon's horn and sphenoidal convolutions, and right hemisphere hemiatrophy and cavitation. Bourneville identified two periods in this case, as in the majority of cases of status: the convulsive and the meningitic. In the convulsive period, the increasingly rapid succession of the series of seizures, associated with a rise in body temperature, heralded the second. The two periods could, as in this case, be separated by some sort of temporary respite. The meningitic period might be brief or prolonged. It might be marked by decubitus, by violent agitation, or by contracture; the one constant feature was a dramatic rise in temperature. Temperature therefore should be regarded as the principal prognostic sign. The clarity and succinctness of this meticulous description earned Bourneville the Prix Godard of the Société de Biologie.

Trousseau (1868a,b) at the rival hospital of the Hôtel Dieu had explored, systematically, the various forms of epilepsy in his clinical lectures published 8 years before Bourneville's essay, and again recognised the special nature of status. He distinguished ordinary seizures from those 'which are repeated in rapid succession and end in the death of the patient' – true status epilepticus. He noted changes in the patterns of convulsions during status, and concluded that:

> in that form of status epilepticus where the convulsions are practically
> continuous something specific happens which demands an explanation.
> The patient is in the throes of his grand mal seizures; then, in a second or
> two, he has a slight convulsion in his face, in his neck or his limbs, a
> convulsion which is very fleeting, barely visible but which is repeated thus
> in 2, 3, 4 or 5 hours. A convulsive seizure is certainly continuing; but it
> is important to note that this is no longer a [simple] grand mal seizure; that
> it is something very different, something quite special, which is dependent
> on the particular state of irritation of the brain and spinal cord.

Trousseau also observed that petit mal seizures might, as with grand mal, occur with such frequency 'that one seizure would become confused with the next, simulating a continuous seizure which might persist for 2 or 3 days'; this was petit mal status, in the same sense, argued Trousseau, that convulsive status can be seen in patients with grand mal seizures (no further advances in this subject were made until Lennox uncovered the EEG pattern of petit mal). Indeed, as grand mal and petit mal seizures often occurred in the same individual, Trousseau considered the seizures to be variants of a single underlying diathesis, and strict differentiation was impracticable, a synoptical view of classification that anticipates the much more modern syndromic approach.

Although Trousseau identified petit mal status, his was not the first description of nonconvulsive status. Cases of epileptic fugue and furor, many of which were probably status, had interested physicians for at least the previous 100 years. Prichard[10] in 1822 wrote:

> epileptic delirium generally appears when the patient is expected to revive
> from the comatose state consequent upon a severe fit; but, in other
> instances, it appears without any fit. The face is flushed, and the aspect of
> the patient is like that of a man under intoxication; he attempts to start from
> bed and run about, and, on being witheld, vociferates and endeavours to
> overcome resistance. Sometimes the appearance of maniacal hallucination
> displays itself, but more generally the disorder resembles phrenetic delirium.
> It continues commonly one, two or three days, during which the patient
> requires confinement in a straight jacket, and then gradually subsides, and
> the patient returns to his previous state.

He also described epileptic ecstasy:

> a more unusual circumstance in the history of epilepsy is the appearance of
> a species of somnambulism, or of a kind of ecstasis, during which the
> patient is in an undisturbed reverie, and walks about, fancying himself
> occupied in some of his customary amusements or avocations.

Prichard documented cases, but did not link these to status; that distinction belonged to Sir Samuel Wilks, the great Guy's syphilologist (also the first systematically to employ bromides in the treatment of epilepsy). He recognised epilepsy to be characterised by two essential symptoms: complete loss of consciousness and convulsion. In grand mal status, both features were unmistakable. But there was also a condition associated with epilepsy, as Wilks saw it, in which neither could be detected:

> the patient is in the condition which is popularly called 'lost'; he is scarcely conscious of acts and conversation going on around him, and yet he may continue walking in a given direction, showing that his movements must still, in a measure, be guided by his senses. He is in a kind of dreamland, and is indeed in much the same state as a somnambulist. This condition, under many varieties of form, is called the status epilepticus, although the term is more usually applied to the case where the patient lies for a lengthened period in a kind of trance or stupor, as, for example, in the case of a man lately in the hospital, who, after a succession of fits, lay for hours in a state of lethargy. In the milder forms it is one of great interest from a physiological point of view and seems to point to the possibility of a subconscious state, in which the brain is sufficiently active to control the spinal system and yet not awake enough to excite the feeling of consciousness. In reference to the influence of the brain on the muscles and the necessity of consciousness to preserve their tone, the condition is one full of interest.

> (Wilks 1878)

Epileptic fugue had been the subject of other sporadic reports; an early example was that of Bright (1831) of a child of about 12–14 years old: 'he became delirious, and wandered in the streets in a state of complete unconsciousness from Clapham Common to Shoreditch, and was between four and five hours on the road'; Bright also described patients dying after a succession of seizures without intervening recovery of consciousness. Perhaps the most celebrated epileptic fugue was that presented by Charcot, on 31 January 1888, of a Parisian delivery man who, in nonconvulsive status, had repeated perambulations across and outside Paris (see frontispiece), lasting days at a time. There were only islands of memory of events during the fugues, but passers-by were unaware of anything untoward; he awoke from one fugue to find himself swimming in the Seine. On compelling grounds, Charcot considered these episodes to be epileptic. Hughlings Jackson also described cases of prolonged psychomotor epilepsy (see Taylor 1931 and p. 116). Amongst the other forms of status recognised in the nineteenth century must be mentioned infantile spasm (West syndrome) which was accurately described by West in 1841, and then lay virtually undiscovered for the next 100 years (see pp. 42–3). Cases of what would now be considered the Lennox–Gastaut syndrome, febrile status, postictal confusion, and myoclonic status were described by Jackson and Gowers. Kojewnikoff's classic description of *epilepsia partialis continua* was published in Moscow in 1895 (Kojewnikoff 1895*a,b*) (see p. 85). The early pathological descriptions of patients dying in status and of epilepsy were made by Sommer (1880), Pfleger (1880), Chaslin (1889), Alzheimer (1898) and Bratz (1899), and are discussed in more detail in chapter 4. Thus, by the end of the nineteenth century, convulsive and nonconvulsive status were recognised, and their clinical forms and associations documented.

In 1903, the era of the classic description can usefully be said to end with the writings of L. Pierce Clark[11] and Thomas P. Prout. The latter was a pathologist and the former an alienist, like Bourneville and others before him. Three papers were published in which the clinical and pathological appearances of status epilepticus were explored systematically in a series of 38 patients (Clark & Prout 1903/4). These descriptive papers on status are unequalled in breadth or perspicacity by any published before or since.

They formulated a definition of status, for the 'typical case': status epilepticus is the maximum development of epilepsy, in which one paroxysm follows another so closely that the coma and exhaustion are continuous between seizures. The state is almost always sooner or later accompanied by a marked rise of temperature, pulse and respiratory frequency, which is indicative of the degree of exhaustion. Their detailed clinical description is cited at length, for its discernment and accuracy, and in particular for its documentation of the natural course of status unaffected by antiepileptic drug treatment – an opportunity no longer with us, as modern treatment so profoundly alters the clinical appearance.

Two phases of grand mal status were notable, resembling the phases described by Bourneville, the first convulsive and the second stuporous. These were often preceded by a prodromal period in which could be noticed 'a steady increase in the paroxysmal frequency of seizures', 'a sort of pseudo-status' (the term is used currently in a different sense). They were 'the heralds; aborted, imperfect or incomplete status periods'.

The temporal pace of status was well observed. In the convulsive phase:

> Generally the attacks occur with an interval of one-half hour or a full hour at the onset. Each attack is complete and separate from its predecessor, keeping the peculiar individuality, common to each case of epilepsy. In Jacksonian, or better, partial epilepsy, the single seizure of the status holds to a distinct order of invasion, so long as exhaustion is not extreme and the definite order of muscular involvement is continued throughout the status. At first, consciousness is completely regained between paroxysms; a little later, as the periods between attacks shorten, consciousness is but partly regained, and finally the comatose state is not rallied from between attacks, and the stupor deepens into profound coma. In all cases in which a definite order of muscular involvement obtains, the subsequent coma is less profound and the status in consequence is less severe. As the attacks culminate in their greatest frequency, the period of rest between convulsions may be entirely omitted and some one part of the body may remain continuously in spasm; the part last involved in convulsion not ceasing from agitation before the muscles engaging in the initial stage of the next paroxysm begin again to sweep the rounds of the muscular invasion of the subsequent fit. The spasm may be incessantly clonic, or there may be a slight lessening of paroxysmal intensity, thus marking the end and the begining of isolated discharges; this overlapping is almost always seen in the convulsive stage of fatal status. With the increasing frequency of attacks the paroxysms usually diminish in intensity; the tonic period, if present at the beginning, may be obviated or omitted entirely in the advanced status. The paroxysms at the end of the convulsion

9

may be localized to a single muscle or a small group of muscles. Generally in status composed of fulminant convulsions, of general and simultaneous involvement, the end of the convulsive stage sees only slight general or fibrillary tremors throughout the whole body. As the exhaustion increases after the first few attacks there is elevation of temperature, increased pulse rate and respiratory frequency. The pulse and temperature may surmount to a great height, the temperature to 107 or 108 F., and pulse to 160 or 200 per minute. At last the convulsions lessen in frequency and the stuporous stage is ushered in with the coma of collapse, which picture is analogous to that of the coma of a dynamic fever, such as typhoid . . .

[The stuporous state] is but the resultant exhaustion from the convulsive stage; exhaustion, as it were, being piled on exhaustion. The mouth is foul, the tongue is dry and fissured, and the skin is covered with cold clammy sweat; swallowing becomes difficult or impossible. The urine is usually voided and stools may be passed involuntarily. The patient may die of asphyxia in the paroxysms, although as a general rule he passes a few hours in profound coma, in which stage, until death or convalescence, slight convulsive tremors may occur. Such convulsive phenomena are but mere phantoms of the former severe convulsions. Therefore one sees how purely arbitrary the clinical division of status into two stages may appear; in the one convulsion, and in the other coma, predominates. All the deep and superficial reflexes are abolished in the coma; the respiration becomes loud, noisy and stertorous in character; the temperature and pulse may undergo marked alteration depending upon the frequency and intensity of the foregoing symptoms. Death may terminate the stuporous stage at any time. If recovery is to occur, coma wears away, and is slowly replaced by stupor which in turn may be followed by mild delirium or hallucinations, which semi-exhausted state is finally replaced by a more or less rapid convalescence and the patient resumes the pre-status condition in a week or ten days. Generally, if recovery does not follow more or less promptly, a low muttering delirium supervenes, extensive sloughing of the nates follows and life itself is more or less suddenly terminated. The foregoing constitutes the usual clinical picture of a case of typical status epilepticus.

The duration of the episodes of status recorded by Clark & Prout was very variable, but most cases continued for 2–9 days, and prognosis was not related to duration (a view no longer tenable). They found, as their predecessors had done, that their 'typical' cases of status were characterised by specific clinical signs. Reflexes, deep and superficial, were lost 'as soon as the comatose stage in the convulsive period becomes continuous between paroxysms and invariably remain absent throughout the stuporous stage. They can again be elicited just before consciousness is regained; their return being often the first indication that consciousness will reappear'. Various changes in the eyes were noted. The pupils usually dilated during the early part of the convulsive period, contracting to normal after the paroxysms, but with deepening stupor they dilated and remained insensible to light. A change in the shape of the pupils, to an ellipse or 'wavy outline', at the onset of convulsions consisting of a general tremor was not unusual; they might also dilate with inspiration and constrict with expiration. A more or less persistent lateral nystagmus was characteristic of the later stages of status, and 'when not in motion, the eyeballs are rolled upwards and internally'. In the later stages of status the skin was covered by cold, clammy sweat 'in striking contrast with the real heat of the body shown by axillary or rectal temperature; urticaria was common as were subcutaneous haemorrhages'. Trophic disorders were of great importance: extreme bodily wasting – the usual loss of weight was about three or four pounds for each day of continuous convulsions – and the persistent forming of bed-sores, the most marked trophic abnormality. Desquamation of the skin, more or less complete, might follow convalescence; growth of hair and nails could also be disturbed. The patient in typical status usually sweated profusely, saturating the bedding in a few seconds. There was a distinctive pattern to be observed in the sweating. 'At first the sweat is like that of an individual undergoing great muscular exertions, but in the latter stages it is very clammy, and its solid constituents increase'. As Bourneville had already emphasised, in grand mal status body temperature usually rose after the first severe seizure, with a steep rise after the sixth or seventh. This could have prognostic significance: 'other things being equal, it may be stated that there exists a direct ratio between the number and severity of the convulsions and the resultant fever'. Pulse rate generally followed a course parallel to the fever curve, but was dependent on the frequency and severity of the seizures – and as such was thought to offer a more accurate index of the degree of exhaustion. The respiratory curve in general followed the temperature and pulse curves. Respiratory exhaustion marked the last phase of status but was not synonymous with death. Even though Cheyne–Stokes respiration was usual in all severe status, many patients had it but none the less recovered.

Not only did Clark & Prout describe grand mal status (typical status) but they also recognised other forms: status periods composed entirely of tetanoid or statuesque attacks; general clonic spasm, rhythmical throughout and without Jacksonian order of invasion; rapidly recurring series of myoclonic spasms 'constituting a status myoclonicus' (two cases, the first of whom had remained perfectly conscious, while the second had been comatose); nonconvulsive forms, much less frequent but none the less well recognised

> composed of delirium, stupor or coma, cough or hiccough, and a variety of
> psychic states which have for their basis cortical discharges resulting in
> more or less complete physical and psychical exhaustion; status comprising
> only psychic seizures, absences or vertigo, with or without a fever curve.

One case (now clearly identifiable as complex partial status) had 760 typical seizures in 12 hours, and the same case, a few days later, had a period of 500 psychic seizures, with subnormal temperature, 'a most unexplainable and interesting freak in the psychic phenomena of epilepsy'. Also recognised was the presence of 'status hystericus', 'which closely simulates true status epilepticus in many of its phases'. In 5 years' observations, 38 cases were of the idiopathic grand mal class, only 2 of the 'psychic variety'. While grand mal status usually ended in death, it was a rarity for 'psychic' status to do so.

In the previous 20 years, new methods for histological and morbid anatomical examination had evolved, which provided Clark & Prout with a scientific basis for a detailed discourse on the aetiology, pathology and mechanisms of status in their third paper. The morbid anatomy of seven cases was examined in detail. Status, it was concluded, as the maximum expression of epilepsy would provide a clue to the underlying causes of epilepsy itself. Aetiologies uncovered included infantile cerebral palsy, trauma, cerebral and meningeal haemorrhage. Developmental defects were regarded as particularly important from an aetiopathological standpoint, and they noted that over one third of cases had infantile cortical lesions. A sequence of pathological changes was found in status (and in the epileptic controls). The first lesion appeared in the nucleus of the nerve cell. The nuclear membrane and karyoplasmic network disappeared, and the karyoplasm became finely granular as a direct consequence of the destruction of the network, and the nucleolus, its anchorage thus destroyed, became a free body within the nucleus. Secondary changes then followed: the chromatin granules disappeared, and finally all trace of the nucleus, leaving the nerve cell as nothing more than a 'shapeless mass of vacuolated protoplasm'. Many neurones disappeared altogether from the cortex, especially from its second and third layers. The cortex was thereafter invaded by leucocytes, particularly the large mononuclear type, with marked phagocytic properties. The neuroglia then proliferated in place of the destroyed nerve cells, more particularly in the outer cortical layer, the proliferation being largely proportional to the duration and severity of the epilepsy. Clark & Prout were in no doubt that while there were a vast number of 'toxic and autotoxic' pathogenic agents in epilepsy, 'the hereditary instability of the cerebral cortex is the real basis of the causation of epilepsy'. They also noted that 'one attack of status paves the way for another, and there is no limit to the number of status periods that may occur before death supervenes', and considered that each repetition of the seizure phenomenon of epilepsy increases and accentuates the abnormal behaviour of cell function. This in turn tends to perpetuate the instability of the brain as a whole, and sets in train a series of degenerative changes whose logical termination is fatal status epilepticus. They considered that neither the subdivision of status into several varieties nor the drawing of a distinction between status and serial seizures served any useful purpose. Serial attacks they saw as 'nothing more than stepping stones to status', and convulsive and nonconvulsive forms merged into each other. Status was an entity which was the maximal expression of epilepsy and separate from epileptic seizures.

These observations are controversial even today, as we will see, and the questions raised in these papers have with few changes been the agenda for research over the rest of the century. Clark & Prout's remarkable study earned them the Stevens Triennial Prize at Columbia University, Ohio, for original research. But the three papers, published in the *American Journal of Insanity*, never entered the mainstream of neurological, or psychiatric, literature. Any subsequent references made to them were at best marginal. Their perceptions, particularly as far as the pathology of status was concerned, were not followed up. Little attention was paid to clinical status in the next 30 years. Such reports as appeared, in a desultory fashion, were confined to idiopathic grand mal status; they added little to the classical clinical descriptions and nothing to pathology.

Era of electroencephalography

'Practical methods of measuring . . . by physio-psychological means would be of the highest value', was how Clark & Prout thought epilepsy would best be advanced. A prescient statement, for, 20 years later, Berger's invention of the EEG provided just such a measure. EEG transformed the study of epilepsy, and, at a stroke, attention was diverted along physiological routes which dominated research for the next 50 years. 'The EEG demonstrates the pathological physiology of epilepsy to be a paroxysmal cerebral dysrhythmia', Gibbs & Lennox concluded definitively, from their study of 400 patients from 1935 to 1937, and the point is unarguable (Gibbs, Gibbs & Lennox 1937). The clinical seizure was 'but the outward manifestation of a disordered rhythm of brain potentials'. The impact of EEG on, and its enormous contribution to, all aspects of status is clear from the subsequent chapters of this book. The very success of EEG had also, however, negative effects, at least as far as status was concerned. An unfortunate consequence was the almost complete cessation of pathological or aetiological research, which had 30 years previously opened up such promising lines of enquiry. EEG also placed the emphasis on individual seizures (and the interictal state) rather than on status as a distinct entity (the severest expression of epilepsy). Anatomical research progressed only where linked to EEG, notably in the contribution made by Penfield[12] and his associates in Montreal. Their crucial achievement was to utilise the EEG (and stimulation and other experimental methods of localisation) during neurosurgery to identify the anatomical correlates of the main seizure types and the features of their clinical expression. In *Epilepsy and the functional anatomy of the human brain* (1954), Penfield & Jasper set out a scheme for the definition, classification and localisation of seizure types. Brief reference only was made to status epilepticus (under the heading, 'Unclassified Miscellany'); defined narrowly, as 'the state of frequently recurring, generalized convulsive seizures between which the patient is apt not to recover consciousness'. More enthusiasm was shown in regard to *epilepsia partialis continua*, 'a motor variant of some interest', first described by Kojewnikoff[13] (1895*a,b*). Penfield & Jasper also identified recurrent sensory phenomena, which were found to be 'at least as common as continuing circumscribed movement'. Thus, whilst the early work on EEG greatly enhanced understanding of the physiological basis of seizures, status remained steadfastly ignored. Perhaps the reason is mundane, simply that the muscle artifact caused by continuous convulsive movements obscures the scalp EEG recording?

An early triumph for EEG, was the discovery of *petit mal status*. Lennox[14], in 1945, described a form of sustained or recurrent petit mal seizures, and identified the EEG correlate of spike and wave discharges at 3 Hz. In 1960, in his eccentric work on epilepsy, he described his own experience (with the Gibbs) of 1039 cases of petit mal, of whom 27 (2.6%) had had a history of petit mal status alone or in combination with grand mal. Lennox's treatment of status was

13

somewhat uneven. Petit mal status was discussed, at some length, in his chapter on petit mal, but grand mal, or convulsive, status did not figure in his chapter on convulsive seizures. Instead, it formed a short chapter on its own, headed simply 'status epilepticus'. Lennox here defined 'status' as:

> a word used to distinguish a period in which symptoms are unduly severe, critical, or prolonged. Usually, as in status asthmaticus or status choreicus, the symptoms are continuous. A status of epilepsy might be termed 'discontinuous epilepsy' because, in the case of convulsions, these recur at irregular intervals of many minutes or hours. Attacks are strung like red beads on a black cord of continuing unconsciousness. In serial seizures such a connecting symptom is lacking . . .

What sets a seizure in motion? There was no answer to Lennox's rhetorical question and, as he acknowledged, 'the cessation of the seizure is almost equally strange'. He resorted to analogy: 'the brain batteries have run down and require time for recharging'. And he extended this curious thought to cover status: 'On occasion, however, and fortunately such occasions are unusual, the interval between seizures is seemingly too brief for the brain to recoup its energy, and the person has a long series of seizures while in a state of continued coma, with brain potentials, as recorded by the EEG, almost quiescent'. Lennox admitted that other forms of status might exist, variants, so to speak, of the principal grand mal and petit mal forms. 'Periods of tonicity without clonic movement may wax and wane and be the counterpart of the convulsive status', also 'a long period of automatism' lasting for hours or days, with islands of memory throughout this period, might be called a status', although 'a status of psychomotor seizures' as such, according to Lennox, had not been described (not in fact so, see Clark & Prout 1903/4).

However, in the *Revue neurologique* for 1956, Gastaut, Roger & Roger had published just such a description. This was of a a 56 year old nurse, admitted to hospital in a fugue state sustained apparently for some 2 months. The following year, she had a second such fugue, heralded by identical symptoms – loss of sleep and appetite for 15 days, irrational weeping and irritation, knocking repeatedly on doors with her fist. The epileptic character of the fugue was demonstrated by her EEG, and the clinical and EEG pattern was of psychomotor status epilepticus secondary to an irritative lesion of the left hemisphere.

Whilst only modest progress had thus been made in the EEG description of status, much greater were the achievements in the EEG study of epilepsy. Clinicoelectrographical descriptions of many different seizures types had been made, and the attention of clinicians was now turning to the thorny question of classification.

Les Colloques de Marseille, and the definition and classification of status epilepticus

This brings us to 1962, and the Xth Marseilles Colloquium (the tenth European electroencephalography meeting) in which the modern conceptual basis of status epilepticus – at least of its clinical forms – was formulated. This meeting was devoted to status (the first ever so to be). It was of great importance in the development of the theory of status, as here was put in place a system of classification of status that is perhaps only now being re-evaluated. Gastaut and his colleagues, leaning heavily on EEG data, proposed a comprehensive definition and, for the first time in the modern history of status, a systematic classification. A total of 103 participants presented 237 cases, with both clinical and EEG findings, 'of abnormally prolonged or serially repeated seizures, most of which did not correspond to the definition of status epilepticus accepted at that time' (Gastaut *et al.* 1967).

The conference (lead by Gastaut) proposed to extend the traditional 'historical' definition (corresponding to grand mal status) to an 'etymological definition', consistent with the meaning of status in the Latin, 'a manner of being fixed and durable': a condition characterised by an epileptic seizure which is so frequently repeated or so prolonged as to create a fixed and lasting epileptic condition. Implicit in this, as Gastaut (1983) recalled later, was not merely the notion that status epilepticus might take a variety of forms, but the specific hypothesis that there were *as many types of status as there were types of epileptic seizure*. At the time of the Marseilles Colloquium of 1962, the first version of the International Classification of Seizures was in preparation, also under the direction of Gastaut. In 1964, the proposed classification both of seizures and of status was presented to the XIIIth Colloquium, again at Marseilles, and an approved version of the *International Classification of Seizure Type* was eventually published in 1970. Gastaut *et al.* edited the proceedings of the 1962 conference on status, published this in 1967, and laid out a classification of status which paralleled the *International Classification of Seizure Type*. The definition and classification were subsequently included in the *WHO dictionary of epilepsy* (Gastaut 1973), and detailed in the *Handbook of clinical neurology* (Roger, Lob & Tassinari 1974) and *Handbook of electroencephalography and clinical neurophysiology* (Gastaut & Tassinari 1975).

The proposed definition of status epilepticus accepted by the conference, and enshrined in subsequent publications was 'a term used whenever a seizure persists for a sufficient length of time or is repeated frequently enough to produce a fixed or enduring epileptic condition'. This definition has been widely accepted, with little by way of modification. Gastaut's subsequent suggestion that the 'fixed and enduring epileptic condition' should last at least 30–60 minutes in order to qualify as status was also adopted as a clinical expedient.

The first *International Classification of Seizure Type* (Gastaut 1969, 1970) identified three main categories of seizure type, to be distinguished by both clinical and EEG features: partial, subdivided into elementary (simple) and complex; generalised, subdivided into convulsive and nonconvulsive; and unilateral, the features of which were similar in character to generalized seizures but their expression was confined 'principally' to one half of the body. Status was similarly classified, and the observations on 213 cases of status assembled at the Marseilles Colloquium were shepherded into these three categories in strict correspondence. When the *International Classification of Seizure Type* was published in 1970, status was mentioned only in an addendum, perhaps in recognition of the potential difficulties of categorisation; these inherent difficulties are expanded upon in subsequent chapters.

The first *International Classification of Seizure Type* used six criteria (clinical form, interictal EEG, ictal EEG, anatomical substrate, age, and aetiology, and dropped Gastaut's original proposal to include also interictal neuropsychiatric changes, response to treatment and pathophysiology (Gastaut 1969). In 1981, a revision was proposed, and officially adopted in 1982 (Commission on Classification and Terminology of the International League Against Epilepsy 1981). The original scheme was preserved, but partial seizures were subdivided into 'simple' and 'complex' according to whether or not consciousness was retained or lost, the unilateral category was abolished and a category of 'unclassified epileptic seizures' introduced. Of the original six taxonomic criteria, three (anatomical substrate, aetiology, age) were deleted, as being 'largely based on historical or speculative information rather than ... direct observation'. Types were now to be defined solely on the basis of clinical and EEG signs, ictal and interictal. Status remained of marginal interest, stored in the category of 'Addenda', defined as before as a 'seizure which persists for a sufficient length of time or is repeated frequently enough that recovery between attacks does not occur'. A precise definition of its characteristic features remained elusive. Most authors followed Gastaut in choosing, as the essential criterion, the duration of the prolonged or repeated seizure activity of more than 30 or more than 60 minutes. There was no agreement as to how 'recovery between attacks' could be defined. The issue of consciousness was evaded, and Jacksonian status and epilepsia partialis continua were included. Gastaut (1967) himself readily acknowledged that most of these criteria are of only relative value: 'what do we know precisely about the physiopathogenesis of seizures and the interictal symptoms observed in epileptics?'.

In 1985, the Commission on the Classification and Terminology of the International League Against Epilepsy proposed a new approach to classification, to complement and ultimately supersede the seizure type classification (the proposal was officially accepted in 1989). The new classification was of the *Epilepsies and Epileptic Syndromes*. This was necessary as clinical research had identified forms of epilepsy which did not fit easily into seizure type categories. Here was a chance to recognise status as an independent entity with its own subtypes and categories, but this opportunity was sadly neglected. Although a few syndromes that might conform to the widened definition of status were included (e.g. EPC, electrical status epilepticus during slow wave sleep, Landau–Kleffner, Lennox–Gastaut, West syndromes) no synoptic view of status was taken. Indeed, again, status is mentioned only in passing, despite its importance and frequency.

The last major review of status epilepticus was an international conference on status held in Santa Monica in California in November 1980 (was this itself a sign of the decline of French hegemony in matters of status?), the proceedings of which were subsequently published in 1983 (Delgado-Escueta *et al.* 1983). In his prologue to the conference, Booker (1983) commented on the lack of interest in status, much as the editors of the Marseilles Colloquium of 1962 had done, and

Clark & Prout at the turn of the century, and Bourneville in 1876. He noted that of 35 000 citations of epilepsy to 1978 collected by the National Institute of Neurological and Communicative Disorders and Stroke, only 215 were primary or secondary references to status (in fact the correct figure is 370). The new review was to remedy this. Booker posed a series of questions that are still relevant today. Agreement, he argued, has to be reached on the following: What, precisely, is status? How can it be classified? How frequent is it? How can it be comprehensively defined? What are its causes? Do unique biochemical or pathophysiological mechanisms exist not present in individual epileptic attacks? Alternatively, is status similar to an isolated seizure with simply a more intense or prolonged mode of initiation, or loss of the inhibitory processes of termination? Do different mechanisms underlie the different types of status? Do drugs actually cause status (Hunter's (1959/60) original concept)? To what extent is animal experimentation valid and referable to human status? What is the best therapy, pharmacological and other? What are the consequences of status, and in particular what factors induce the brain to consume its own substance?

Fundamental, to Booker, was the question of definition; this had to be explored and agreed upon before other topics were approached. Unfortunately, his challenge was scarcely addressed. Neither the editors nor contributors dwelt on definition, but stated the Marseilles 'formula', and then followed essentially the same classification scheme (Gastaut himself contributed the chapter on classification). Gastaut acknowledged that a 'physiopathogenic classification' was desirable, but he saw it in terms of a further subdivision of types – of a distinction, for example, between the short-spaced series and the single prolonged seizure in status. Thus, the seizure type classification was maintained with, as an afterthought, status uncomfortably clinging on. Indeed, the frontispiece of the book, an illustration of video-telemetry, was captioned: 'there are as many types of status epilepticus as there are types of seizures described in the international classification of epileptic seizures (H. Gastaut)'. The conference dealt rather briefly with 'electroclinical correlations', with most enthusiasm directed towards quite other things. Much more space was devoted to the mechanisms of brain damage in status (24 chapters) and to treatment (20 chapters); both issues were too little developed to attract much attention at Marseilles, and the published proceedings surveyed most of the progress made since the 1967 Colloquium. Thus far had epilepsy research moved on in the intervening years. Booker's questions though are still central to the study of status, still in large part unanswered, and still fundamental to successful clinical management of status; these questions are the starting point for this book.

Notes

1. Sakikku (all diseases) is a medical diagnostic series of 40 tablets. The XXV/XXVIth tablet contains the earliest known historical mention of epilepsy. Two duplicate tablets exist, in Neo-assyrian and Neo-babylonian script; the latter now lies in the British Museum and was translated in 1989 by J.V. Kinnier Wilson, who, to complete the

epileptic circle, is the son of S.A. Kinnier Wilson (1878–1937), the leading neurologist of his generation at the National Hospital, Queen Square. This quotation is taken from Kinnier Wilson & Reynolds (1990).

2. Thomas Willis (1621–1675), the *first inventor of the nervous system*, coined the term neurology and was to the brain what Harvey was to the heart. He was author of numerous important neurological and anatomical tracts, and was first also to describe myasthenia, narcoplepsy paracusis, spinal accessory nerve, and first division of the fifth nerve. He recorded epidemic typhoid, and introduced the term reflex, and described the eponymous circle.

3. Louis Florentin Calmeil (1798–1895), psychiatrist, pupil of the great Esquirol, whose thesis for the University of Paris was entitled De l'épilepsie, étudiée sous le rapport de son siège et son influence sur la production de l'aliénation mentale. In addition to first recording 'état de mal' in the thesis, he was also the first to introduce the term 'absence'.

4. Richard Hunter (1923–1981), was psychiatrist to the National Hospital, Queen Square, an original and brilliant thinker, a bibliophile with an unrivalled historical medical collection, and son of the formidable psychoanalyst Ida McAlpine, whose shadow was said to hover behind all his consultations.

5. Hans Berger (1873–1941) was an assistant to Binswanger, and Professor of Psychiatry and Rector of the university at Jena. He worked in secret on EEG, and made his first recording in 1924. His work was first published in 1929, and initially ridiculed and ignored. Due recognition had to wait until he was invited by Lord Adrian, an English neurophysiologist and Nobel laureate, to preside at a celebrated symposium on the electrical activity of the brain in Paris in 1938. The second world war took its toll and he committed suicide in 1941.

6. The National Hospital for the Paralysed and Epileptic (now the National Hospital for Neurology and Neurosurgery), the first specialised neurological hospital in the world, opened in 1860. This was an auspicious event for epileptics, and in the 1870s as many as 50% of the inpatients and a greater proportion of the outpatients had epilepsy. Over a 50 year period, a succession of physicians and surgeons were appointed who were the glory of British neurology, and gave to the hospital international stature:

John Hughlings Jackson (1835–1911), 'father of British Neurology'. His main interest was epilepsy, and he coined the phrase 'psychomotor seizures, uncinate seizures' and gave his name to Jacksonian seizures. His also was the famous definition of epilepsy as: an occasional, sudden, excessive rapid and local discharge of the 'grey matter'. He was editor of *Brain*, a prolific author, and a quiet, unassuming man (the antithesis of Charcot, who greatly admired him).

David Ferrier (1843–1928) was educated in Edinburgh, and first a general practitioner. He then worked with Jackson and Sherrington, and became a staff physician to the National Hospital in 1880. His work helped to establish the motor and sensory area, and he was instrumental in localising cases for early brain surgery, and was present at the operation on James B. He was an animal experimentor who was taken to court by antivivisectionists, and at once became famous throughout England for his defence of his case.

William Richard Gowers (1845–1915) was educated at London and Oxford and became a physician at the National Hospital in 1880. He wrote intensively on many aspects of neurology, including his textbook of neurology, which became the 'bible' to generations of neurologists in all parts of the world. His works on epilepsy have never been bettered. His breadth of knowledge was legendary, and, perhaps to support his huge written output, he was a great enthusiast for shorthand.

Victor Alexander Haden Horsley (1857–1916), appointed at age 29 as surgeon to the National Hospital, Queen Square, was a great and pioneering neurosurgeon. He carried out the first brain operation for epilepsy in 1886 on James B, whose case was presented at a famous meeting of the British Medical Association in Brighton with both Jackson and Charcot present, and later also operated upon his son after his first epileptic seizure. He then suddenly abandoned his neurosurgical work, became an antiviviectionist and political activist, campaigned for women's suffrage, and crusaded against alcohol. He died in Mesopotamia from heatstroke having volunteered for the Tigris campaign.

Edward Henry Sieveking (1816–1904), one of the older generation, who joined the staff of the National Hospital in 1864. His major work was *Epilepsy and epileptiform seizures, their causes pathology and treatment*, and it was he who translated Romberg's *Treatise of Neurology* into English.

William Aldren Turner (1864–1945) was born in Edinburgh, neurologist to the War Office and medical board. He was especially interested in spas and antiques. He published a textbook on nervous diseases as well as his famous work on epilepsy *A study of epilepsy, the idiopathic disease.*

Walter Stacy Colman (1864–1934) was educated at Edinburgh and University College London, before becoming assistant physician to the National Hospital in 1898. His particular interest was in the improvement of mental hospitals, and he helped to found the Chalfont Centre for Epilepsy. He was a keen archaeologist and freemason.

7. The Salpêtrière had a colourful history. Originally an arsenal, then an asylum, then a women's prison, it became a hospital during the nineteenth century. Neurology developed there to create order out of the 'pandemonium of human infirmities' as mental and nervous disorders were seen. It was made famous by the succession of remarkable and gifted neurologists and psychiatrists who attended there, and became a mecca of neurology, in the time of Charcot:

Etienne Dominique Esquirol (1722–1840) was the first of the great French psychiatrists to practise at the Salpêtrière. He was responsible for the establishment of seperate institutions and wards for epileptics (actually to prevent the sight of an epileptic fit causing epilepsy in other insane but non-epileptic cases). He popularised the terms grand mal and petit mal.

Philip Pinel (1745–1826) was part of the new wave of psychiatrists whose enlightened attitude to mental disease allowed the systematic and sympathetic study of epilepsy. Through his teaching and writing, he had an important influence on the development of thought about epilepsy throughout the nineteenth century in both France and England.

Jean-Martin Charcot (1825–1893) was a dominating and intimidating figure, frequently likened to Napoleon, initially a neuropathologist and then the greatest French neurologist of the nineteenth century. He made contributions to the study of syphilis, polio, motor neurone disease, aneurysms, diphtheria, and gave his name to Charcot–Marie–Tooth disease. His greatest legacy was to the field of hysteria and to epilepsy, however, and his extensive writings were renowned throughout Europe and beyond. At the Salpêtrière, he held open clinical demonstrations which were theatre in the purest sense, and to which all of fashionable society came. His medical influence was great and at his feet were physicians and students from many countries of the world.

8. Desiré Magloir Bourneville (1840–1909) was a physician and scholar, revered by all of France; he was chief of the paediatric service at the Bicêtre. On Saturdays at the Bicêtre, he held open days which rivalled Charcot's at the Salpêtrière, where the public of Paris could visit to see the inmates performing exercises and dances to the accompaniment of a band composed of idiots, epileptics and spastics. He was the leading continental authority on mentally handicapped children. He gave his name to Bourneville disease, edited Charcot's *Leçons*, and founded the *Archives de Neurologie*.

9. Armand Trousseau (1801–1867) was a contemporary of Charcot and physician at the Clinique Medicale de l'Hôtel Dieu in Paris. An original and great neurologist, amongst other contributions he coined the term aphasia.

10. James Cowles Prichard (1786–1828) was one of the first nineteenth century neurologists to write a textbook on neurology (*A treatise on diseases of the nervous system*, 1822),

and refined the term aura (which originated from Galen in the second century) and gave it its modern meaning.

11. L. Pierce Clark (1870–1933) was First Assistant Physician to the Craig Colony for Epileptics in New York, and an early American alienist. Interestingly, he spent at year in Europe with Prout, working with Marburg and Hughlings Jackson; is it fanciful to think that their interest in status derives from this time in London?

12. Wilder Penfield (1891–1977) graduated from Johns Hopkins, and studied under Sherrington, Holmes, Cushing and Horsley. Founded the Montreal Neurological Institute, and through his papers on cerebral localisation had a profound influence on twentieth century neurology. A pioneer surgeon for epilepsy who initiated the famous surgical programme which still fourishes at Montreal, he also wrote fiction and was the author of papers on cultural, sociological and historical subjects.

13. Alexie Kojewnikoff (1836–1902) was educated in Moscow and Europe, a pupil of Charcot, who on returning to Russia became dozent in nervous and mental diseases at Novo-Ekaterininskii hospital, and first alienist of the Moscow faculty. In addition to his research on epilepsy, he worked on lathyrism, spastic diplegia and wrote a manual of nervous diseases, famed for its brevity and lucidity.

14. William Lennox (1884–1960) was educated at Harvard and worked at the Massachusetts General Hospital. He popularised the newly developed EEG techniques with the Gibbs, and his major volume on epilepsy, written with his daughter Margaret, became a classic. He was also an active eugenecist.

CHAPTER 2

Definition, classification and frequency of status epilepticus

If the clinician, as observer, wishes to see things as they really are, he must make a tabula rasa of his mind, and proceed without any preconceived notions whatsoever.

(Charcot 1889)

Definition of status epilepticus

With Charcot's wise counsel, let us start with definitions. We have seen, in chapter 1, how theoretical constructs of status evolved, and how the subject was last seriously considered at the Marseilles Colloquium in 1962. The exegesis of status arrived at is one which has been widely adopted. It is the basis of the WHO *dictionary* definition of status as 'a condition characterised by epileptic seizures that are sufficiently prolonged or repeated at sufficiently brief intervals so as to produce an unvarying and enduring epileptic condition' (Gastaut 1973; an 'etymological' definition, which was an extension of the 'historical' definition confined to grand mal status). It has been carefully worded in order to incorporate what was seen at Marseilles as the increasing proliferation of 'enduring epileptic conditions', all with a compelling claim to be included in the family of status. When Bourneville recognised the special nature of prolonged seizures, his concern was only tonic–clonic convulsions (*état de grand mal*), and definition was relatively simple. With the subsequent identification of nonconvulsive status, epilepsia partialis continua, neonatal status, absence status, myoclonic status, and childhood status syndromes, the definition had to be widened. The WHO formula, excellent though it is, is indubitably imprecise; a little dissection is in order.

1. What is an epileptic seizure? The usual definition emphasises transience and implies a clinical event. Status is by its nature prolonged (fixed and enduring), and some nonconvulsive episodes may exceptionally last even weeks or months. In many conditions 'seizure activity' is covert (e.g. subclinical seizures, nonconvulsive status, or even the later stages of tonic–clonic status). Quite how electrographic changes occurring without obvious clinical seizures fit into this rubric is unclear. It is not an insignificant point, for if electrographic change in the absence of clinical change is accepted, many apparently interictal 'epileptic' states could be included under this definition of status (see Trimble &

21

Reynolds, 1986). Moreover; the emphasis on a 'seizure' leads inexorably to classification by seizure types, which as discussed below is a poor way to approach the nosology of status. Other clinical states, associated with active epilepsy, exist that have prominent encephalopathic, psychiatric or psychological features. In some it may be impossible to decide whether or not the seizure activity is contributing to the clinical symptoms; some are 'boundary conditions', and are discussed in chapter 3.

2. For how long must the condition persist, before considered to be 'enduring'? This is another unanswerable question, as individual seizures show wide ranges of variation and fluctuation. Again, the question is perhaps easiest to address with tonic–clonic status, but even here fruitless arguments have raged about whether or not there should be a lower limit of 60 or 30 or even 20 minutes of seizure activity before status is pronounced to be present. More important would be to decide whether or not status is simply the repetition or prolongation of seizures, or forms a separate entity, related to but distinct from ordinary epileptic attacks. There is increasing neurophysiological, neurochemical and clinical evidence to support this latter contention, as is clear throughout this book. Even if, for operational purposes, a minimum time limit must be set for convulsive status, how can it be accurately measured when the onset of status is preceded by increasingly frequent serial attacks and when the end of a tonic–clonic seizure is so diffuse (think of the prolonged EEG changes and the postictal confusion), and how are the effects of therapy allowed for? These questions have no simple answer.

3. What is unvarying? Here again strict definition is difficult. Many seizures show marked variation, and no attempt has been made to define limits to these fluctuations. Physiological work shows a progression in signs during prolonged seizures, and even if the clinical appearances are static there are profound and progressive biochemical and electrographic changes. It would indeed be fair to say that status is *never* unvarying in the strictest sense. The mode of progression and fluctuations in both tonic–clonic and complex partial status are discussed in detail in chapters 3 and 4.

4. When is a seizure 'recurrent' and when is it 'prolonged'? The distinction between continuous and discontinuous forms of status has generated controversy for years, particularly in relation to absence and complex partial status. It is a problem made even more difficult when one considers neonatal status or boundary conditions.

As the term status now incorporates conditions of great diversity, many of which are poorly understood, it is perhaps fruitless to seek a single or unitary definition; an inability to provide absolute definitions in medicine is, after all, not a problem confined to status epilepticus. If status defies single definition, we must make do with less satisfactory operational definitions, with the implication that we really know what status is, even if it cannot be defined. This is nevertheless a poor substitute for definitive clinicopathophysiological definition, which remains an important but elusive objective.

In this book the following operational definition is suggested:

> Status epilepticus is a condition in which epileptic activity persists for 30
> minutes or more, causing a wide spectrum of clinical symptoms, and with
> a highly variable pathophysiological, anatomical and aetiological basis.

This definition acknowledges that status is not simply rapid repetition of seizures, but a condition (or group of conditions) with distinctive pathophysiological features. Very importantly, it avoids the term epileptic seizure and thus the difficulties of definition and classification of seizures. It allows the incorporation of conditions which do not conform to a 'seizure type', and conditions where there is continuous electrographic ictal activity causing persisting symptoms but no discrete seizures, thus including many types of nonconvulsive status. Excluded, however, are cases exhibiting persistent electrographic activity in the total absence of clinical symptoms, as might occur for instance with interictal spiking. A minimum limit of 30 minutes is set (this has some physiological justification, see chapter 4) to render the definition clinically useful. No distinction is made between recurrent or prolonged seizures, nor is the activity required to be enduring or unvarying. The diversity of clinical features of status is also recognised, as is the highly variable patho-anatomical and aetiological basis.

As will become evident, such a definition allows a liberal interpretation of what can be counted as status, deliberately so, in an attempt to encourage thought about the principles of status, unemcumbered with arbitrarily restrictive criteria. I believe that the definition conforms to the spirit of status, without being over-inclusive or overexclusive, although there exist (as is usual in epilepsy) a range of boundary conditions where the distinction between epilepsy and either functional (psychiatric) or organic (encephalopathic) symptoms is difficult to make.

Classification of status epilepticus

The admission that *there is no satisfactory definition of status* is an ominous start for the taxonomist; but one scarcely avoidable. Any honest classification scheme must be of necessity tentative and provisional. It is a premise in this book that the adherence to the currently fashionable *seizure type classification* ('there are as many types of status as there are seizure types') is unsatisfactory and restrictive. Nevertheless, this classification or minor variants has been followed in all recent reviews (see for instance Dunn 1988; Lacey 1988; Shields 1989; Bleck 1991; Leppik 1986, 1990; Hauser 1990); an example of this classification scheme is shown in table 2.1. The disparagement of the *seizure type classification* is justified on various counts, given below; in formulating an alternative classification, the following points should be acknowledged:

1. There are types of status in which no overt 'seizure' occurs, including many nonconvulsive epileptic confusional states, some cases of myoclonic status in coma, some cases of tonic status, the boundary states, some neonatal status, and childhood syndromes of status such as electrical status epilepticus during

23

Table 2.1. *Seizure type classification of status epilepticus*

Generalised status epilepticus
Tonic–clonic status epilepticus
Tonic status epilepticus
Clonic status epilepticus
Myoclonic status epilepticus
Absence status epilepticus
Atonic and akinetic status epilepticus

Partial status epilepticus
Elementary partial status epilepticus
Complex partial status epilepticus

Unilateral status epilepticus

Note: This is one example of a number of similar classifications in common use that were derived from the time of the Xth and XIIIth Marseilles Colloquia on Status Epilepticus and on the Classification of Seizure Type.
From Gastaut 1983.

slow wave sleep (ESES) or the Landau–Kleffner syndrome. It is selfevident that such conditions are not easily categorised into seizure types.

2. Some seizure types are manifest only in certain clinical contexts. Tonic status is an example, which is seen almost exclusively in the Lennox–Gastaut syndrome, mixed with other expressions of status. Where it occurs outside the syndrome (e.g. in neonatal status or occasionally in other situations) it assumes atypical forms with probably different pathophysiology. Myoclonic status is another example, categorised best by its occurrence in coma, mental handicap, or in the progressive myoclonic epilepsies; in each the form, prognosis, course, treatment and probably pathophysiology of the myoclonus are distinct. To categorise by clinical context in these circumstances rather than by seizure type gives physiological coherence to the clinical appearance.

3. The basic pathophysiology of many types of status (especially of syndromic, nonconvulsive or childhood forms) is not well understood, there are few experimental models available, little is understood about the neurochemical basis, and there are few detailed stereoencephalographic (SEEG), imaging or pathological studies. To an extent, classification is therefore arbitrary. It is this very arbitrariness that requires a classification to be fully in accord with *observed forms*, rather than one that is essentially a *theoretical scheme* (e.g. of seizure type) imposed upon these forms.

4. Although the definition of status is firmly embedded in EEG, subclassification should not depend simply on EEG appearances, as these are often nonspecific (in the same sense that a haemoglobin measurement is a relatively nonspecific indicator of haematological diseases). EEG provides a visual record that is only

an indirect measure of underlying neurochemical or anatomical mechanisms of the epilepsy. A tendency to overemphasise EEG has to an extent driven nosology into a cul-de-sac, and status particularly has suffered from this (see for instance the syndromic mire into which the classification of childhood epilepsies has sunk; Hajnšek & Dürrigl 1970; Roger *et al.* 1985, 1992). A more synoptical approach is needed, where genetic, anatomical, pathological and aetiological features are accounted for, in addition to electrographic and clinical appearances; such a 'biological approach' is not currently feasible, but should be the goal of future taxonomy.

5. A classification should acknowledge the importance of the patient's age and level of cerebral development, as this is critical in defining the clinical type (incorporating, as it were, patient as well as illness variables). The form, convulsive or nonconvulsive, which status takes in young children is characteristically much less well differentiated (more fractionated) than in adults or older children, and the clinical appearances of status in childhood are dependent more on age than on any other factor. The evolution over time of one type of status into another as the child grows older is further evidence of the relevance of cerebral development.

An appreciation of the level of cerebral development is also important in considering status in the mentally handicapped. These people form a subpopulation with diffuse brain damage whose cerebral development is arrested, and who fail to achieve adult levels of cerebral maturity. Status may begin in childhood and persist into adult life, with clinical appearances which are very atypical, and are determined more by the degree of arrested cerebral development than by other clinical factors (for instance, aetiology). A nosological approach in this situation based on seizure type (or syndrome) makes little sense.

A new classification of status epilepticus

It is to be hoped that the future revisions of the International League Against Epilepsy (ILAE) syndromic classification schemes will address the problems of status. It is the contention of this book that a definitive classification of status should not be based upon seizure type alone, but on other features, the most important of which are age and level of cerebral maturity of the subject, pathophysiological mechanisms of the epilepsy, and clinical features (such as anatomy, EEG findings, aetiology, and clinical form as appropriate).

A new classification scheme has been devised here, given in table 2.2, which follows these principles. This is a provisional classification, necessarily primitive and incomplete, to which future modifications are inevitable, and desirable. Its major subdivision is based upon age. Within each age group, there is a mixed classification based upon:

1. *Clinical and EEG seizure type* (e.g. tonic–clonic status, simple and complex partial status). This categorisation is valid particularly in symptomatic status of late childhood and adult life.

Table 2.2. *Revised classification of status epilepticus*

	Status seizure type
Status epilepticus confined to the neonatal period	
Neonatal status epilepticus	Subtle, tonic, clonic, myoclonic, electrographic, nonepileptic, apnoeic, unilateral, other fragmentary
Status epilepticus in neonatal epilepsy syndromes	
Early infantile encephalopathy	Tonic
Neonatal myoclonic encephalopathy	Erratic, myoclonic
Benign familial neonatal seizures	Clonic
Benign neonatal seizures	Clonic, apnoeic
Status epilepticus confined to infancy and childhood	
Infantile spasm (West syndrome)	Salaam attacks
Febrile status epilepticus	Convulsive or hemiconvulsive
Status epilepticus in the childhood myoclonic syndromes	
Cryptogenic and symptomatic childhood myoclonic epilepsy	Myoclonic
Severe myoclonic epilepsy in infants	Myoclonic, myoclonic–absence
Myoclonic status in nonprogressive encephalopathy	Myoclonic, myoclonic–absence, electrographic
Myoclonic–astatic epilepsy	Absence, myoclonic, astatic, myoclonic–astatic
Status epilepticus in the benign childhood partial epilepsy syndromes	
Benign rolandic epilepsy	Complex partial
Benign occipital epilepsy	Complex partial
Electrical status epilepticus during slow wave sleep (ESES)	Electrographic
Syndrome of acquired epileptic aphasia	Electrographic
Status epilepticus occurring in childhood and adult life	
Tonic–clonic status epilepticus	Tonic–clonic, subtle
Absence status epilepticus	Typical absence (and atypical absence, complex partial)
Epilepsia partialis continua (EPC)	Simple partial
Myoclonic status epilepticus in coma	Myoclonic
Specific forms of status epilepticus in mental retardation	Atypical absence, tonic, minor motor, electrographic
Myoclonic status epilepticus in other epilepsy syndromes	
Primary generalised epilepsies	Myoclonic and myoclonic–absence
Progressive myoclonic epilepsies	Myoclonic
Nonconvulsive simple partial status epilepticus	Simple partial

26

Table 2.2. (*cont.*)

	Status seizure type
Complex partial status epilepticus	Complex partial
Boundary syndromes	
Electrographic status epilepticus with subtle clinical signs	Electrographic
Prolonged postictal confusional states	Electrographic
Epileptic behavioural disturbances and psychosis	Electrographic
Status epilepticus confined to adult life	
De novo absence status epilepticus of late onset	Absence

2. *Pathophysiology and epilepsy syndrome* (e.g. epilepsia partialis continua, febrile status, West syndrome, acquired epileptic aphasia, childhood epilepsy syndromes, Landau–Kleffner syndrome, myoclonic status of coma). These syndromic categories are perhaps the best defined of all status variants.

3. *Clinical phenomenology* crossing seizure type and syndromic boundaries (e.g. neonatal status, absence status, *de novo* absence status of late onset, status in mental handicap). Here are recognised syndromes which do not fit neatly into either a syndromic or seizure type categorisation, yet are relatively well defined from a clinical or pathophysiological perspective.

4. *Boundary conditions* the inclusion of which in status will be controversial, but which conform to wider definitions of status (e.g. postictal confusion, sub-clinical status, epileptic behavioural disorder).

The divisions are based on pathophysiological, aetiological or anatomical data where possible, fields which should be greatly advanced by current developments in magnetic resonance imaging (MRI). Subdivision on purely EEG grounds is avoided.

Frequency of status epilepticus

If one cannot easily define a condition or indeed satisfactorily classify it, clearly any estimate of its frequency must be of doubtful validity; this is the position with status. Until very recently, all computations of frequency were restricted to tonic–clonic status, but even here only the vaguest guesses at incidence or prevalence were possible. Hunter (1959/60) contrasted the increasingly frequent references to status in the second half of the nineteenth century with the paucity of earlier reports, and inferred that the condition became common only with the appearance of effective antiepileptic drugs (bromides). Clark & Prout (1903/4) thought the condition 'rare', and Turner (1907) that it was 'more frequent than is generally supposed', quoting a frequency of 5% in his 280 personally observed patients. Lennox (1960) found 10% of his 1271 patients seen before 1940 had one or more periods of status, over half of whom had had two or more attacks. He confirmed the view of all those before him that status was more common in the mentally defective and in those in institutions.

A number of more recent studies have attempted to quantify the frequency of status in various selected clinical populations. These surveys were (with few exceptions) retrospective record reviews, with all their inherent inaccuracies. Cases are very likely to have been missed, especially those which were mild, those which were treated outside neurological services, and those with other primary diagnoses. The case ascertainment of short-lived status episodes poses a particular problem. Although all seizures over 30 minutes (or 20 or 60 minutes, depending on the definition employed) should be included, one suspects that very often seizure duration is not recorded, and that many relatively short status episodes are categorised as seizures not status, and overlooked.

Status epilepticus as a proportion of hospital admissions

Hunter (1959/60) found 1.3% (30 of 2303 cases) of all epileptic admissions to the National Hospital, Queen Square (a specialised neurological hospital) over a 10 year period were with status. Rowan & Scott (1970) identified retrospectively 42 cases of major status admitted to the London Hospital (a general hospital) over a 20 year period (which was 0.01% of all admissions). Oxbury & Whitty (1971*a*) found 3% (86 of 2500 cases) of status amongst patients with epilepsy admitted to the United Oxford Hospitals over a 20 year period, and Goulon, Lévy-Alcover & Nouailhat (1985) 3.5% of all admissions (282 of 7955 patients) to two neurological intensive care units over 8 years. In a single year, epilepsy accounted for 2.4% (1574 of 66 017 visits) of all visits to the casualty department of a university hospital in Helsinki and status for 5.4% of all epileptic seizures (85 patients, 0.13% of all casualty visits; Pilke, Partinen & Kovanen 1984).

Status epilepticus as a proportion of all epileptic cases

Turner's (1907) estimate that a history of status had occurred in about 5% of his clinic cases was roughly confirmed by subsequent studies, at least until recent times. Janz (1961) recorded status in 3.7% (95 of 2588) of epileptic cases visiting his clinic over a 13 year period, Lennox (1960) 10% (127 of 1271) of patients, Heintel (1972) 7.2% (39 of 541) of cases, and Celesia *et al.* (1972) 2.3% (27 of 1166) of patients of whom about half were over 40 years. In children the incidence is higher. Aicardi & Chevrie (1970) found status in 16% of children with the diagnosis of epilepsy before the age of 16 years. Yager, Cheang & Seshia (1988) identified status in 13% of all children (52 of 412 patients) presenting with seizures to an emergency department of a children hospital (69% had tonic–clonic status), and Hauser (1990) in 24% of all children presenting with nonfebrile seizures.

The timing of status epilepticus

Tonic–clonic status can occur either as the initial epileptic event or as an intercurrent episode in established epileptic patients; this is an important distinction as the aetiology and implications of status in the two situations may be very different (see table 3.8). In children, status is commonly the first epileptic event,

76% of 432 cases, for instance, in two series (Aicardi & Chevrie 1970; Phillips & Shanahan 1989). This reflects the high incidence of acute aetiologies and febrile status (5% of febrile seizures present in status). In adults, the data are conflicting, not least because of selection bias. Older studies show most cases occurring in existing epilepsy (e.g. 61% (221 of 362 patients): Janz 1961; Oxbury & Whitty 1971*a*; Heintel 1972; Aminoff & Simon 1980), but these were from specialist neurological practices. A more recent survey, based on intensive care unit admissions, found only 29% (81 of 282) of patients in status to be established epileptics (Goulon *et al.* 1985). In a study of status presenting to an urban hospital in the 1980s, Lowenstein & Alldredge (1993) found that 44% (67 of 152) of cases of status had no previous history of epilepsy, and Hauser (1990) reported that status accounted for 12% of all newly diagnosed cases of epilepsy presenting to hospital with a first epileptic event. In 30% of the 342 elderly patients presenting with status after the age of 60 in a hospital-based investigation from Taiwan, the status was the initial epileptic manifestation (Sung & Chu 1989*a*). In established patients, status can develop at almost any time during the course, but earlier in symptomatic than idiopathic cases. Indeed, idiopathic epilepsy rarely presents as status, and, if status does develop, it is usually only after many years of epilepsy (mean of 15 years after the onset in the cases of Heintel (1972)). Presentation with status in an adult often indicates focal structural cerebral pathology.

Factors influencing the frequency of tonic–clonic status epilepticus

Age is a the major determinant of status. All studies have shown greater frequencies of status amongst patients with epilepsy starting in childhood. About 70% of neonatal seizure disorders assume the proportion of status, and about 5% of all febrile convulsions. In the series of Aicardi & Chevrie (1970), 16% of all children with epilepsy below the age of 15 years had a history of status, and 30% of these had febrile status; extrapolating this to a general population, a population frequency of 4–8 children per 1000 may be expected to develop status before the age of 15 (Hauser 1983). There is no particular sex ratio bias. Since the first reports of status, the condition has been clearly recognised to be commoner in institutions than amongst the general clinic epileptics. Turner (1907) realised that epileptics with *mental handicap* were much more likely to suffer status and this has been amply confirmed subsequently; the risk of status in many categories of mental handicap is very high. Hunter (1959/60) and Janz (1961) also pointed out that, amongst the outpatients with epilepsy, those with *symptomatic epilepsy* were more likely to have a history of grand mal status than those with idiopathic epilepsy (9% compared with 1% amongst the cases of Janz), a tendency endorsed by every succeeding investigation (e.g. Rowan & Scott 1970; Aicardi & Chevrie 1970; Oxbury & Whitty 1971*a*; Aminoff & Simon 1980). An excess of patients with *frontal lobe pathology* in status was first observed by Whitty & Taylor (1949), and confirmed by Oxbury & Whitty (1971*a*), reporting frontal lesions in 87% and 50%, respectively, of cases with focal cerebral damage. The predominance of frontal lobe pathology in status was explored comprehensively by Janz (1960, 1964) in patients with tumours or head injury and postsurgery. Of 27 status-precipitating

29

tumours 20 (74%) were found to be in the frontal lobe; 47% (20 of 43) of anteriorly placed tumours caused status compared with 9% of posteriorly placed tumours (Janz 1964). Similarly, 94% (15 of 16) of open-head injuries precipitating status involved the frontal lobe. Janz also quotes postmortem studies of status where 78% had frontal lobe pathology, and reports of post leucotomy patients of whom almost half had status. These findings pre-dated modern imaging, and current MRI experience suggests that frontal lesions occur in a similar preponderance of cases. Interestingly, a propensity for frontal lobe lesions to produce complex partial status has also been recognised recently (see pp. 128–9). The reasons for the prediliction of status for the frontal lobe is not known, although the well-established ease and speed of spread of epileptic discharges unilaterally and bilaterally from frontal lobe foci may be relevant.

Population estimates of the frequency of status epilepticus

The validity of these statistics is uncertain, not least because almost all are derived from hospital records reviewed retrospectively. One wonders how often the duration of an epileptic fit is actually recorded, or indeed even measured, and yet this will determine the accuracy of these figures; this is particularly important where definition includes seizures lasting only 20 or 30 minutes, where underreporting in retrospective reviews will be a serious issue in epidemiological studies. The importance of definition of minimum time for status is shown in studies of febrile status, where 20 minute seizures are 10-fold more common than 60 minute seizures.

On the basis of such (potentially dubious) data, however, Hauser (1990) has computed impressive figures for the incidence and prevalence of status in newly diagnosed patients, those with established epilepsy, febrile convulsions and acute symptomatic seizures (see table 2.3):

1. Patients with newly diagnosed epilepsy (excluding acute symptomatic seizures): 12% present with status. This figure derives from one limited prospective study of newly diagnosed patients (Hauser 1990), and is not a well-supported statistic (see Sander *et al.* 1990, for a critique). In children, higher figures are usually quoted (e.g. 40% of all epilepsies in the first year of life), as they are in retrospective hospital adult series (39% of 362 cases) and in late onset status (30% of 342 cases). Hauser calculated an annual incidence of about 80 per 1 000 000 persons in the general population.
2. Patients with established epilepsy: 0.5–1% will develop status per annum. The basis of this figure (unreferenced in Hauser's paper) is unsupported to my knowledge by published data. The hospital series discussed above provides widely varying estimates of the occurrence of status in patients with epilepsy, which are often higher than this figure. No prevalence surveys have been conducted, however, nor any population-based studies. On the basis of these figures, an annual incidence can be calculated of 40–80 per 1 000 000 persons in the general population.

30

3. Febrile convulsions: 2–4% of the population will have at least one febrile seizure by the age of 5 years; in 5% of these, seizures are of more than 30 minutes' duration and a further 0.5% of more than 60 minutes' duration (figures are derived from several well-conducted studies, see Hauser 1990). On this basis, the annual incidence of febrile status (>30 minutes) can be calculated to be 20–40 per 1 000 000 persons in the general population.
4. Acute symptomatic seizures: one third to one half of all patients of status in hospital series present as acute symptomatic seizures, in those without a history of epilepsy. Hauser estimated that this contributes about 40–80 cases per 1 000 000 persons in the population per year. The basis of this figure is unclear and unreferenced.

In table 2.3 are computations based on these figures, for the total US population and for the UK population (assuming an age structure approximately similar to that in the USA) and a similar general population of 1 000 000 persons. As the frequency of status is strongly age dependent, total numbers would be expected to be higher in developing countries where a greater proportion of cases are in the younger age groups, and also where more symptomatic epilepsy occurs. Clearly, all such figures are approximations only, and are based on what are highly unreliable data. On the whole, as the bias is towards underreporting for all the reasons discussed above, these statistics should be considered as minimum estimates; the true figure may be much higher. The statistics are, furthermore, concerned only with tonic–clonic status, and other forms are very common. The following have been ignored:

5. Typical absence status: a history of absence status is said to occur in 5–10% of all patients with generalised absence (petit mal) seizures. On this basis, assuming the prevalence of absence epilepsy to be about 100 per 1 000 000 persons, and assuming an annual occurrence of about 1% in patients with petit mal, an annual incidence of absence status can be calculated to lie between 1 per 1 000 000 persons in the general population.
6. Complex partial status: common and probably much more so than convulsive status at least in adults, although published statistical evidence on this point is entirely lacking. It is my impression, based on specialist adult practice, that at least 15% of patients with active complex partial epilepsy have a history of nonconvulsive status episodes. Assuming an annual incidence of status of 1.5% of all complex partial cases, the annual incidence of complex partial status in the general population can be calculated to be 35 per 1 000 000 persons.
7. Neonatal status: occurs in about 10 per 1000 live births. On the basis of this figure, assuming about 12 000 live births per annum per 1 000 000 persons, an annual incidence can be calculated of 120 per 1 000 000 persons in a Western general population.
8. Nonconvulsive status in a mentally handicapped population: assuming a mental handicap prevalence of about 1% in the population, a rate of epilepsy of about 20% in the mentally handicapped population, and an annual incidence of nonconvulsive status of about 5–10% in these patients, the annual incidence

31

Table 2.3. *Approximate annual incidence of status epilepticus in a general population, and in the USA and the UK*

	General population of 1 000 000 persons (*n*)	US population (250 million persons approx.) (*n*)	UK population (50 million persons approx.) (*n*)
1. Newly diagnosed epilepsies, presenting with convulsive status epilepticus	80	20 000	4000
2. Established epilepsy, convulsive status epilepticus	40–80	10 000–20 000	2000–4000
3. Febrile status epilepticus	20–40	5000–10 000	1000–2000
4. Acute symptomatic seizures	40–80	10 000–20 000	2000–4000
5. Typical absence status epilepticus	1	250	50
6. Complex partial status epilepticus	35	8750	1750
7. Neonatal status epilepticus	120	30 000	6000
8. Nonconvulsive status in the mentally handicapped	100–200	25 000–50 000	5000–10 000
9. Other status epilepticus syndromes	5–10	1250–2500	250–500
Total number of cases of status (per annum)	441–646	110 250–161 500	22 050–32 300
Total number of cases of convulsive status epilepticus (per annum)	180–280	45 000–70 000	9000–14 000

1–4 are derived from Hauser 1990; for further explanation, see the text.

of status can be calculated to be 100–200 per 1 000 000 persons in the general population.

9. Other status syndromes: West syndrome, the neonatal and childhood status syndromes, epilepsia partialis continua, simple partial status, and absence status in the elderly are rare, and can contribute to the annual incidence of status no more than 5–10 cases per 1 000 000 persons in the general population (at a conservative and approximate estimate).

The boundary syndromes have not been included in these calculations, but are relatively common. Nevertheless, a total annual incidence of status can be arrived at (in extremely approximate terms) of about: 500 (441–646) cases per 1 000 000 persons in a general population; 25 000 (22 050–32 300) persons in the UK per year; a frequency of status of about 7% (2.5% convulsive status) of all epileptic cases each year. Though it will be palpably clear from the above comments that these statistics are very approximate, none better exist, a quite unsatisfactory state of affairs, requiring early remedy.

CHAPTER 3

Clinical forms of status epilepticus

As is evident from chapter 2, the classification of status is fraught with difficulties. Objections to a simple seizure-type classification were elaborated upon, and a provisional hybrid scheme was proposed based upon a wider range of clinical criteria. As the level of cerebral maturity and development is perhaps the single most important determinant of the clinical form of status, the primary subdivision of this classification scheme is by age. In this chapter, the clinical forms of status are described and categorised according to this scheme, dealing successively with status in the neonatal period, early childhood, late childhood and adult life.

Status epilepticus confined to the neonatal period

Neonatal status epilepticus

The neonatal brain is immature, myelination is limited, cellular migration unfinished and synaptic connections incomplete. It is consequently not surprising to learn that the appearance of 'status epilepticus' differs greatly from those in later childhood or adult life, both from the clinical and electrophysiological points of view, and that the aetiological and anatomico-pathological bases are also distinct. Kellaway & Hrachovy (1983) made an important contribution to the 1980 International Conference on Status Epilepticus. It is noteworthy, however, that their text was devoted largely to seizures rather than status, reflecting the lack of distinction possible in the immature brain, where seizure activity is inchoate and disordered and where the physiological processes underlying both the evolution and cessation of seizure activity are not well formed. Since other seizures, if they occur, are beyond the limits of detectability, any discussion of clinical status is necessarily limited to motor phenomena. The EEG too is of limited help in neonatal status, as varying and nonspecific features are frequent.

Frequency

There is no doubt that neonatal seizures are of serious import and common, although their exact frequency is uncertain because of difficulties in detection and definition. The incidence is usually said to vary between 5 and 16 per 1000 live births (up to 23% in premature infants), mortality is high and morbidity even higher (see Kellaway & Hrachovy 1983; Anonymous 1989; Brett 1991; Aicardi 1992*a,b*; and pp. 301–2). The proportion of cases which amount to status is

34

unknown, but is high. Status in this critical phase of infantile development is ominous, not only because it is at times indicative of cerebral disease, but also because the seizures may possibly damage the developing brain. In neonatal rats, seizures have been shown to inhibit DNA, RNA, protein, and cholesterol synthesis, and result in diminished brain weight and cell numbers; similar damage is likely in human infants also (Wasterlain 1978; Dwyer & Wasterlain 1983; Wasterlain & Dwyer 1983).

Definition

Neonatal seizures are rarely isolated events, much more frequently they are repeated or continuous over hours or days. Definitions of status in the neonatal period vary, but a common formula is that of Monod & Dreyfus-Brisac (1972) 'a repetition of clinical or even subclinical seizures, which occur for at least one hour in a baby having abnormal neurological symptoms between seizures'. Cukier, Sfaello & Dreyfus-Brisac (1976) accepted electrographic seizures, and defined status by the presence of recurring electrographic seizure discharges, lasting 10 seconds or more over several hours, associated with an abnormal neurological state and unconsciousness. These definitions are necessarily imprecise, evading the questions of how neurological symptoms or unconsciousness (let alone seizures) can be reliably ascertained in the newborn, and how recurring seizures can be clinically differentiated from status.

Clinical forms

The clinical form of neonatal status is very different from that at other ages. The seizures are very often 'quite anarchic, polymorphic and poorly organised' (Dreyfus-Brisac & Monod 1977). Some seizures resemble isolated fragments of seizures seen in older individuals (e.g. clonic movements, tonic spasm), and it can be easily postulated (less easily proven) that such fragmentary states are due to the poor synaptic connectivity and immature cortical architecture of the newborn brain, preventing synchronisation of epileptic activity and seizure propagation. To what extent electrographic phenomena at cellular level are also different is not known. There is no doubt that most neonatal seizures are *epileptic* in nature, especially those with paroxysmal electroencephalographic (EEG) changes (e.g. clonic seizures). Controversy abounds, however, about other seizures, especially some forms of subtle or tonic seizure, that are less clearly epileptic. Although epilepsy without scalp EEG change is a common experience, the frequent lack of EEG abnormality in these seizures has led to the suggestion that subcortical mechanisms (release phenomena), not epilepsy, may be responsible. Stimulus sensitivity, graduated forms and spatial and temporal summation support this view (Kellaway & Hrachovy 1983; Camfield & Camfield 1987). Repeated clinical (clonic and subtle) and electrographic seizures have also been observed in an infant with complete atelencephaly (Danner, Shewmon & Sherman 1985). There is little experimental evidence to illuminate the issue, and nowhere in status is the neurophysiological basis of the epilepsy so obscure. This is not simply a semantic problem, as prognosis differs in nonepileptic and epileptic seizures, and

Table 3.1. *Neonatal status epilepticus: the relation of seizure type to aetiology in a series of 82 cases*

Cause	Total $n = 82$ (%)	Clonic $n = 14$ (%)	Myoclonic $n = 17$ (%)	Tonic $n = 13$ (%)	Automatisms $n = 22$ (%)	EEG sz only $n = 11$ (%)	Other[a] $n = 5$ (%)
Hypoxic–ischaemic encephalopathy	46.3	7.1	64.7	53.8	54.5	54.5	20.0
Infection	17.1	21.4	—	38.5	22.7	9.1	—
Hypoglycaemia	4.9	7.1	5.9	—	18.1	9.1	20.0
Cerebrovascular	21.9	57.1	5.9	7.7	18.1	27.3	20.0
Miscellaneous	9.8	7.1	23.6	—	4.5	—	40.0

EEG sz, electroencephalographic seizures.
[a] Includes focal tonic (2), infantile spasms (2), and apnoea (1).
From: Mizrahi & Kellaway 1987, with kind permission.

treatment varies. The clinical appearances of status in the newborn are highly dependent on the level of cerebral maturity, and clinical forms differ in the premature and term infant and evolve as the child ages.

A number of 'seizure types' are recognised (table 3.1; see Mizrahi & Kellaway 1987).

SUBTLE (MINIMAL) SEIZURES: a particularly noteworthy form in the neonatal period, both in premature and term infants. They may be missed by the casual observer, so slight are their manifestations, which can take the form of jerks, spasms and automatisms. Characteristic features include slight jerking or deviation of the eyes, fluttering of the eyelids, orofacial movements, apnoea, autonomic changes, rowing, pedalling, swimming or boxing movements, brief myoclonic movements of the trunk or limbs or tonic spasm. These may continue for hours or days. The EEG may or may not reveal an epileptic basis, showing high voltage slow activity, rhythmic activity or burst suppression. Apnoeic seizures with EEG correlates are relatively common.

TONIC SEIZURES: a common neonatal seizure type, and especially in the premature. They differ totally in clinical and EEG appearances from the tonic seizures in older children or adults (see pp. 105–7), and from infantile spasm. The motor form is a rapid extension of all four limbs (or flexion of the upper and extension of the lower limbs), often with apnoea and upward deviation of the eyes, and tremor of the extended limbs. The seizures are sometimes stimulus sensitive. The EEG shows paroxysmal electrographic high voltage slow or burst suppression activity in about 15–30% of patients, but in other cases no EEG abnormalities occur.

CLONIC SEIZURES: either focal or multifocal (erratic, migratory, fragmentary seizures), comprise random or organised jerking of the limbs, which may spread or fluctuate. They can resemble fragments of tonic–clonic convulsions, and the flitting movements may be misconstrued as a 'tonic–clonic' convulsion by the inexperienced. Multifocal clonic seizures rarely occur in preterm infants and require a higher level of brain maturation than do tonic seizures. Focal clonic seizures are commoner in term infants but also occur in preterm infants. The EEG in clonic seizures is regularly abnormal, with focal or multifocal paroxysmal activity, sharp waves or spikes.

OTHER SEIZURE TYPES: fully developed generalised tonic–clonic or clonic seizures (or status) do not occur in the neonatal period, nor does complex partial or absence status in the sense applied to childhood or adult patients. True myoclonic seizures and status occur in term and preterm infants, and are especially common in children with developmental brain disorders. Strictly unilateral status was studied in 21 neonates (8% of all cases) by Bour *et al.* (1983) and was found to be due to anoxia, cardiac surgery or structural lesions in all cases. Status took the form of hemiclonic movements and vegetative (autonomic) signs, and EEG was useful in establishing the diagnosis. The unilateral nature of the seizures reflects the poor connectivity of the neonatal brain, but neither clinical nor EEG features are aetiologically or prognostically specific. Persisting focal clonic seizures are, however, usually indicative of focal cerebral damage. The frequency of clonic status in the neonatal period is falling because of better perinatal care.

Electrographic seizures, without obvious clinical signs, also occur in the neonatal period. With cerebral function monitoring in 87 neonates, seizure activity lasting 1 hour or more without clinical signs were found in 14 (16%), two of whom had never had any obvious clinical seizures (Hellström-Westas, Rosén & Svenningsen 1985). Eyre, Cozeer & Wilkinson (1983) found seizure discharges in 45% (9 of 20) of neonates, and Clancy, Legido & Lewis (1988), in 41 neonates with frequent seizures, could not detect clinical correlates in 79% (310 of 393) of electrographic discharges. Infantile spasms exceptionally may start in the neonatal period. As mentioned above subtle and tonic seizures are probably not always 'epileptic', and other movement disorders may also be confused with seizures. These include: jitteriness and tremor (Volpe 1977); toxic or withdrawal 'seizures' (from maternal medication); and some of the abnormal movements in hypoxic–ischaemic encephalopathy, neonatal intracranial haemorrhage or inborn errors of metabolism, where the EEG may be inactive or discontinuous (*tracé paroxystique*). It may be quite impossible to decide, particularly when EEG changes are absent, whether or not a clinical manifestation is epileptic.

Electroencephalography

The EEG in neonatal status is variable, and waveforms include: short-lived repetitive paroxysmal activity; spikes or sharp waves, usually focal or multifocal and of varying polarity; bursts of alpha, delta or beta activity; and periodic lateralised epileptic discharges (PLEDS). Symmetrical synchronous generalised activity is

37

Table 3.2. *Causes of neonatal status epilepticus*

Hypoxic–ischaemic encephalopathy

Acute cerebrovascular event
Subarachnoid haemorrhage
Intraventricular haemorrhage
Intracerebral haemorrhage
Subdural haemorrhage
Cerebral infarction

Intracranial infection
Meningitis (e.g. group B streptococcus, *E. coli*)
Encephalitis (e.g. herpes simplex virus, toxoplasmosis, Coxsackie B virus, rubella, cytomegalovirus)
Abscess

Cerebral malformations
Neuronal migrational and other developmental defects (e.g. agyria, pachygyria, polymicrogyria, macrogyria, corpus callosal agenesis, anencephaly, holoprosencephaly, lissencephaly)
Neurocutaneous disorders (e.g. Sturge–Weber, neurofibromatosis, tuberose sclerosis)
Chromosomal anomalies (e.g. Down's, trisomies 13 and 18)

Metabolic causes
Hypokalcaemia (e.g. primary, perinatal asphyxia, small for gestational age, diet, diabetic mother, septicaemia, hypomagnesaemia, malabsorption)
Hypoglycaemia (e.g. premature, small for gestational age, perinatal asphyxia, meningitis, transfusion, galactosaemia, fructosaemia, leucine sensitivity, pituitary hypoplasia, pancreatic tumour, glycogen storage disease)
Hyponatraemia (e.g. inappropriate therapy, inappropriate antidiuretic hormone secretion)
Inborn errors of metabolism (e.g. aminoaciduria, urea cycle defects, organic acidurias, pyridoxine deficiency)
Bilirubin encephalopathy
Hypomagnesaemia

Benign and familial syndromes
Benign familial neonatal convulsions
Benign neonatal convulsions
Benign neonatal sleep myoclonus

Toxic or withdrawal convulsions
Toxins (e.g. mercury, hexachlorophene)
Drugs (e.g. penicillin, anaesthetics)
Drug withdrawal (e.g. maternal barbiturate, alcohol, narcotics)

Specific epileptic encephalopathies
Ohtahara syndrome
Neonatal myoclonic encephalopathy
Early infantile epileptic encephalopathy

Derived from: Kellaway & Mizrahi 1987; Brett 1991; Aicardi 1992*a*.

Table 3.3. *Changing trends in the main aetiological factors in neonatal seizures over two decades*

	Presumptive cause				
	221 neonates 1958–68		210 neonates 1969–79		
Aetiological factor	(*n*)	(%)	(*n*)	(%)	
Asphyxia	25	(11.3)	51	(24.3)	$p < 0.01$
Cryptogenic intracranial haemorrhage	11	(5.0)	25	(11.9)	$p < 0.02$
Traumatic intracranial haemorrhage	22	(10.0)	9	(4.3)	$p < 0.02$
Late-onset hypocalcaemia	29	(13.1)	6	(2.9)	$p < 0.01$

There were no differences in the frequency of the following causes (percentage of causes in the two decades in brackets): cerebral infections (14.5, 11.9), recognised cerebral dysgenesis (6.3, 8.6), early-onset hypocalcaemia (7.7, 13.8) or other metabolic disturbances (19.9, 26), postmaturity (4.5, 2.4), familial neonatal seizures (2.3, 3.8), drug withdrawal seizures (2.7, 1.9), or other miscellaneous (4.1, 5.7) or cryptogenic cases (27.6, 22.9).
From Lombroso 1983, with kind permission.

rare. Patterns over time also change, in localisation and duration, even in the same infant. Seizures are often localised to one hemisphere, maximal over occipital and central, rather than over temporal or frontal, regions. The discharges may spread over the hemisphere only slowly, and clinicoelectrographic correlations are loose (Monod & Dreyfus-Brisac 1972; Plouin *et al.* 1981). Clinical seizures in neonates often have no scalp EEG change, and although some such phenomena may not be 'epileptic', it is also evident that true epileptic status can occur without obvious EEG change (Radvanyi-Bouvet *et al.* 1985; Hellström-Westas *et al.* 1985). Focal clonic and myoclonic seizures almost always show ictal EEG changes, but subtle and tonic seizures do not.

Causes

There are often multiple potential causes of status in a newborn (table 3.2), and this complicates statistical analysis. As status may be difficult to differentiate from other seizure forms (which anyway have similar causes) none of the large series has been confined specifically to status (see for instance Rose & Lombroso 1970; Dreyfus-Brisac & Monod 1972, 1977; Rossier, Caldera & Le-Oc-Mach 1973; Combes *et al.* 1975; Eriksson & Zetterstöm 1979; Lombroso 1983; Dulac *et al.* 1985; Fenichel 1985; Dreyfus-Brisac *et al.* 1981; Kellaway & Hrachovy 1983; Volpe 1987; Mizrahi & Kellaway 1987). The spectrum of causes of status has changed over recent decades, as neonatology and treatment have improved (see table 3.3).

In most modern case series, neonatal hypoxic–ischaemic encephalopathy, metabolic disorders, intracranial haemorrhage and infection are the most common identifiable causes, accounting for up to 80% of cases. The seizures in hypoxic–

ichaemic encephalopathy are usually clonic in form and, when perinatal in origin, present in the first 12 hours, reach maximum severity at 24–48 hours, and resolve after 72 hours. As perinatal care improves, the frequency of ischaemic–hypoxic encephalopathy should lessen. Neonatal infection is the next most frequent cause (meningitis with group B streptococcus or *Escherichia coli*; abscess; meningoencephalitis due to herpes simplex, toxoplasmosis, Coxsackie B, rubella, cytomegalovirus) accounting for up to 50% of cases, usually after the first week of life. Intracranial haemorrhage may be intraventricular (especially in premature infants), subarachnoid, subdural or intracerebral, and may result from coagulation defects. The advent of modern imaging has shown cerebral infarction to be commoner than was previously thought (14% of one series of 50 full-term infants with seizures, Levy *et al.* 1985). Hypocalcaemia and/or hypomagnesaemia account for about 10–55% of cases (about one third in modern series), causing seizures usually in the first 5–10 days of life, and hypogylcaemia for 3–39% of cases, presenting in the first 3 days of life. Other metabolic causes or inborn errors of metabolism are rare. Pyridoxine-dependent status may even start in intrauterine life. Congenital anomalies, especially disorders of neuronal migration, account for 1–8%. No cause is found in up to one third of patients, and these cryptogenic cases have been specifically studied by Plouin *et al.* (1981).

The treatment and prognosis of neonatal status are described on pp. 288 and 301–3.

Status epilepticus in neonatal epilepsy syndromes

A number of electroclinical childhood 'syndromes' of status have been delineated in the neonatal period (albeit with the usual controversy surrounding epilepsy classification). Perhaps the best documented and most important are the following.

Early infantile epileptic encephalopathy

This is also known as EIEE; Ohtahara's syndrome; early infantile epileptic encephalopathy with suppression-bursts (Ohtahara *et al.* 1987). It may develop in the neonatal period, although more commonly the seizures become manifest at about 3 months of life. The affected children develop increasingly frequent fits, with characteristic tonic spasms (flexor, extensor or asymmetrical), and with a burst suppression pattern on the EEG. Severe mental retardation, cerebral palsy and seizures result. The clinical picture can evolve into that of the Lennox–Gastaut syndrome, and a range of pathological aetiologies (including malformations of the central nervous system) have been found to underlie the condition.

Neonatal myoclonic encephalopathy

This is a severe epileptic encephalopathy in which erratic fragmentary myoclonus is the predominant seizure type, and also massive myoclonus, partial motor and tonic spasms (Aicardi & Goutières 1978; Aicardi 1992*b*). There is often a familial tendency, and identified causes include nonketotic hyperglycinaemia, D-glyceric acidaemia, methylmalonic acidaemia, propionic acidaemia, and hemimegalencephaly or other malformations may be identified (Aircardi 1992*b*). Transitional cases are encountered, difficult to classify, with some features of EIEE.

Benign familial neonatal seizures

Seizures usually begin on the second or third day of life of this autosomal dominant condition, have a benign prognosis, and seldom amount to status (Plouin 1985).

Benign neonatal convulsions

This is an ill-defined syndrome in which repetitive seizures occur at day 4–6 of life ('fifth day fits'), continue for a few days and then remit. The EEG in about 60% of cases shows spikes on a relatively normal background (theta point alternant), amounting to electrographic status in some cases; the EEG disturbance can be continuous up to day 12 of life. A similar status EEG pattern may also be seen in other cases of symptomatic neonatal status (Plouin 1992). The aetiology, if indeed there is a unitary cause, is unclear and the prognosis is good.

The treatment and prognosis of status in the neonatal epilepsy syndromes are described on pp. 288 and 303.

Status epilepticus confined largely to infancy and childhood

By common consent, the frequency of status is greatest in children. The highest incidence is in the neonatal period, and frequencies then fall, to plateau after the first 5 years of life (Aicardi & Chevrie 1970, 1983; Phillips & Shanahan 1989; Shields 1989; Chevrie 1991). With age, the spectrum of epileptic activity broadens. Convulsive seizures in the young child are not so fragmentary. Combined tonic and clonic forms appear, approaching the classical grand mal type, and electrographic activity gradually acquires differentiated forms from the age of about 6 months (Harris & Tizard 1960; Massa & Niedermeyer 1968). Problems of electroclinical correlation, however, remain formidable. Behavioural phenomena characteristic of nonconvulsive seizures may present in the young child but their interpretation is difficult, and is complicated by the lack of EEG definition. The emergence of more definitive epileptiform features becomes clearer with age, as the central nervous system grows and matures. Tonic–clonic status is undoubtedly the form most commonly described in older children, but whether the majority of such episodes are true tonic–clonic status or are more fractionated is quite uncertain; but the latter seems more likely. A divergence in the types of status manifest in children in whom cerebral development is normal or abnormal also becomes evident as the brain matures.

There have been a small number of case series of childhood status, the earliest and definitive being that of Aicardi and Chevrie (1970). A total of 239 cases of childhood status (less than 15 years of age), reviewed from clinic records of 8 years, were identified. Of these 43% were tonic–clonic and 38% unilateral clonic seizures; 37% of all cases occurred in the first year of life, and 85% before the fifth birthday. In 77%, the status was the first epileptic manifestation, especially in the younger patients. Some 53% were idiopathic (and half of these were febrile

Table 3.4. *The effect of age on the causes of status epilepticus in children*

Cause	All episodes ($n = 218$)	No. of cases by age		
		<1 yr old ($n = 60$)	<3 yr old ($n = 139$)	>3 yr old ($n = 79$)
Acute aetiology	87 (40)	45 (75)	65 (47)	22 (28)
Chronic encephalopathy	32 (15)	2 (3)	16 (12)	16 (20)
Epilepsy	43 (20)	0 (0)	13 (9)	30 (38)
Febrile convulsion	50 (23)	12 (20)	41 (29)	9 (11)
Idiopathic	6 (3)	1 (2)	4 (3)	2 (3)

Acute: cerebral infection, trauma, cerebrovascular disease, tumour, metabolic disorder.
Chronic encephalopathy: congenital or perinatal condition.
Epilepsy: pre-existing epilepsy (with or without fever).
Figures in parentheses are percentages.
Derived from Phillips & Shanahan 1989.
193 of 218 were first episodes of status.

status), and identifiable causes were found in 47%, with a higher frequency in the youngest children and often in patients with no previous history of epilepsy. A similar survey by Phillips & Shanahan (1989), of 218 episodes in 193 patients over 4 years from intensive care records, makes an interesting comparison (table 3.4). Again the majority (73%) of episodes occurred within the first 5 years of life, and 28% in the first year. In the first year, the majority of cases (75%) were in the context of an acute illness, a proportion which fell with age (47% in the first 3 years, and 28% in older children). Twenty-three per cent of the children had idiopathic febrile status, without a prior history of epilepsy, a figure similar to that found by Aicardi & Chevrie (28%) in 1970.

Infantile spasm (West syndrome)

Dr W.J. West, a general practitioner in Tonbridge in Kent, first described a 'peculiar form of infantile convulsion', in his previously healthy 4 month old son, and this epileptic condition bears his name (West 1841). West's is a classic description, worth quoting at length:

> The child was ... a remarkably fine, healthy child when born and continued to thrive til he was four months old. It was at that time that I first observed slight *bobbings* of the head forward, which I then regarded as a trick, but were, in fact, the first indications of disease; for these *bobbings* increased in frequency, and at length became so frequent and powerful as to cause a complete heaving of the head towards the knees, and then immediately relaxing into the upright position, something similar to the attacks of emprosthotonus: these bowings and relaxings would be repeated alternately at intervals of a few seconds, and repeated from ten to twenty or more times at each attack, which attack would not continue more than two or three minutes; he

sometimes has two, three or more attacks in the day; they come on whether sitting or lying; just before they come on he is all alive and in motion, making a strange noise, and all of a sudden down goes his head and upwards his knees; he then appears frightened and screams out: at one time he lost flesh, looked pale and exhausted, but latterly he has regained his good looks, and independent of this affliction, is a fine grown child, but he neither possesses the intellectual vivacity or the power of moving his limbs, of a child of his age... he has no power of holding himself upright or using his limbs, and his head falls without support.

Leeches, cold applications to the head, calomel purgatives, antiphlogistic treatment, lancing of the gums and warm baths were tried, but the frequency of attacks increased to 50–60 per day. Sedatives, syrup of poppies, conium and opium were then given. The child was seen by Sir Charles Clarke (who called the condition 'salaam convulsion'), Sir Astley Cooper, Dr Locock and Dr Maunsell to no avail, and, at 7 months, the attacks evolved into what were probably tonic seizures. West's remarkable description has not been bettered, yet the condition sank into obscurity again until the hypsarrhythmia pattern was identified (Gibbs & Gibbs 1952), and adrenocorticotrophic hormone (ACTH) was shown to ameliorate the spasms (Sorel & Dusaucy-Bauloye 1958).

Frequency and clinical form

Infantile spasm is rare, with an incidence of about 0.25–0.42 per 1000 live births and there is a family history of epilepsy in about 7–17% (Van den Berg & Yerushalmy 1969; Lacey & Penry 1976; Westmoreland & Gomez 1987; Cowan & Hudson 1991). The spasms rarely develop before the age of 3 months, 90% start in the first year of life, and peak incidence is at 4–6 months. Neurological deficit is often noticed before the onset of spasms (up to 80% of patients), which are often accompanied by further mental regression. The spasms take the form of sudden brief contractions of the head, neck or trunk, usually in flexion (where salaam is a good description), but sometimes in extension or commonly both. There may be a cry, and the arms rise upwards or sideways. Some attacks are less dramatic, and take the form of simple head nodding, elevation of the eyeballs or shoulder shrugging. The attacks last a second or so, and cluster with rapid repetition. It is not uncommon for dozens of spasms each separated by a few seconds to occur in a short cluster, usually lessening in severity and in frequency over time. One reported infant had over 700 spasms in 1 hour (Coulter 1986). Clusters may be repeated many times a day, and hundreds of attacks can occur in a day. The spasms are usually generalised, but may be asymmetrical or even unilateral, and are most frequent on awakening or before sleep.

Electroencephalography

The interictal EEG shows the highly characteristic pattern of hypsarrhythmia (originally described by Gibbs & Gibbs (1952)); in its fully developed form, a disorganised and chaotic succession of high voltage slow waves with intermingled multifocal asynchronous spike and sharp waves. These changes are virtually continuous, although altered in non-REM (non-rapid eye movement) sleep, and sometimes remitting in REM sleep. The typical EEG occurs in about two-thirds of EEG in infantile spasm. A burst suppression variant (with poorer prognosis) has been described (Hrachovy, Frost & Kellaway 1984). Modified forms with relatively normal background activity, focal features or synchronous spike–wave activity occur in some 40% of patients, and a unilateral form may occur rarely. Ictally, 11 different patterns have been described (Kellaway *et al.* 1979): the commonest is the electrodecremental pattern, and others include spike, spike–wave, slow wave activity with superimposed fast activity, and attenuation. The hypsarrhythmia may diminish during a series of spasms, recurring when the series subsides. Occasionally the ictal EEG shows no change, and EEG seizures can occur without any clinical event. The hypsarrhythmia may evolve from other abnormal EEG patterns, and resolves gradually usually in parallel with the clinical improvement.

Causes

The syndrome has numerous causes (table 3.5), of which tuberous sclerosis, brain dysgenesis, chronic acquired lesions and cerebral maldevelopment are the commonest. Metabolic and degenerative causes are rarer. No specific cause can be found in about 40%, but only about 10–15% of cases are free of pre-existing mental, developmental or neurological abnormalities (cryptogenic cases). Prenatal causes account for about 20–60%, perinatal causes account for 15–40% and postnatal causes for 10% of patients. The condition can evolve from pre-existing epileptic or nonepileptic encephalopathies, for instance from *Ohtahara's syndrome* or *neonatal myoclonic encephalopathy*. In these and other severe cases the infantile spasms can be viewed as further nonspecific evidence of profound cerebral malfunction and the clinical findings in an individual patient thus essentially reflect the cause. A small group of idiopathic cases also exists, with a mild condition and a good prognosis (Dulac *et al.* 1986). If no clues are present a careful screening for the cutaneous manifestations of tuberous sclerosis should be carried out.

The underlying physiological disturbance is uncertain, but the discharges arise from brain stem or cortical structures, on a developmental, neurochemical or even immunological basis (Lacey & Penry 1976; Hrachovy *et al.* 1985, 1987; Hrachovy & Frost 1990).

As with all the 'syndromes' of status in childhood, there are related and overlapping epileptic conditions. These include: *early myoclonic encephalopathy* and *Ohtahara's syndrome*, which can exhibit EEG patterns of burst suppression which evolve into hypsarrhythmia; *periodic lateralised spasms* associated with focal brain lesions; and partial seizures which are rare in infancy, and can also evolve into a classical West syndrome.

The treatment and prognosis of infantile spasm are described on pp. 288 and 303–4.

Table 3.5. *Causes of infantile spasm (West syndrome)*

Disorders of cerebral development
Neuronal migrational and other developmental defects (e.g. heterotopia, agyria–
    pachygyria, corpus callosal agenesis, dysplasia, hemimegaencephaly, holoprosencephaly,
    microcephaly, macrocephaly, porencephaly, schizencephaly)
Neurocutaneous syndromes (e.g. tuberose sclerosis, Sturge–Weber syndrome,
    neurofibromatosis, incontinentia pigmentia and linear naevus syndrome)

Metabolic and degenerative disorders
Metabolic disorders (e.g. phenylketonuria, nonketotic hyperglycinaemia, pyridoxine
    deficiency, Leigh's disease, histidinaemia, hyperornithinaemia-hyperammonaemia,
    homocitrullinaemia, maple syrup urine disease, leucine-sensitive hypoglycaemia)
Degenerative disorders of uncertain aetiology (e.g. poliodystrophies, leucodystrophies,
    Alper's disease, Sandhoff disease, Tay–Sachs disease)

Perinatal or postnatal chronic acquired cerebral lesions
Hypoxic–ischaemic encephalopathy and cerebral infarction
Haemorrhage (intracranial, subarachnoid, subdural)
Infection (meningitis, encephalitis, abscess, intrauterine infection)
Cerebral trauma
Cerebral tumour
Maternal toxaemia
Metabolic and endocrine disorders
Infantile spasms evolving from neonatal seizure syndrome (e.g. Ohtahara syndrome or
    neonatal myoclonic encephalopathy)

In approximately 40% of cases, no cause is found (of whom 10–15% show some
preceding developmental disturbance).

The condition is best viewed as an age-specific epileptic response to cerebral injury,
and it can thus be due to many conditions which affect the brain.

Derived from Westmoreland & Gomez 1987; Brett 1991; Aicardi 1992*a*.

Febrile status epilepticus

Between the ages of 6 months and 6 years, children are very prone to epileptic
convulsions during febrile illnesses. In Western populations, 2–5% of children
have suffered a febrile convulsion by the age of 5 years, the peak incidence being
between 18 months and 3 years of age (Van den Berg & Yerushalmy 1969; Aicardi
& Chevrie 1970; Nelson & Ellenberg 1981; Wallace 1988). Most children have
a short convulsion which does not recur, and are otherwise neurologically normal.
A minority have an identifiable pre-existing developmental or neurological abnormality. A proportion have seizures that are repetitive or persist for 30 minutes or
more; this is febrile status epilepticus.

Febrile status is one of the commonest forms of convulsive status epilepticus
in young children. The seizures are clonic or tonic–clonic in form and may often
be unilateral, a characteristic feature not seen in older children, or focal (Aicardi
& Chevrie 1970). Febrile status can be followed by a Todd's paresis, or occasionally by permanent neurological deficit. Most prolonged convulsions happen in

children under the age of 18 months, especially before the age of 13 months (about 30% of all febrile convulsions in children under 13 months are prolonged; Lennox-Buchthal 1974), and after the age of 2 years, the proportion of febrile convulsions that amounts to status is low. Febrile status is also more likely in children with pre-existing neurological or developmental problems, and prolonged seizures are more likely to exhibit focal features. Status or serial seizures (more than one seizure per episode of fever), and seizures with focal features (complex febrile seizures) carry a poorer prognosis than do 'simple febrile seizures'. Febrile status is a medical emergency, requiring urgent treatment as delay in controlling the seizures can result in permanent cerebral damage, subsequent chronic epilepsy, developmental retardation and focal neurological deficit.

The treatment and prognosis of febrile status are described on pp. 288–9 and 304–6.

Status in childhood myoclonic epilepsies

Cryptogenic and symptomatic childhood myoclonic epilepsies

The classification of the myoclonic epilepsies of childhood is a mire of confusion and muddle, in which one dabbles at one's peril. A simplistic view is taken here, in which the epilepsies are divided into crytpogenic, symptomatic and syndromic categories. Cryptogenic myoclonic epilepsy refers to those cases (the majority) in which no cause for the epilepsy is identifiable. Myoclonic status is common in this condition, particularly in those patients with coexisting mental retardation. Symptomatic myoclonic epilepsy may be the result of various prenatal pathologies, and less often perinatal injury (e.g. hypoxic–ischaemic encephalopathy, perinatal haemorrhage). Although accounting for only a small proportion of cases, myoclonic status is also a frequent symptom of hereditary metabolic diseases, including: neuronal ceroid lipofuscinosis (four variants – early infantile (Santavuori-Hagberg), late infantile (Jansky-Bielschowski), juvenile (Spielmeyer-Vogt), late childhood (Kuf's)); sialidosis; Tay–Sachs and Sandhoff diseases (GM_2 gangliosidosis); Gaucher's disease type 3; mitochondrial disease; nonketotic hyperglycinaemia and D-glyceric acidaemia; and Lafora body disease. Other hereditary metabolic disorders may produce status, although not specifically myoclonic in type (adrenoleucodystrophy, for instance, frequently results in clonic or tonic–clonic status).

In addition to these cryptogenic and symptomatic myoclonic epilepsies, there are three relatively well-defined myoclonic syndromes in childhood. The first is the syndrome of *benign myoclonic epilepsy in infants* (Dravet & Bureau 1981), which has excellent prognosis and in which status does not occur. In the two other myoclonic syndromes, however, status is common.

Syndrome of severe myoclonic epilepsy in infants

This is a severe infantile myoclonic syndrome in which status is common (Dravet *et al.* 1982; Dravet, Bureau & Roger 1985; Dravet *et al.* 1992). The onset is frequently with febrile clonic seizures in the first year of life. A progressive and severe epileptic disorder develops, characterised by clonic, myoclonic, atypical absence and partial seizures, and psychomotor retardation. Myoclonus is prominent, may be massive and is often induced by photic stimuli, and there is often a family history. Status can take the form of obtundation, with erratic small myoclonias, persisting for hours or days, sometimes triggered or perpetuated by variations in the intensity of ambient light. The EEG during the status shows continuous slow activity with spike–wave bursts of varying topology.

Syndrome of myoclonic status epilepticus in nonprogressive encephalopathy

Dalla Bernardina *et al.* (1992) differentiate this syndrome from other severe myoclonic epilepsies on the basis of its clinicoelectrographic features. Typically, signs of a severe encephalopathy, characterised by hypotonia and abnormal movements, pre-date the epileptic manifestations. Myoclonus and absence develop in the first year of life, and the epilepsy then evolves to be characterised by prolonged periods of myoclonic status. During these episodes, the children appear obtunded and ataxic, and show continuous myoclonias. The EEG shows frequent spike and spike–wave bursts, with electrographic status often recorded during slow wave sleep. Electrographic status may also occur during wakefulness, without overt clinical signs. In most reports of children, though, the aetiology of this epileptic encephalopathy is obscure, although cases with Prader–Willi syndrome, Angelman syndrome, and fetal or neonatal anoxia have been described (Dalla Bernardina *et al.* 1992). The boundaries between this syndrome, and those of the other myoclonic epilepsies in childhood, the myoclonic forms of Lennox–Gastaut syndrome, minor epileptic status (Brett 1966) and other childhood encephalopathies are difficult to define.

Syndrome of myoclonic–astatic epilepsy

The nosological position of this epileptic syndrome is also fraught with contention. As the name suggests, it is characterised by myoclonic and astatic or myoclonic–astatic seizures. The condition is said to account for 1–2% of all childhood epilepsies (Doose *et al.* 1970; Doose 1985). Doose classifies the status as primary generalised absence (petit mal) status, a disputatious view because of its clinical context and prognosis. Furthermore, when severe, the condition is very similar to the Lennox–Gastaut syndrome, leading some to doubt whether myoclonic–astatic epilepsy exists as a separate entity (Gastaut 1982; Henriksen 1985). In the 117 cases described by Doose (1985), the onset is between 2 and 5 years, 74% were male, the EEG showed bilateral synchronous irregular and regular 2–3 Hz spike or polyspike and wave, with a slow background. One third of patients have a family history, and no other specific cause is found.

About 40% of patients exhibit episodes of absence status, during which the child appears apathetic, hypokinetic or stuporous; there is fine irregular twitching of the extremities, facial muscles and eyelids, which may be palpated if not seen.

The expression is blank, drooling occurs and speech is slurred, sparse or absent. There can be head nodding, and the status may be interrupted by astatic seizures (Doose *et al.* 1970; Doose 1983, 1985). During periods of status, the child may be unable to keep the head upright, and feeding may be difficult. Status typically develops on awakening and may last hours or even days. Pure myoclonic status is rare. The EEG shows 2–3 Hz spike–waves, and polymorphic irregular hypersynchronous activity. This EEG pattern is activated by non-REM sleep, and may dominate the sleep record. Occasionally, the status is myoclonic in form with repetitive polyspike EEG discharges. The level of consciousness correlates much more closely with the EEG changes than in secondarily generalised absence status (e.g. of the Lennox–Gastaut variety).

Differentiation from the Lennox–Gastaut syndrome may be difficult, and transitional cases possibly exist. Doose (1985, 1992) listed the following criteria useful for distinguishing the syndrome of myoclonic–astatic epilepsy: genetic predisposition, normal premorbid development, absence of an underlying neurometabolic or degenerative disorder, lack of neurological deficits, generalised seizures (myoclonic, astatic, myoclonic–astatic, grand mal), rarely partial seizures, no atypical absence or daytime tonic seizures, and primary generalised EEG patterns without focal abnormalities.

The treatment and prognosis of status in the childhood myoclonic epilepsies are described on pp. 289 and 306.

Status epilepticus in the benign childhood epilepsy syndromes

Benign rolandic epilepsy (benign epilepsy of childhood with rolandic spikes)

This is a well-defined childhood syndrome accounting for up to 15% of all childhood epilepsies. Four cases of nonconvulsive status have been described in this condition (Fejerman & Di Blasi 1987; Boulloche *et al.* 1990; Colamaria *et al.* 1991), characterised by tonic deviation or weakness of the face, speech arrest, sialorrhea, drooling of saliva, swallowing difficulties, oromotor 'apraxia' and partial loss of awareness. The EEG shows continuous secondarily generalised or bilateral centrotemporal focal spike or slow spike–wave complexes. Colamaria *et al.* (1991) pointed to the similarities of this form of status with the *anterior operculum syndrome* (*Foix–Chavany–Marie syndrome*), with bilateral ictal discharges in the lower rolandic region. The response to treatment is good, and status does not adversely affect outcome in this benign syndrome. Occasional patients show the EEG pattern of ESES (see next section) during slow wave sleep, without neuropsychological deficit, witness to the nosological overlap in the childhood epileptic syndromes (Dalla Bernardina *et al.* 1978; Aicardi & Chevrie 1982).

Benign occipital epilepsy

Prolonged seizures, often lasting several hours, are characteristic in this syndrome (Kuzniecky & Rosenblatt 1987; Panayiotopoulos 1989). In one series, nonconvulsive (or convulsive) status was reported in 14% (9 of 62) of childen, often as the first epileptic manifestation (Kivity & Lerman 1992).

The treatment and prognosis of status in the benign childhood epilepsy syndromes are described on pp. 289 and 306–7.

Electrical status epilepticus during slow wave sleep

This term was first introduced by Patry, Lyagoubi & Tassinari (1971), who described six children with almost continuous slow spike–wave EEG complexes during non-REM sleep. Five of the six children had epilepsy (atypical absence or rare nocturnal seizures), all were mentally retarded, and four had severe speech disturbance. Tassinari *et al.* (1977*b*) reported further patients and named the syndrome 'electrical status epilepticus during sleep' (ESES), and in subsequent reports described 19 personal patients and reviewed 25 other cases from the literature (Tassinari, Terzano & Capocchi, 1985; Tassinari, Bureau & Thomas 1992). Morikawa *et al.* (1985) reported a further five patients, contrasted these with Lennox–Gastaut cases, and designated the syndrome 'continuous spike–wave discharges during sleep' (CSWS). The International League Against Epilepsy (ILAE) *Classification of the epilepsies and epileptic syndromes* lists the syndrome under the title 'Epilepsy with continuous spike–waves during slow wave sleep'. There have been at least 60 subsequent case reports (Kellermann 1978; Dalla Bernardina *et al.* 1978, 1989; Billard *et al.* 1981; Beaumanoir 1983; De Marco 1988; Kobayashi *et al.* 1988), and the condition has been the subject of several reviews (Morikawa *et al.* 1989; Jayakar & Seshia 1991; Yasuhara *et al.* 1991; Tassinari *et al.* 1992).

Morikawa *et al.* (1989) reported the syndrome to be present in 0.5% of 12 854 children with epilepsy over a 10 year period, although a higher frequency might be found if routine sleep records were more often obtained. The diagnostic criterion is the presence on the EEG of spike–wave discharges occupying at least 85% of non-REM sleep. There is no consensus about the number of EEG records required to show these changes, nor the period of time over which these should be observed (Patry *et al.* 1971; Morikawa *et al.* 1985; Tassinari *et al.* 1985). The EEG changes are essentially generalised, but some authors have included cases with relatively focal abnormalities, and some with sharp waves not spike–wave. During REM sleep and wakefulness, spike–wave discharges may occur but to a much lesser degree. The aetiology is unknown, although about 20–30% of cases have identifiable brain pathology (e.g. previous meningitis, birth asphyxia, cytomegalovirus infection), 3% of children have a family history of epilepsy, and 15% a history of febrile convulsions (Morikawa *et al.* 1989). Therefore, as with many other epilepsy syndromes, definitions are ambiguous, pathophysiological mechanisms obscure, and causes diverse.

The clinical signs of the core syndrome include seizures, mental retardation and infrequently other neurological features. Seizures are almost invariable, usually developing between the ages of 1 and 14 years (mean about 5 years), and may be focal motor, tonic–clonic, absence, atonic or complex partial in form. Tassinari *et al.* (1985) divided their 18 cases into three categories; those with rare motor seizures usually nocturnal, those with mainly nocturnal unilateral partial seizures and daytime absence seizures, and those with rare nocturnal seizures and day time atypical absence seizures with atonic or clonic components. Whether such a classification is useful is debatable. Other case reports have shown a mixture of epileptic types, both diurnal and nocturnal, and (with the exception of tonic seizures) almost all clinical epileptic manifestations seem to occur. Some patients have episodes of overt absence or focal motor status. The striking sleep-related EEG abnormalities which define the syndrome, however, are not usually associated with any overt clinical seizure activity. Over half of the recorded cases have normal intellectual function prior to the development of ESES (68% of the 49 patients of Tassinari *et al.* (1985) and Morikawa *et al.* (1989)), but in most cases mental processes deteriorate during the status, sometimes to a very severe extent. In 11 patients who had normal functioning before ESES (Tassinari *et al.* 1985), overall IQ scores fell to between 45 and 78. The regression seems particularly to affect language functioning, and mutism may develop (De Marco 1988). Other reported intellectual deficiences include impairment of memory, temporal and spatial orientation, hyperkinetic or aggressive behaviour, and psychosis. A proportion of cases (44% of the patients of Tassinari *et al.* 1985) exhibit neurological signs of varying nature, prior to the development of ESES. Drug treatment may or may not abolish the ESES, although overt seizures are usually helped (see Jayakar & Seshia 1991; Yasuhara *et al.* 1991).

The relationship of ESES to other syndromes of 'status' has been the subject of some debate. There are similarities with the Landau–Kleffner syndrome. Both occur at about the same age, include striking abnormalities of speech, multiple seizure types, and severe EEG disturbances, especially in slow wave sleep. However, in the Landau–Kleffner syndrome, the typical electrographic changes of ESES are manifest only occasionally, the neuropsychological disturbances are more specific, and the course is somewhat different. The Lennox–Gastaut syndrome too has features which overlap, including psychological deterioration, multiple seizure types and frequent spike–wave bursts on the EEG. The typical nocturnal ESES pattern is rare in the Lennox–Gastaut syndrome, and more usually the sleep EEG pattern is dominated by polyspikes rather than spike–wave. Tonic seizures do not occur in typical cases of ESES, and the temporal course and prognosis of the two syndromes differ. A patient of complex partial status with ESES has been reported (Sacquegna *et al.* 1981); ESES has also been recorded in atypical benign partial epilepsy (Aicardi & Chevrie 1982; Kobayashi *et al.* 1988), and is occasionally seen in other epilepsies. The condition is quite possibly underreported, and the wider use of sleep studies in severe epileptic patients would undoubtedly reveal hitherto unsuspected cases. In a proportion of patients (both children and adults) with severe epilepsy, EEG abnormalities are greatly enhanced during sleep, and in some cases these sleep abnormalities are of 'status' proportions. How common this is amongst the generality of epileptic patients is uncertain, but I have encountered occasional adult patients in whom sleep abnormalities of the ESES type are uncovered unexpectedly. The ESES pattern might simply be an extreme of a spectrum of sleep-activated EEG changes.

On EEG grounds, the epileptic discharges certainly resemble those of status, yet are not accompanied by overt seizures. Thus, as with the Lennox–Gastaut and Landau–Kleffner syndromes, the nosological position of ESES in regard to status is uncertain. Without a more detailed understanding of the underlying physiology, it is not clear whether the EEG findings are epiphenomena of specific encephalopathy, whether the EEG changes are responsible for the regression and cerebral damage (and if they are not, what is?), or whether treating the EEG will prevent mental deterioration. These are all important unresolved questions.

The treatment and prognosis of status in ESES are described on pp. 289–90 and 307.

Syndrome of acquired epileptic aphasia (Landau–Kleffner or Worster-Drought syndrome)

This disorder of childhood in which persisting aphasia develops in association with severe focal EEG abnormalities was first described by Landau & Kleffner (1957) and Worster-Drought (1971). Since then over 200 cases have been reported (Gascon *et al.* 1973; Sato & Dreifuss 1973; McKinney & McGreal 1974; Shoumaker *et al.* 1974; Giovanardi Rossi, Pazzaglia & Frank 1976; Deuel & Lenn 1977; Deonna *et al.* 1977; Foerster 1977; Lou, Brandt & Bruhn 1977; Rapin *et al.* 1977; Beaussart & Faou 1978; Cooper & Ferry 1978; Koepp & Lagenstein 1978; Lanzi & Bojardi 1978; Petersen *et al.* 1978; van Harskamp, van Dongen & Loonen 1978; Mantovani & Landau 1980; Billard *et al.* 1981; Holmes, McKeever & Saunders 1981; Toso *et al.* 1981; Dugas *et al.* 1982; Rodriguez & Niedermeyer 1982; Dulac *et al.* 1983; Bishop 1985; Msall *et al.* 1986; Ansink, Sarphatie & van Dongen 1989; Deonna, Peter & Ziegler 1989; Hirsch *et al.* 1990; Loonen & van Dongen 1990; Maquet *et al.* 1990; Marescaux *et al.* 1990; Deonna 1991; Beaumanoir 1992; Paquier, van Dongen & Loonen 1992; Pascual-Castroviejo *et al.* 1992). It is an uncommon condition, usually without a family history and with a male prepondance (about 2:1). The aetiology, pathogenesis and pathophysiology are unknown (Landau 1992). Two temporal lobectomy specimens have been examined showing nonspecific gliosis only (Cole *et al.* 1988), biopsy material from a further atypical case suggested encephalitis (Lou *et al.* 1977) but this has not been confirmed by others. Isolated cerebral arteritis was reported in four children, on the basis of angiographic irregularity in the territory of the carotid artery (Pascual-Castroviejo *et al.* 1992), although this is generally a rather unreliable radiographic sign. Maquet *et al.* (1990) reported bitemporal blood flow changes on positron emission tomography (PET); an observation which does not much further advance understanding of the condition. I have observed a patient, with accompanying complex partial and generalised seizures, with widespread EEG and cognitive changes, in which magnetic resonance imaging (MRI) (but not computed tomography (CT)) revealed an anterior temporal neocortical benign tumour; to what extent local temporal pathology could be responsible for the totality of the clinical picture is uncertain.

The syndrome usually occurs in children who have previously developed normally. The aphasia may develop in a subacute or gradual fashion, with deficits evolving in some patients over weeks and in some over several years. Verbal comprehension is invariably affected, usually in combination with a motor aphasia. In some patients the speech disorder has been attributed to an auditory agnosia (word deafness) rather than aphasia, and can extend to familiar noises, as the patients become increasingly incapable of attributing semantic value to acoustic signals (Rapin *et al.* 1977; Beaumanoir 1985). Speech can be sparse, amounting at times to almost total mutism. The aphasia may fluctuate, and transient but complete remission of all symptoms may occur (Mantovani & Landau 1980; Sawhney *et al.* 1988). Other inconstant clinical features include hyperkinesis, personality disturbances and intellectual deficits; some of these additional features may be secondary to the loss of language, but the predominant deficit in all cases is of speech. Overt epileptic seizures are manifest in only about 70% of patients, and are usually mild. Overt status epilepticus of various types occurred in about 15% of cases in the literature review of Beaumanoir (1985). The epilepsy, but not the EEG disturbance, is controlled by anticonvulsant treatment.

The EEG shows repetitive high voltage spikes or spike–wave discharges, in a generalised focal or multifocal distribution, which is activitated in slow wave sleep and may attain the continuous or nearly continuous activity of electrographic status. These abnormalities are not specific and occur in other clinical settings. The EEG disturbances usually involve the dominant temporal region, and it is tempting to postulate that the speech disturbance is directly due to electrographic activity. Some have demonstrated a correlation of EEG abnormalities and language disorder (Shoumaker *et al.* 1974; Cole *et al.* 1988), and there is a general but not absolute temporal association between the evolution and resolution of EEG abnormalities and the aphasia. ESES has been observed in a proportion of cases, with accumulating evidence that this too specifically affects language functioning, although the temporal relationship between ESES and language functions in the Landau–Kleffner syndrome is not very close (Dulac, Billard & Arthuis 1983; Paquier *et al.* 1992).

The pathophysiology of the syndrome is unclear. A number of neuropsychological explanations have been proposed, matched in audacity only by the lack of supporting evidence. Pervading all is the argument that the enduring aphasia is caused by the electrographic disturbance ('bio-electric status'); the fluctuation (even to temporary complete remission), the correlation with EEG changes, and the eventual parallel resolution of epilepsy, EEG disturbance and aphasia all support this contention. In this sense the condition can be categorised as a form of 'status epilepticus', albeit in the absence of overt seizures.

The treatment and prognosis of the syndrome of acquired epileptic aphasia are described on pp. 289–90 and 307.

Status epilepticus occurring in late childhood and adult life

Tonic–clonic status epilepticus

Tonic–clonic status epilepticus (the modern sobriquet for the more lovable grand mal status epilepticus) is the classic clinical form, first described by Calmeil and subsequently the subject of repeated study; this early clinical literature is discussed in chapter 1. Indeed, until quite recently, the term status epilepticus was used to refer exclusively to grand mal status, and other forms were either not recognised or not so categorised. The clinical form of tonic–clonic status was well defined in the nineteenth century, and the EEG in the post-war years; both were well summarised by Roger *et al.* (1974) in their study of 100 cases collected for the Xth Marseilles Colloquium. The original descriptions of clinical phenomenology are unequalled in their detail and accuracy, and are given in summary on pp. 5–6 (Bourneville's description) and pp. 9–10 (that of Clark & Prout). In this section, aspects covered in more recent work are emphasised.

Clinical features

PREMONITORY (PRODROMAL) STAGE As noted by Clark & Prout in 1903/4, in established epileptics, tonic–clonic status is often preceded by a premonitory stage of some hours during which seizure activity increases from its usual level. Seizures develop with increasing frequency or severity. In those with generalised epilepsy, progressive myoclonic jerking may occur, and in others subclinical seizure activity produces mental changes or confusion. The clinical deterioration is an augury, often stereotypic, and the danger of impending status is only too well recognised. In patients not previously subject to epileptic seizures, however, the status may start abruptly.

MOTOR ACTIVITY: Motor activity in established tonic–clonic status evolves though several stages; termed the convulsive and meningitic stages by Bourneville and the convulsive and stuporous stages by Clark & Prout. At the onset of status, the repeated tonic–clonic convulsions have the same tonic then clonic form as isolated seizures, although Gastaut *et al.* (1967) also emphasised a third postictal phase of tonic spasm (of trunk and limbs, with trismus) not seen in isolated grand mal. In the Marseilles series (Roger *et al.* 1974), the average duration of the tonic and clonic stages was 90 seconds, shortening as the status progressed to less than 1 minute, and seizures recurred in fully established status at a mean frequency of 4–5 per hour; however, higher frequencies are not uncommonly encountered (to over 20 fits per hour in my own experience). In the pretreatment era enormous numbers of seizures were noted: Clark & Prout (1903/4) recorded 488 attacks in 24 hours leading to 1000 in 3 days in one case that ended fatally, and 3000 in 4 weeks in another. Kinnier Wilson (1940) recorded a girl aged 13 who experienced 3231 major seizures in 17 days, of which 2258 were observed in 6 consecutive days, and who then made a perfect recovery. As time passes, the convulsions change their form. Usually, the tonic phase becomes prolonged and the clonic jerking less pronounced and less severe. Indeed, eventually, clonic jerking may be almost completely absent (as noted by many authorities, including Bourneville (1876); Clark & Prout (1903/4), and Kinnier Wilson (1940)), a state now designated subtle status epilepticus. The physiological basis for this striking diminution of motor phenomena is unclear; biochemical alterations at synaptic or cellular level, systemic disturbances, or sedative drug therapy might all contribute. A focal onset of the motor activity can be clear during individual seizures, and this is of course an important clinical signal of localised cerebral disorder. Other neurological signs present during the episode of status depend to a large extent on the underlying cause. Plantar responses may be extensor, either unilaterally (66%) or bilaterally (33%) (Roger *et al.* 1974).

AUTONOMIC CHANGES: Autonomic changes can be profound and dominate the clinical picture. These include tachycardia, cardiac arrythmia, hypertension, apnoea, pupillary enlargement, hypersecretion and sweating. The corneal and pupillary responses, both during and between attacks, are abolished. Salivation and tracheobronchial secretions may embarrass respiration. Status causes massive excitation of the sympathetic nervous system, resulting in adrenaline and noradrenaline release (12 and 40 times baseline levels, respectively, 10 minutes after a single seizure; Simon 1985). This causes an initial rise in systemic, pulmonary and left atrial blood pressures, which subsequently falls in spite of persisting elevation of catecholamine level, due to mechanisms as yet unclear. The high catecholamine levels contribute to cardiac dysfunction, arrhythmia and tachycardia (Benowitz, Simon & Copeland 1986).

STAGING OF PHYSIOLOGICAL CHANGES: It is usual to divide the physiological changes in tonic–clonic status into two phases: phase I is the early (compensated) stage and phase II the late (decompensated) stage (Brown & Hussain 1991*a,b* Walton 1993). The move from phase I to phase II is usually said to occur after about 30 minutes of continuous seizures. It is for this physiological reason that 30 minutes is chosen as the minimum time limit when status is defined (see fig. 3.1 and table 3.6). Whilst staging the process helps to conceptualise physiological changes, great variation is seen in clinical practice. The rate and extent of physiological change is critically dependent on the aetiology, the site and the severity of the seizures, and the therapies deployed.

HYPOXIA: There is a greatly increased demand by cerebral tissue for oxygen. The cellular metabolic rate during the first stage of grand mal status is phenomenally raised, shown both in experimental studies and human PET studies (Franck *et al.* 1986*a,b*), and is compensated for by greatly increased cerebral blood flow (up to 400%), with greater glucose and oxygen delivery. Experimental studies show a decrease in cerebrovascular resistance, and the increased perfusion initially parallels the increased cerebral metabolic rate. It is postulated, however, that as cerebral autoregulation is lost in the transition from phase I to phase II, these compensatory

Table 3.6. *Physiological changes in tonic–clonic status epilepticus*

Phase I: compensation

During this phase, cerebral metabolism is greatly increased due to seizure activity, but physiological mechanisms are sufficient to meet the metabolic demands, and cerebral tissue is protected from hypoxia or metabolic damage. The major physiological changes are related to the greatly increased cerebral blood flow and metabolism, massive autonomic activity and cardiovascular changes.

Cerebral changes	Metabolic changes	Autonomic and cardiovascular changes
Increased blood flow	Hyperglycaemia	Hypertension
Increased metabolism	Lactic acidosis	Increased cardiac output
Energy requirements matched by supply of oxygen and glucose (increased glucose and oxygen utilisation)		Increased central venous pressure
		Massive catecholamine release
Increased lactate concentration		Tachycardia
		Cardiac arrhythmia
Increased glucose concentration		Salivation
		Hyperpyrexia
		Vomiting
		Incontinence

Phase II: decompensation

During this phase, the greatly increased cerebral metabolic demands cannot be fully met, resulting in hypoxia and altered cerebral and systemic metabolic patterns. Autonomic changes persist, and cardiorespiratory functions may progressively fail to maintain homeostasis.

Cerebral changes	Metabolic changes	Autonomic and cardiovascular changes
Failure of cerebral autoregulation; thus cerebral blood flow becomes dependent on systemic blood pressure	Hypoglycaemia	Systemic hypoxia
	Hyponatraemia	Falling blood pressure
	Hypokalaemia/ hyperkalaemia	Falling cardiac output
	Metabolic and respiratory acidosis	Respiratory and cardiac impairment (pulmonary oedema, pulmonary embolism, respiratory collapse, cardiac failure, arrhythmia)
Hypoxia		
Hypoglycaemia	Hepatic and renal dysfunction	
Falling lactate concentrations	Consumptive coagulopathy, DIC, multiorgan failure	
Falling energy state	Rhabdomyolysis, myoglobulinuria	Hyperpyrexia
Rising intracranial pressure and cerebral oedema	Leucocytosis	

DIC, disseminated intravascular coagulation.

Note: the physiological changes listed above do not necessarily occur in all cases. The type and extent of the changes depend on aetiology, clinical circumstances and the methods of therapy employed.

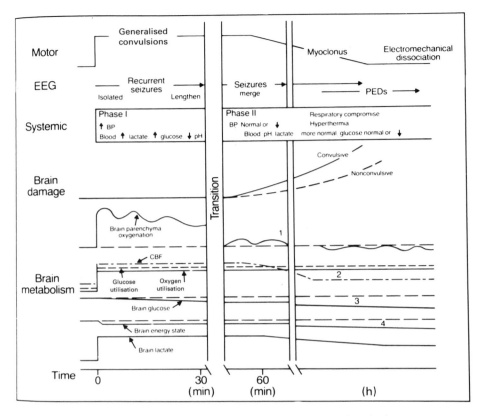

Fig. 3.1. Diagram of the temporal changes which occur as tonic–clonic status epilepticus progresses. Motor activity lessens, EEG evolves (see fig. 3.2) and profound physiological changes occur, both systemically and cerebrally. In the first 30 minutes or so, physiological changes are largely compensatory, but as the seizures continue these compensatory mechanisms break down. The biphasic evolution is emphasised. PED, periodic epileptic discharge. 1, loss of reactivity of brain oxygen tension; 2, mismatch between the sustained increase in oxygen and glucose utilisation and a fall in cerebral blood flow; 3, a depletion of cerebral glucose and glycogen concentrations; 4, a decline in cerebral energy state. (From Lothman 1990, with kind permission.)

mechanisms are lost. Cerebral perfusion then becomes largely dependent on systemic blood pressure, hypotension develops and cerebral blood flow decreases. This results in cellular hypoxia, which is possibly particularly severe in the epileptic tissue where metabolic rates are highest.

Human studies are lacking (DeGiorgio *et al.* 1992), although impressive experimental evidence both from primate and non-primate experiments shows local ischaemia developing as status becomes prolonged (see Meldrum 1983; Franck *et al.* 1986*a,b*; Siesjö & Wieloch 1986). How hypoxia damages tissues is uncertain, but possible mechanisms include intracellular acidosis, ATP depletion, rupture of lysosomes, free radical release, or cellular oedema. Even if oxygen and gluose are adequately supplied to epileptic tissue, cellular damage can result from the endogenous release of the excitatory amino acids (glutamate and others) mediating the seizure discharges (see pp. 165–74). The mechanism of excitotoxic damage is not fully established, but is possibly related to intracellular calcium ion flux (for a more detailed debate of these issues, see pp. 170–3). The increased demand for oxygen is not confined to cerebral tissue. Convulsing muscles create huge metabolic demand, at a time when spontaneous ventilation may be impaired or paralysed, due to ventilatory muscle spasm, unconsciousness or respiratory obstruction.

Within 30 minutes or so, most patients in major convulsive status have measurable systemic hypoxia; indeed, to a degree almost always greater than clinically suspected. Assisted ventilation should therefore be instituted early, much earlier than would be usual in respiratory failure from other causes. Cerebral hypoxia is an important antecedent of cerebral damage, especially in the young, and is responsible for substantial morbidity.

HYPERCAPNIA: Raised carbon dioxide levels are common in status. Of the 18 patients reported by Aminoff & Simon (1980) 13 had carbon dioxide levels exceeding 60 mmHg, although at what stage of the status hypercapnia developed is unclear. High carbon dioxide levels may predispose to pulmonary oedema and occasionally carbon dioxide narcosis is life threatening. Usually, however, hypercapnia is of no great clinical importance.

BLOOD PRESSURE: In phase I of convulsive status, blood pressure is invariably elevated, due mainly to catecholamine release (Blennow *et al.* 1978; Simon 1985; Benowitz *et al.* 1986), and occasionally levels rise close to those of an hypertensive encephalopathy. Hypotensive therapy, however, is rarely required. The adrenal catecholamine release is due to neuronal stimulation, and can be blocked by spinal anaesthesia (Anton, Uy & Redderson 1977). Marked tachycardia can also occur in both ictal and interictal periods. Indeed, ictal tachycardia is sometimes the only sign of individual seizures occurring in comatose ventilated patients during status epilepticus. As phase II physiological changes develop (after about 30 minutes), blood pressure begins to fall, and may remain normal or slightly low for some time before hypotension develops. In prolonged status, hypotension is common, and is due to secondary cerebral, metabolic and endocrine changes, drug therapy, or possibly desensitisation of catecholamine receptors (Morin & Westerlain 1983).

BLOOD SUGAR CHANGES: At the onset of status, the massive release of catecholamines, insulin and glucagon results in glycogenolysis and moderate hyperglycaemia (Meldrum & Horton 1973; Kreisman *et al.* 1981). There is some experimental evidence that hyperglycaemia may contribute to cerebral damage in status, as in human stroke, by enhancing metabolism and thus inducing cellular excitotoxicity (Melamed 1976; Blennow *et al.* 1978; Pulsinelli *et al.* 1983), and routine administration of glucose to patients who are not hypoglycaemic should therefore probably be avoided.

As seizures continue, however, hypoglycaemia may develop, due to exhaustion of glycogen stores, hepatic damage, rebound hyperinsulinaemia and other endocrine factors (Meldrum & Horton 1973; Meldrum & Nilsson 1976; Meldrum *et al.* 1979; Horton *et al.* 1980; Benowitz *et al.*, 1986). The low blood sugar exacerbates the cellular metabolic disturbance induced by falling oxygen levels and failing cerebral blood flow.

ACIDOSIS: Lactic acidosis is almost invariable in major status epilepticus, from its onset. Potential mechanisms include lactate production from neuronal and muscle activity, the acceleration of glycolysis, tissue hypoxia, impaired respiration, and catecholamine release. In a series of 70 cases immediately following the cessation of status, 84% had serum pH below normal (pH 7.35), in 33% the pH was below 7.0, and in one patient a level of 6.18 was recorded (Aminoff & Simon 1980). Lactate levels may be very high and serum potassium levels low. Other metabolic or respiratory acidosis is less common. Magnetic resonance spectroscopy has demonstrated an approximately 30% fall in levels of phosphocreatine in brain, low cerebral pH, and normal ATP levels in paralysed rabbits (Petroff *et al.* 1984). The administration of bicarbonate has been advocated (Wasterlain 1974), in the hope (not proven in clinical studies) of preventing shock, and mitigating the effects of hypotension and low cerebral blood flow. Generally, though, bicarbonate infusion is of uncertain benefit, and best avoided unless the acidosis is extreme. If bicarbonate is needed a dose of 100 mequiv. can be given by injection, and blood gases monitored (Wasterlain *et al.* 1993). More effective is the rapid control of respiration and abolition of motor seizure activity, which probably contributes more to lactic acidosis than any other factor. Acidosis is not a great problem in well-ventilated patients and, unlike changes in blood pressure or temperature, it does not worsen as the duration of status increases. Acidosis was not thought to be an important cause of status-induced cerebral injury in paralysed and ventilated primates (Meldrum & Brierley 1973), and, in human adult status at least, it is unlikely to be a major cause of cellular damage (only 5% (3 of 59) of acidotic patients reported by Simon (1985) sustained cerebral damage). Nevertheless, elevation of cerebrospinal fluid (CSF) lactate level has been shown to correlate with a poor outcome from status (Calabrese *et al.* 1991). In children, the metabolic risks of prolonged convulsions may be more severe. Simpson, Habel & George (1977) measured arterial and CSF acid–base variables, and lactate and pyruvate levels in 22 infants and children and found signs of cerebral hypoxia in 7, with repetitive or prolonged convulsions (greater than 30 minutes).

HYPERPYREXIA: An increase in body temperature is common in status epilepticus, due to convulsive muscle activity, massive catecholamine release, and possibly other central mechanisms. Hyperpyrexia can occasionally be severe and prolonged, in which case the outcome is poor – a fact noted from the first reports of Bourneville (1876) and Clark & Prout (1903/4). Hyperpyrexia is associated with cellular damage in experimental status especially of the cerebellum (Meldrum & Brierley 1973), and also results in permanent cerebral damage in humans. In a series of 75 patients, temperatures over 107 °F (42 °C) were recorded in two who were in status for over 9 hours; both patients sustained cerebral damage (Simon 1985).

INTRACRANIAL PRESSURE AND CEREBRAL OEDEMA: As is commonly observed in intensive care settings, all epileptic seizures transiently elevate intracranial pressure. In status, however, persistingly high intracranial pressure may develop quickly. In phase II, the combined effects of systemic hypotension and intracranial hypertension can result in a compromised cerebral circulation and cerebral oedema. In adults severe cerebral oedema is unusual even in patients dying in status, but in children oedema is more common and severe, and oedema can impair cerebral circulation to the extent that watershed infarction results (Brown & Hussain 1991*a*). Intracranial pressure monitoring is advisable in prolonged severe status, especially in children, when raised intracranial pressure is suspected. The need for active medical or surgical therapy is largely determined by underlying pathology, being more often necessary in encephalitis or trauma, for instance, than in drug-induced status or status following drug withdrawal.

Focal cerebral oedema is sometimes manifest as low density on MRI or CT scanning, which may last for days and can be easily mistaken for other pathologies (Sammaritano *et al.* 1985; Kramer *et al.* 1987; Bauer *et al.* 1989; Riela, Sires & Penry 1991). The structural imaging findings have been correlated with single-photon emission tomography (SPECT) and intensive EEG monitoring in one patient (Bauer *et al.* 1989), and with angiography in another (Lee & Goldberg 1977). The exact mechanism underlying the production of focal oedema is not known, but must be closely related to vascular changes; possibly focal lactic acidosis or hypoxia, causing vasodilatation and blood–brain barrier breakdown. How often such focal oedema can be detected in focal status is quite unknown. In acute status in patients without prior epilepsy or cerebral disturbance, underlying vascular or inflammatory pathologies are a commoner cause of transient focal imaging abnormalities than is epilepsy-related focal oedema, and this can complicate diagnosis. Certainly, before assuming a change to be seizure related, other causes should be excluded; this is a problem, sometimes not acknowledged in published work, which bedevils all imaging studies.

PULMONARY OEDEMA: Pulmonary hypertension and oedema are frequent in status, even in the presence of systemic hypotension, and are probably the result of direct seizure-related autonomic effects. Pulmonary artery pressures rose to 685% of control values in one experimental study, falling to normal after 15 minutes, long before systemic arterial pressure fell (Bayne & Simon 1981). Such pulmonary artery pressures are well in excess of the osmotic pressure of blood, the oedema fluid can therefore be both an exudate or transudate, and the high pulmonary arterial pressures can cause stretch injury to lung capillaries (Simon *et al.* 1982;

Simon 1985). Pulmonary oedema worsens outcome, and is a common finding in patients dying in status.

CARDIAC ARRHYTHMIA AND OTHER CARDIAC DYSFUNCTION: Cardiac arrhythmias in status epilepticus have several possible mechanisms including direct autonomic effects of seizures, catecholamine release, hypoglycaemia, lactic acidosis, electrolyte disturbance, or cardiotoxic therapy. Seizure-related autonomic effects are sometimes caused by simultaneous discharges in sympathetic and parasympathetic fibres. Intravenous sedatives depress cardiac function, and the drug effects can be potentiated by pre-existing compromise of cardiac function. Arrhythmias and cardiovascular collapse are frequently encountered in experimental status models (Meldrum & Horton 1973; Meldrum, Vigouroux & Brierley 1973; Horton *et al.* 1980), as well as in humans, yet there have been only a few formal haemodynamic studies of either. Young *et al.* (1985) studied bicuculline-induced seizures in neonatal pigs, and observed initial systemic and pulmonary hypertension, followed by progressive hypotension and falling cardiac output. Echocardiology revealed decreasing left ventricular contractility, and increased lactate and reduced glucose, triglyceride and ATP levels were measured in cardiac muscle. Low or high output cardiac failure, cardiac arrhythmia and pulmonary hypertension might result from such changes, and undetected cardiac dysfunction contributes to morbidity and mortality in status. Cardiac hypertrophy has been demonstrated after status in rats, but the relevance of this observation to human status is uncertain (Rubinstein, Walton & Treiman 1992).

RHABDOMYOLYSIS AND MYOGLOBINURIA: Rhabdomyolysis, caused by the violent convulsive movements, can develop early in status (Winocour *et al.* 1989) and worsen as status continues. Anoxia due to compromise of the muscular vascular supply in the decubitus comatose patient can contribute to muscle damage. Occasionally the rhabdomyolysis is severe, and the resulting myoglobinuria may precipitate renal failure (Grossman *et al.* 1974; Singhal, Chugh & Gulati 1978). Rhabdomyolysis can be prevented in the ITU by artificial ventilation and muscle paralysis.

DISSEMINATED INTRAVASCULAR COAGULATION AND MULTIORGAN FAILURE: Disseminated intravascular coagulation (DIC) is a rare but serious complication of status. The exact mechanism is uncertain, but is probably related to rhabdomyolysis and thromboplastin release by muscle injury, hyperpyrexia, myoglobinuria, renal or hepatic failure, sometimes in the context of multiorgan failure. One reported patient had few haemorrhagic features and a self-limiting condition (Fischer *et al.* 1977), but a poor outcome is more usual. There has been inconclusive speculation about the role of drugs (e.g. lamotrigine or valproate) in the precipitation of disseminated intravascular coagulation and multiorgan failure in status.

METABOLIC DISTURBANCE AND RENAL AND HEPATIC FAILURE: Electrolyte disturbances in status have various causes. Hyperkalaemia is a particular problem, exacerbated by rhabdomyolysis, but nevertheless also common in paralysed patients. Acute tubular necrosis due to myoglobinuria or dehydration, and occasionally fulminant renal failure may occur. Hepatic failure due to other physiological disturbances, drug treatment or the underlying cause of the status is a relatively frequent complication. Valproate therapy possibly induces hepatic failure in some cases, and its use in status should be circumspect. Intractable status and acute hepatic failure leading to death are features of Alper's disease, usually unsuspected premortem. My own experience suggests that this is an unusual but not rare occurrence, and one in which valproate therapy is possibly implicated. A recent familial case was found to have cytochrome c oxidase deficiency, dying after receiving valproate therapy. This is the first time that an underlying metabolic disturbance has been recognised (Bourgeois & Aicardi 1992).

OTHER PHYSIOLOGICAL CHANGES: Leucocytosis is frequent in status, even in the absence of infection. In a series of 80 patients (Aminoff & Simon 1980) the white cell count at the time of presentation was increased in 50 (62%), and was above $20\,000/mm^3$ in 15%, with a predominance of polymorphonuclear cells. In the 65 patients without an alternative explanation for CSF changes, CSF leucocytosis was also present in 12 (18%), and was above 70 cells/mm^3 in 2 (3%) (Aminoff & Simon 1980). I have occcasionally encountered counts in excess of 100 cells/mm^3. This rise is usually early and is transient; a persisting elevation implies an additional cause. Vomiting, urinary or bowel dysfunction, sweating, salivation, and tracheobronchial secretion are common autonomic effects. Inhalation and asphyxia may occur because of secretions or vomit. Other systemic effects include loss of weight, trophic abnormalities and bed-sores. The skin changes of status were detailed by Clark & Prout (1903/4): and include the 'tâche cérébrale' of Trousseau, the 'meningitic streak' of Bourneville, or the 'dermographism' of Feré & Lamy which were said always to accompany severe status, whereas the 'white and blue oedema' of Sydenham and Charcot are seen only in hysteria.

Electroencephalograpy

Although tonic–clonic status is a common condition, detailed studies are surprisingly rare. Gastaut could find only six records in over 100 000 EEGs from the clinic in Marseilles, and the analysis for the Xth Marseilles Colloquium included only 45 well-documented (clinically and electrographically) records, from 28 different centres, and 67 incomplete records. The definitive EEG study is that of 100 patients in tonic–clonic status published by Roger *et al.* (1974) after the Colloquium. The classic EEG pattern of grand mal seizures is usual in the early stages. This includes flattening (desynchronisation) at the onset of the seizure followed by a recruiting rhythm of about 10 Hz increasing in amplitude, interrupted by bursts of high voltage slow activity during the clonic phase, and then followed by postictal slow activity (Gastaut *et al.* 1974). The EEG silence which commonly follows an isolated seizure was seen in only 46% of the series. This might indicate that failure of inhibition is a fundamental part of the underlying physiological alteration in status. A focal EEG onset to the seizures in status is commonly detectable. Lennox (1960) noticed that the EEG changes as the status progresses, the brain potentials eventually becoming 'almost quiescent', and periodic lateralised epileptiform discharges (PLEDS) are a common finding in end-stage status (Snodgrass, Tsuburaya & Ajmone-Marsan 1989). More recently, a distinctive five-phase temporal evolution in EEG patterns during status has been postulated (Treiman, Walton & Kendrick 1990, on the basis of a review of 60 EEG records; fig. 3.2):

1. EEG changes of discrete seizures.
2. Merging seizures with waxing and waning of amplitude and frequency of EEG rhythms.
3. Continuous ictal activity.
4. Continuous ictal activity punctuated with low voltage 'flat' periods.
5. PLEDS on a 'flat' background.

The time period of this evolution is not specified, and how consistently this pattern occurs is unclear; certainly I have encountered cases which do not seem to have followed this sequence. There is no doubt, however, that the EEG evolves over time in status, in parallel to the clinical evolution, and both the clinical and EEG features of early and established tonic–clonic status are very different (fig. 3.3).

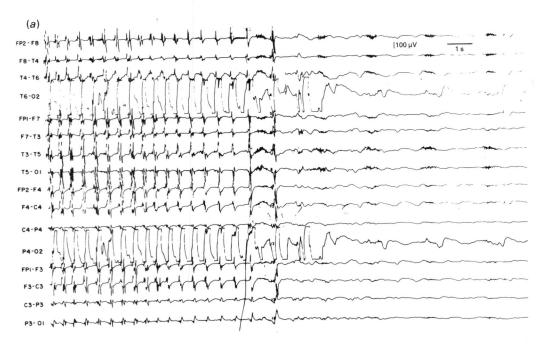

Fig. 3.2. The progression of EEG during tonic–clonic status epilepticus. The EEG shows a progressive evolution in five stages: (*a*) discrete seizures with interictal slowing;

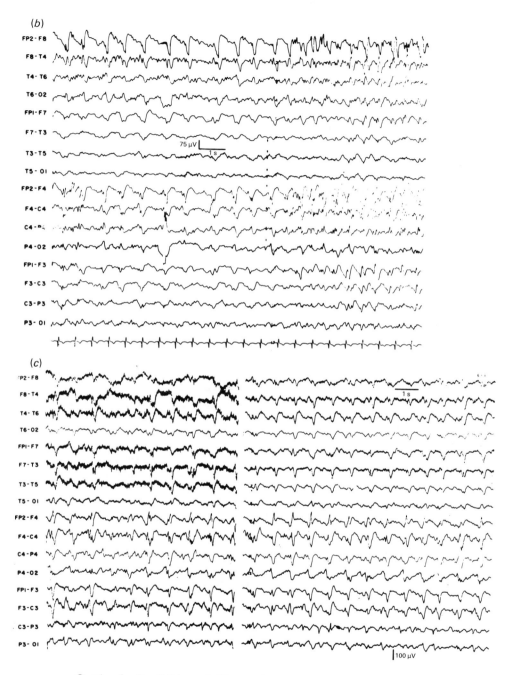

Caption for fig. 3.2 (*cont.*). (*b*) merging of decrete seizures, with waxing and waning between seizures; (*c*) continuous ictal discharge (examples 16 minutes apart);

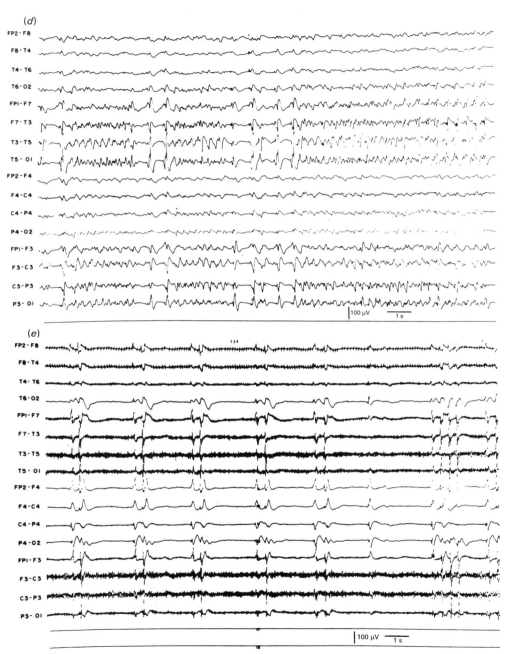

Caption for fig. 3.2 (*cont.*). (*d*) continuous ictal discharges with flat periods; (*e*) periodic lateralised epileptic discharges on a flat background. (From Treiman *et al*. 1990, with kind permission.)

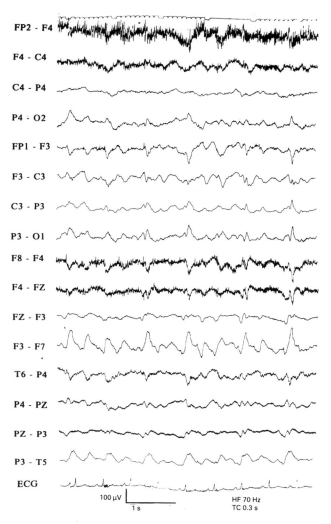

Fig. 3.3. EEG from a 31 year old female who developed tonic–clonic status epilepticus a week after an episode of fever and abdominal pain. Despite intensive treatment, including anaesthesia and full intensive care unit support, she remained in electrographic status for 2 weeks. Extensive investigation failed to reveal a cause for the status. Volumetric magnetic resonance imaging on recovery showed both hippocampi to be very small, without change in size over the next 4 months. On recovery she showed severe amnesia and intellectual deficit, which improved considerably over the next 6 months. The EEG was recorded during the second week of status, and shows the periodic lateralised epileptiform discharges (PLEDs) typically seen in the late stages of status. ECG, electrocardiograph. (With thanks to Dr Shelagh Smith, National Hospital for Neurology and Neurosurgery, for preparing this illustration.)

Changes in the underlying cause of status (for instance, encephalitis, head trauma), systemic physiological changes and drug treatment all greatly affect EEG, and to what extent a consistent sequence of EEG changes occurs due to inherent underlying progressive pathophysiology is not known. The nature of PLEDs in end-stage status has been the subject of controversy, with argument that the pattern simply reflects severe cerebral dysfunction rather than epileptic activity. Support for an epileptic basis to the EEG pattern is provided by the finding of hypermetabolism during PLED activity in rats, using 2-deoxyglucose autoradiology (Treiman 1993), and the claim (on the basis of limited evidence) that anticonvulsant drugs can abolish the EEG pattern. This is an important issue, for if PLEDs do represent ongoing seizure activity, effective antiepileptic therapy might prevent seizure-induced cerebral damage. The same five electroencephalographic stages were observed in status in Sprague-Dawley rats over a short time course, in which no anticonvulsant therapy was administered, and it is arguable that these changes represent the 'natural history' of status, perhaps reflecting neuronal damage (Treiman *et al.* 1990); this proposition requires confirmation.

Causes

There have been no population-based studies, and our knowledge of the range of causes of tonic–clonic status derives largely from hospital or clinic surveys, a selection of which are summarised in table 3.7. Before accepting the findings uncritically, however, certain limitations from such studies should be acknowledged.

1. All are highly selected, some from ITUs (Goulon *et al.* 1985; Phillips & Shanahan 1989), others from specialist neurological inpatient services (e.g. Janz & Kautz 1963; Aicardi & Chevrie 1970; Heintel 1972; Sung & Chu 1989*a*) and Roger's cases (Roger *et al.* 1974) were the best-documented 100 reported by 28 epilepsy experts to the Marseilles Colloquium (Roger *et al.* 1974). None was of unselected populations.
2. Most were retrospective reviews.
3. Most were of restricted age groups, which profoundly effects the frequency and disposition of status. The influence of age is shown in table 3.7. In childhood febrile idiopathic and congenital causes are predominant, in adult life acquired cerebral and metabolic disorders, and in the elderly metabolic and cerebrovascular diseases.
4. The aetiology of status is often multifactorial. Thus, status in patients with underlying structural lesions may be precipitated by acute events (metabolic disturbance, alcoholism, etc.), and the distinction between 'precipitating factor' and 'cause' is only relative, a problem not acknowledged in some reports.
5. Related to this is the distinction which should be drawn between those cases in which status occurs as an intercurrent event in established epilepsy, and those in which it is a first epileptic event. A minority of cases occur in existing epileptics (e.g. 29% of 282 patients, Goulon *et al.* 1985; 33% of 239 patients, Aicardi & Chevrie 1970; 23% of 193 patients, Maytal *et al.* 1989; 29% of 193

cases, Phillips & Shanahan 1989; 35% of 52 cases, Yager *et al.* 1988; 46% of 100 cases, Roger *et al.* 1974). The 'causes' of status in pre-existing epileptic and previously nonepileptic cases are different (see table 3.8). This distinction has not always been made in the published literature.

6. In the more recent published series, not all included cases were of grand mal status; other types accounted for 57%, 27%, 29%, 50% and 29% of the patients of Aicardi & Chevrie (1970), Sung & Chu (1989*a*), Celesia (1976), Yager *et al.* (1988), and Maytal *et al.* (1989), respectively.

For all these reasons, the distribution of causes in unselected populations is unknown. It seems likely that hospital series overrepresent structural and serious neurological lesions, and under-represent acute precipitants; but these issues will not be resolved without population-based investigation.

It is usually taught that almost any grey matter central nervous system (CNS) disturbance can cause epilepsy and, by extension, status. Whilst this may be (indeed is likely to be) true, the reported causes of status in the published case series are relatively limited in number. There are differences in the patterns of aetiology in status and in epilepsy (e.g. the higher incidence than expected of status in cerebral tumour, trauma and infection; Heintel 1972), implying that the underlying physiology of status is not simply that of epilepsy (and that status is merely a severe form of epilepsy) but rather that there are more fundamental differences. A comparative study of aetiology would be informative, giving clues to underlying pathophysiological mechanisms, but unfortunately none is available. The propensity for frontal lobe structural lesions (of any sort) to cause status is discussed on pp. 29–30. In a study from a large general hospital in an American inner city, comparison was made between the causes of adult status in the 1970s and 1980s. Surprisingly little difference was found, and in both decades the commonest causes were: poor antiepileptic drug compliance/drug withdrawal (in the 1980s: 31%, 48 of 154 cases), alcohol-related status (28%, 43 of 154 cases), drug toxicity or abuse (9%, 14 of 154), CNS infection (8%, 12 of 154). Cerebral tumour, trauma, refractory epilepsy, stroke, metabolic disorders and cardiac arrest accounted for the rest (Lowenstein & Alldredge 1993). Of those with a history of prior epilepsy (87 of 154 cases), the commonest causes were anticonvulsant drug withdrawal (39 cases, 45%) and alcohol (25 cases, 29%). In the 67 patients without a history of epilepsy, the most frequent aetiologies were: alcohol (14 cases, 21%), drug toxicity (12 cases, 18%) and infection (6 cases, 9%). How representative such a sample is of the generality of status can only be guessed, drawn as it is from a deprived inner city area with a high incidence of alcoholism, drug abuse and violence.

CEREBRAL TRAUMA: Open-head injuries are more likely than closed head injury to result in status, often in the acute phase (Oxbury & Whitty 1971*a*), as is head injury complicated with intracerebral haemorrhage. In early seizures due to trauma, 10% present as status epilepticus. Status in trauma damaging large areas of brain, contusion, or depressed fracture also carries a poorer prognosis. Neurosurgery may also cause status; the risk of epilepsy after burr hole is about

Table 3.7. *The causes of status epilepticus in 1679 patients from 13 case series*

Sources	n	Percentage of cases								
		Cerebrovascular	Tumour	Trauma	Infection	Congenital/ perinatal	Acute metabolic, toxic, anoxic	Other	Febrile	Idiopathic/ cryptogenic
Childhood										
Alcardi & Chevrie 1970	239	0	0	1	12	21	14	0	28	24
Yager et al. 1988	52	2	4	0	19	23	15	4	21	12
Philips & Shanahan 1989	218	1	1	5	14	14	14	6	29	16
Maytal et al. 1989	193	2	1	4	8	23	6	9	24	24
All ages										
Janz 1960	95	4	25	24	3	3	0	7	0	34
Rowan & Scott 1970	43	7	5	26	5	16	4	2	5	21
Oxbury & Whitty 1971a	86	15	22	8	10	5	2	9	0	28
Heintel 1972	83	13	20	20	7	8	8	2	0	19
Roger et al. 1974	56	12	20	39	0	0	0	17	0	12
Adults										
Aminoff & Simon 1980	98	15	4	3	4	0	34	24	0	15
Hauser 1983	132	13	3	17	14	0	0	15	5	32
Goulon et al. 1985	282	20	5	9	7	3	37	13	0	7
Elderly adults										
Sung & Chu 1989a	102	35	8	21	3	0	10	11	0	13
Total/%	1679	10%	7%	10%	9%	10%	14%	9%	12%	19%

Table 3.8. *The causes of status epilepticus as the presenting symptom of epilepsy, or as an intercurrent event in established epilepsy[a] (in 554 patients from 5 case series)*

	Status as presenting symptom of epilepsy (%) ($n = 327$)	Status as an intercurrent event (%) ($n = 227$)
Cerebral trauma	12	17
Cerebral tumour	16	10
Cerebrovascular disease	20	19
Intracranial infection	15	6
Acute metabolic disturbance	12	5
Other acute event	14	3
No cause found	11	41

[a] Excluding precipitating causes.
From Janz 1961; Oxbury & Whitty 1971a; Aminoff & Simon 1980; Goulon *et al.* 1985; Dunn 1988.

9–13%, after craniotomy for glioma 19%, craniotomy for intracranial haemorrhage 21%, and for meningioma removal 22% (the site of the structural lesion, the presence or absence of neurological deficit, and the prior occurrence of seizures are both important factors influencing this risk). After surgery for aneurysm the risks of epilepsy fall to between 4% for carotid ligation and to 20% for craniotomy for a posterior communicating aneurysm (see Shorvon 1992). The proportion of patients developing status after surgery for these various conditions is not known.

CEREBRAL INFECTION: A wide variety of infectious causes of status has been listed by Heintel (1972), but in routine adult practice the commonest are bacterial meningitis, abscess, and severe viral encephalitis, usually herpes simplex. Infectious illnesses (with or without fever) may also precipitate status in established epileptic cases, especially in children. Human immunodeficiency virus (HIV) infection is another recently defined cause of status (Holtzman, Kaku & So 1989), as is cerebral malaria (Phillips & Solomon 1990). Chronic encephalitis is discussed on pp. 85 and 95–6.

CEREBRAL TUMOUR: Almost any cerebral tumour may cause status, but the propensity to do so is greater in axial rather than extra-axial tumours and in those which are rapidly growing. Thus, the relative incidence of status compared to isolated seizures is lower in oligodendroglioma and meningioma and higher in astrocytoma or malignant glioma. The site of the tumour is also important, and status is more common in supratentorial than in subtentorial tumours, in superficial rather than deeply placed tumours, and is particularly common in tumours of the frontal cortex.

CEREBROVASCULAR DISEASE: Intracerebral or subarachnoid haemorrhage, angiomata, and cerebral infarction or embolism are all important causes of status, although the exact frequency is uncertain, nor is it possible to say whether or not these conditions cause status proportionally more commonly than they do ordinary epilepsy. Sung & Chu (1989*b*) found seizures in 4.6% (64 of 1402) of patients admitted with intracranial haemorrhage. Status occurred in 11 (17% of those with epilepsy) and was the initial presentation of the haemorrhage in 6 (9%). The same authors (Sung & Chu 1990) also reviewed 118 patients with CT evidence of thrombotic stroke, of whom 13% had had status, occurring in the acute phase in 4 (5%). Arteriovenous malformation and cavernous angiomata cause epilepsy (the latter an increasingly recognised cause of focal seizures), although status seems rare. In a survey of 1000 patients with acute stroke, 44 had early seizures (within 2 weeks of the onset of stroke) and 2 status epilepticus (0.2% of all strokes and 5% of those with epilepsy). Similarly, in 90 cases of postinfarction epilepsy, Gupta *et al.* (1988) recorded status in 8% of all initial seizures after acute stroke, and Cocito, Favale & Reni (1982) in 5 (23%) of 22 selected cases with carotid arterial occlusive disease. In general, large lesions, those that are cortically placed and acute lesions seem more likely to result in status (and other epileptic seizures) than do small, chronic, or deep vascular lesions, features rather similar to those associated with status in cerebral tumour.

FEBRILE STATUS EPILEPTICUS: In children, the causes of status are very different from those in adults. After the neonatal period, fever is the commonest cause of status in the first 2 years of life (see pp. 45–6), often occurring in children with pre-existing neurological problems. Fever precipitates status in adults much less commonly.

METABOLIC CAUSES: Almost any metabolic disturbances can result in status, more commonly in children than in adults and with a differing emphasis at different ages. Acute metabolic changes, especially of serum electrolytes or sugar, are more likely to causes seizures than are slowly developing changes. In the neonatal period, hypoglycaemia, hypocalcaemia and hypomagnesaemia are important causes of status. Status is uncommon in hepatic encephalopathy, unless acute with cerebral oedema. In patients with chronic hepatic failure, status is usually due to associated electrolyte disturbance or cerebral lesion. In Wilson's disease, epilepsy occurs early in about 6% of cases, typically at the onset of therapy when copper concentrations are changing; the condition can also present as status (Dening, Berrios & Walshe 1988). Hyperparathyroidism (Sallman Goldberg & Wombolt 1981), porphyria (Lévy-Alcover & Goulon 1967) and chronic disorders of calcium or magnesium metabolism can also cause status.

TOXIC CAUSES: Toxic exposure to, and the withdrawal of, drugs can result in status. Indeed, it was Hunter's (1959/60) proposition that status became common only in the anticonvulsant era, because of anticonvulsant drug withdrawal. It is now clear, however, that many cases are in drug-naive patients, or in epileptics on stable regimens. The extent to which drug intoxication causes status is not known. The Boston Collaborative Drug Surveillance Program reported 51 cases of drug-induced convulsions amongst 32 812 treated patients, of which 8 were status epilepticus (status reported with isoniazid (3 cases), lidocaine (2 cases) and psychotropic agents, bronchodilators, and insulin (Messing, Closson & Simon 1984)), a gross underestimate of the true frequency. Drugs most implicated in routine practice are the psychotropics, anaesthetic and analgesic agents (e.g. enflurane, lidocaine), anticonvulsants, penicillins, contrast media, and others (e.g. baclofen). Penicillin is a notable cause of status, especially if given intrathecally or, I have observed, parenterally to a patient with a dural abnormality. Interestingly, drugs with anticonvulsant activity have been implicated in status, although this might be due to covert withdrawal. In addition to the conventional anticonvulsants, baclofen (or its withdrawal) is more frequently implicated in status than would be expected (e.g. Hyser & Drake 1984; Messing *et al.* 1984). I have encountered status due to parenteral lignocaine, as have Messing *et al.* (1984), who noted that heart failure may exacerbate the risk. Paradoxically, the general anaesthetics used to treat status (see pp. 262–85) can also cause it, as can the aqueous iodinated contrast media meglumine and metrizamide; the latter in particular seem prone to trigger nonconvulsive status in adults (Buchman, Klawans & Russell 1987). The frequency in which status is induced or precipitated by alcohol (or its withdrawal) is uncertain, but this is probably an important cause in many places. Victor & Brausch (1967) in their earlier classic studies of alcoholism found status in 3.3% of 241 patients, and Simon & Aminoff (1980) considered alcoholism to contribute to 15% of their 98 patients of status. In a recent study addressing this problem, of 82 unselected patients of status epilepticus admitted to the casualty department in a large hospital in Helsinki (a city with a high alcoholism rate), 7.3% were due to alcohol withdrawal, and alcohol abuse preceded status in 35% of patients (some with no previous history of seizures, and some in which other potential causes were also present; Pilke *et al.* 1984). It is not clear whether alcohol-induced and alcohol-withdrawal seizures have similar pathophysiology. Both can be complicated by acute changes in serum osmolarity, blood sugar and anticonvulsant ingestion.

OTHER NEUROLOGICAL CONDITIONS: A wide variety of other neurological conditions occasionally result in status. Multiple sclerosis has been particularly reported to do so, and is also associated with a higher than expected incidence of epilepsy (e.g. Hunter 1959/60; Lévy-Alcover & Goulon 1967; Boudouresques *et al.* 1980; Ghezzi *et al.* 1990). The mechanisms of epilepsy in what is essentially a white matter condition is unclear. Of defined causes reported in the literature, hydrocephalus seems especially well represented; whether or not this results specifically in status is not known, but hydrocephalic epilepsy is not especially common. The issue is complicated by the fact that hydrocephalus may be caused by neonatal haemorrhage or other potent causes of status, and that shunting or shunt infections can also result in seizures. Although myoclonic epilepsy is characteristic of mitochondrial cytopathy, tonic–clonic status is not uncommon and can be the first epileptic or neurological manifestation of the condition; see for example the case of Galan *et al.* (1992). In this patient, the epilepsy remained

71

intractable until 10% glucose, riboflavin and CoQ were added to his therapy. Other oddities resulting in status include, cat scratch fever (Anonymous 1992; Tsao 1992), eye-closure (Ripamonti *et al.* 1991; a warning to the weary!), and near hanging (Dinsmore, Crane & Callender 1985).

CONGENITAL AND PERINATAL CAUSES: Status in early life is most commonly due to prenatal causes, and less often to perinatal and postnatal disorders; the importance of prenatal abnormality being increasingly recognised because of advances in imaging and genetic investigation. Almost any congenital disturbance can result in status, and the most important in numerical terms are probably the disorders of neuronal proliferation and migration.

In a population survey of epilepsy amongst the mentally retarded (299 cases; Forsgren *et al.* 1990), a history of convulsive status was obtained in 19%. Prenatal factors accounted for 35% of the cases of epilepsy, perinatal factors for 9.5%, postnatal factors for 8.8% and multiple factors for 14.9%. In 31.5% no cause could be assigned (table 3.9).

The causes listed above are those identified largely in the traditional manner. In many cases of status, however, no obvious or single cause has been found. In the past decade, progress in developmental neurobiology has elucidated the processes of neuronal formation, migration and maturation, and it is now recognised that disturbances of these processes often result in epilepsy. Many such disorders have been unidentifiable in life and indeed are missed on routine pathological examination.

Such mild developmental abnormalities have now been demonstrated frequently in human idiopathic epilepsies (Meencke & Janz 1984, 1985; Lyon & Gastaut 1985; Meencke 1985; Cook *et al.* 1994*b*). These anomalies are of the microdysgenesis type, largely quantitative alterations of neuronal disposition in cortex and subcortical regions. In primary generalised epilepsy, for instance, Meencke & Janz (1984) have consistently demonstrated unipolar and bipolar cells in the subpial regions, increased cell density in the stratus moleculare, protrusions of nerve cells into the pia, loss of columnar architecture in the cortex, and increased numbers of neurones in the white matter. Microdysgenesis and related anomalies, it is postulated, are a common cause of epilepsy, previously ignored perhaps because of their subtle nature. Indeed, Meencke (1991, 1994) has proposed that the phenomenological expression of secondary and primary generalised childhood epilepsies depends largely on the type and extent of microdysgenesis. He demonstrated microdysgenesis in 38% of 591 brains from patients with epilepsy, compared to 8% in 7374 control brains. In 12.3% of the epileptic brains (and 2% of the controls), the changes were severe. Hardiman *et al.* (1988) similarly found severe neuronal microdysgenesis in 21 (42%) of 50 temporal lobectomy specimens (and none of 33 normal controls). Refinements in MRI techniques are increasingly likely to demonstrate the importance of these conditions. An example is the recent finding of abnormalities of the grey–white interface, indicating subtle cortical organisational disturbances, on magnetic resonance-based fractal analysis, in a high proportion of patients with 'idiopathic' focal epilepsy (Cook *et al.* 1994*a*).

Table 3.9. *Causes of epilepsy in a mentally retarded population*

Cause	Pathogenic period				
	Total (%)	Prenatal (%)	Perinatal (%)	Postnatal (%)	Multiple/additional (%)
Chromosmal	8.4	7.0			1.4
Neurometabolic	3	2.4			0.6
Neurocutaneous	1.7	1.4			0.3
Other hereditary	0.6	0.3			0.3
Multifactorial	8.0	5.0			3.0
Other recognised syndromes (e.g. Rett) or unknown causes	11.1	4.6			4.4
Endogenous intoxication (e.g. phenylketonuria)	0.3				0.3
Premature	1.0	0.3			0.7
Low birth weight	8.0	1.7			6.3
Small for dates	5.7	1.3			4.4
Other pregnancy-related factors	12.7	2.0			10.7
Neonatal asphyxia	18.7	0.7	7.0		12.0
Neonatal hypoglycaemia	1.0		0.7		0.3
Neonatal haemorrhage/ infarct	2.4		0.7		1.7
Infection	11.0	2.0	0.7	4.7	3.7
Trauma	3.0			2.3	0.7
Tumours[a]	1.0				
Autism[a]	4.1				2.4
Others[a]	1.3			0.6	
Not known	28				

[a] Unknown pathogenetic period for all cases.
This was a prevalence survey of all those registered in a northern Swedish county as mentally retarded with active epilepsy (299 subjects; 20% of the mentally retarded). Some persons feature in several categories. This is a point prevalence study, and so the incidence of the conditions causing epilepsy is not known, and may well be very different. Derived from Forsgren *et al.* 1990.

Recent MRI studies have also emphasised the importance of small developmental lesions in epilepsy (Barkovich, Gressens & Evrard 1992; Cook *et al.* 1994*a,b*; Meiners *et al.* 1994; Raymond *et al.* 1994), and abnormalities of the grey–white matter interface have been demonstrated by various methods (Cook *et al.* 1994*a,b*; Meiners *et al.* 1994; Raymond *et al.* 1994).

A consideration of the phases of fetal development provides a good framework for understanding the underlying pathology of such epileptogenic developmental lesions (the reader is referred for more details to the excellent recent reviews by

Aicardi (1992*a*) and Barkovich *et al.* (1992)). In the human fetus, between the first and the sixteenth week after gestation, the neural tube and crest form, close, and basic differentiation occurs. By 32 or 33 days, the prosencephalon has formed and the telencephalon and diencephalon are grossly distinguisable. The proliferation of primitive cells which will form neurones and glia begins at about 4 weeks, from cellular elements situated close to the lumen of the neural tube. Neuroblast proliferation is maximal between 10 and 18 weeks of gestation, and by 20 weeks all neuronal cells are formed. Neuronal migration starts at about 12 weeks, reaches its peak before 20 weeks, but continues through pregnancy, and indeed into the postnatal period (particularly in hippocampus and brain stem neurones). The proto-neurones migrate initially along glial guides (later to transform into astrocytes) that extend from the ventricular ependyma to the pial surface of the neural tube. The cells of layer I migrate first, and remain at the surface of the brain. Other cells migrate in an 'inside out' manner, with the large pyramidal cells destined for layers IV and V migrating before those of the more superficial layers. Glial cell proliferation begins at about 25 weeks. Dendrites, axons and synapses develop rapidly, and this process is continued to about the fourth year of life. Myelin begins to be deposited at about 30 weeks. and myelination continues well into childhood. Sulci develop in the second half of gestation, most gyri are present by 28 weeks, and the final pattern and full laminar structure of cortex is present at term.

Disturbances of these developmental processes result in congenital defects. If disorders occur in the phase of neural tube formation, major defects result (e.g. anencephaly, holoprosencephaly, encephalocoele, dysraphism) and the fetus is often not viable. Disorders of cortical cellular proliferation and differentiation (8–16 weeks) cause microcephaly or megalencephaly, and defects associated with macrocephaly include congenital tumours, tuberous sclerosis, neurofibromatosis type 1, Sturge–Weber, some leucodystrophies, and hemimegalencephaly. Epilepsy is common in most of these conditions. The process of neuronal migration, however, is the most important from the viewpoint of status. Disturbances of migration do not necessarily cause major malformations, but will disrupt the normal organisation of the brain, and common consequences are mental retardation and seizures. A spectrum of disorders caused by disorders of neuronal generation and migration includes forms of agyria, pachygyria, lissencephaly, schizencephaly, heterotopias (diffuse and focal subcortical), polymicrogyria, macrogyria, corpus callosal agenesis, and microdysgenesis (see fig. 3.4). The causes of migrational disturbance are not well understood. Undoubtedly important are genetic factors; several syndromes have a well-defined genetic basis, but most do not. Pre-natal environmental and perinatal factors are also involved and numerous possible causes have been identified. Myelination is delayed after complicated preganancies (e.g. with maternal diabetes, placental insufficiency), or after birth complications (asphyxia), and perintal and postnatal disorders can also affect the later stages of neuronal migration and maturation. Meencke & Janz (1984) postulated that the microdysgenesis they observed in primary epilepsy is a disorder of migration at about the seventh to ninth month of gestation, and emphasised the importance of this period of fetal development in epilepsy.

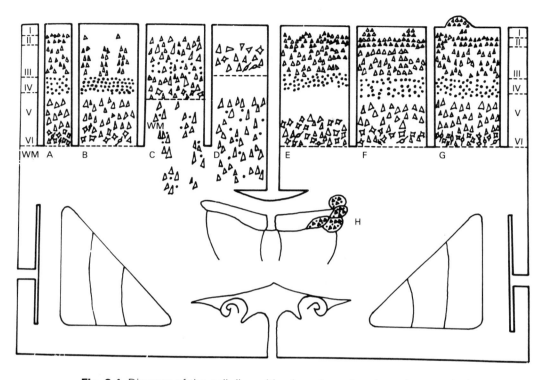

Fig. 3.4. Diagram of the cell disposition in various disorders of neocortical development, of the type that commonly cause epilepsy. A, normal cortical pattern in radial microbrain; B, microcephalia vera; C, Zellweger disease; D, type 1 lissencephaly; E, microgyria; F, atypical microdysgenesis; G, neuronal ectopia within the subarachnoid space; H, periventricular heterotopias; I–VI refer to the neocortical layers in normal brain; WM, white matter; dotted line, inferior limit of neocortex. (Reprinted from Evrard *et al.* 1989, with kind permission.)

Until very recently, disorders of neuronal migration were thought to be rare in epilepsy, but the advent of MRI has allowed the visualisation of previously covert minor alterations of neocortical development, particularly those due to abnormal neuronal migration, in many secondarily generalised and cryptogenic focal epilepsies. It seems likely that such abnormalities will be found in many cases of status, and perhaps such disorders will prove to be the main pathological underpinning of severe epilepsy (and thus status) where other aetiological factors are absent. This is an exciting area of current research.

ITERATIVE STATUS: Repeated attacks of status epilepticus (iterative status) sometimes without other seizure manifestations is a curious pattern occasionally encountered in clinical practice, perhaps more commonly in nonconvulsive than

75

in convulsive status (see Courjon, Fournier & Mauguière 1984). An example of iterative convulsive status is reported in a patient with neuroacanthocytosis (Meirkord & Shorvon 1990), Janz mentions postleucotomy cases (Janz 1983), and iterative status is also a rare manifestation of trauma or tumour (Heintel 1972). De Marco (1991) described a case of secondarily generalised status, of unknown aetiology, which recurred every few months. Shinnar *et al.* (1992) followed 95 children with status for a mean of 29 months, 17% had further attacks, 5% had 3 or more (mainly febrile status), and all the latter showed evidence of neurological impairment.

The treatment and prognosis of tonic–clonic status are described on pp. 175–203 and pp. 293–301.

Absence status epilepticus

Prolonged epileptic states without convulsions were well-recognised curiosities in the nineteenth century. Prichard (1822), Trousseau (1868*a,b*), Hughlings Jackson (see Taylor 1931), Wilks (1878), Colman (1903) and Clark & Prout (1903/4) all described cases. Charcot described epileptic fugues sometimes lasting days in a 37 year old Parisian delivery man, in which he would travel for long distances, once by train out of Paris, and in others complicated traverses across the city (see frontispiece). Charcot himself suggested that these fugues were long epileptic seizures. Though such nonconvulsive epileptic states were thought possibly to be equivalents of petit mal, it was not until the introduction of EEG into clinical practice in the 1930s that further progress in understanding these conditions was made. EEG had an enormous impact on all subsequent developments in epilepsy, and nowhere more so than in shaping concepts of nonconvulsive status.

Distinction between typical and atypical absence status epilepticus and other nosological problems

The identification of the EEG pattern underlying petit mal (now generalised absence) seizures was a landmark in twentieth century neurology. At a single stroke, EEG established itself as a fundamental investigation in epilepsy; indeed, one which, it could be claimed, was nothing less than an extension of the physical examination. The first description of petit mal status came in 1938, within a few years of the clinical introduction of EEG. The patient was a cousin of Lennox who had continuous spike–wave recorded on an EEG following insulin-induced hypoglycaemia, during which she was obtunded and partially unresponsive; Lennox coined the term *petit mal status* in 1945. For a time, all subsequent nonconvulsive status reports were grouped together under the single rubric of petit mal, a unified approach which became evidently untenable when epileptic confusional states without concurrent EEG spike–wave discharges were then described, and when prolonged spike–wave was observed in some patients without overt seizures. A nosological labyrinth resulted, with complicated new terms created to describe the increasingly variable clinical and clinico-EEG phenomena encountered (table 3.10).

Table 3.10. *Some published synonyms of absence status epilepticus (generalised typical and atypical, and complex partial)*

Petit mal status
Spike-and-wave stupor
Etat confusionnel simple
Epilepsia minoris continua
Minor epileptic status
Epileptic twilight state
Prolonged epileptic twilight state
Prolonged behavioural disturbance as ictal phenomenon
Prolonged epileptic twilight state with almost continuous spike–waves
Epileptic twilight state with spike–waves
Absence continuing
Prolonged petit mal automatism
Status pyknolepticus
Centroencephalographic condition of prolonged disturbance of consciousness (CCC)
Ictal psychosis
Transient ictal psychosis
Etat de mal généralisé à l'expression confusionelle
Status psychomotoricus
Borderline petit mal status
Petit mal status like
Transitional petit mal status
Etat de mal frontal polaire
Temporal lobe status
Poriomania

Today, absence status can be best subdivided into at least three separate syndromes, with overlapping clinical and EEG features, and with transitional cases.

Typical absence status: nonconvulsive status, occurring in the syndrome of primary generalised epilepsy. This is the status equivalent of the generalised absence (petit mal) seizure.

Atypical absence status: status that occurs largely in secondarily generalised epilepsy of the Lennox–Gastaut type, and also in other patients with compromised cerebral function.

Complex partial status: nonconvulsive focal status.

This latter condition is now clearly differentiated from the other two syndromes (and is discussed further on pp. 104 and 116–18). The differentiation between typical and atypical absence status on clinical or EEG grounds is, however, contentious. Some authorities, including Gastaut (1983), prefer to lump these together under the rubric 'absence status', on the basis that the clinical and EEG semiology may be indistinguishable (a contention not in doubt), and that aetiology is 'a relative phenomenon'. This line was followed by Porter & Penry (1983), who nevertheless preferred the appellation 'petit mal status' (confusingly in my estimation, as perhaps this term should be confined to absence status in primary generalised epilepsy). Berkovic *et al.* (1987, 1990) also preferred to view the absence epilepsies as a 'biological continuum'. Amongst those taking an opposing position are Gibberd (1972), Doose (1983) and Ohtahara *et al.* (1979); Doose (1983) complicated the matter further by admitting a category of atypical primary generalised cases into the typical absence category ('primary myoclonic–astatic epilepsy'). In my view, typical and atypical absence status should be differentiated, because of the dissimilarity of their general clinical features, natural history, pathological basis, response to treatment and prognosis. There is undeniably, however, considerable overlap, and the clinical and EEG features may be indistinguishable.

Assessment of the published literature of absence status is complicated by three factors. First, as discussed above, is the fact that many authorities have failed to separate typical and atypical absence (e.g. Bendix 1964; Lob *et al.* 1967; Dalby 1969; Hajnšek & Dürrigl 1970; Roger *et al.* 1974; Gastaut 1983). Second, there is the once prevalent view that all generalised spike–wave discharges are centrencephalic (Niedermeyer & Khalifeh 1965). It is now abundantly clear that frontal (and other) focal seizures can produce identical EEG patterns (see Bancaud *et al.* 1974; Bancaud & Talairach 1992), yet undoubtedly some patients with focal status have been included in case series of absence status. Finally, there is the difficulty that exists in regard to patients with electrographic spike–wave status, in whom there are also focal EEG features greater than would normally be accepted for a truly generalised epilepsy, but who have no other focal clinical features. Such cases are not uncommon particularly in adult practice, and conform neither to the classical picture of primary generalised nor that of secondary generalised (e.g. Lennox–Gastaut) epilepsy. These patients are difficult to classify (see, for instance, Hess *et al.* 1971; Niedermeyer *et al.* 1979). Some (perhaps the majority) are cases of complex partial status of frontal origin, but others are transitional cases in which it is not possible to decide whether or not there is a focal or generalised origin.

Of the cases which followed Lennox's early description, some with classical EEG changes would now probably be classified as typical absence status (e.g. Tucker & Forster 1950; Gibbs & Gibbs 1952; Schwab 1953; Vizioli & Magliocco 1953; Mann 1954; Zappoli 1955; Kellaway & Chao 1955; Bornstein, Coddon & Song 1956; Friedlander & Feinstein 1956; Merlis 1960; Dalby 1969; Lipman, Isaacs & Suter 1971; Novak, Corke & Fairley 1971; Andermann & Robb 1972; Richard & Brenner 1980; Nightingale & Welch 1982), but others as complex partial or atypical absence status (e.g. Putnam & Merritt 1941; Goldensohn & Gold 1960; Lennox 1960; Goldie & Green 1961; Niedermeyer & Khalifeh 1965; Brett 1966; Lion 1967; Dalby 1969; Hess *et al.* 1971; Lugaresi, Pazzaglia & Tassinari 1971; Moe 1971; Geier 1978; Fincham *et al.* 1979; Niedermeyer *et al.* 1979; Bauer, Aichner & Mayr 1983; Fujiwara *et al.* 1988). The published literature should be approached with these provisos in mind. The following sections concentrate on typical absence status (and transitional forms). Atypical absence and complex partial status are considered further on pp. 104 and 116.

Frequency and clinical features

Lennox (1960) reported a history of petit mal status in 27 (2.6%) of his 1039 petit mal patients, Livingston *et al.* (1965) a history of petit mal status in 11 (9.4%) of 117 patients with petit mal, and Loiseau & Cohadon (1970) in 5.8%. Dalby (1969) reported petit mal status in 21 (6.2%) of his series of 346 patients with 3 Hz spike–wave and 15 (9.3%) of the 160 patients with a history of petit mal absences. As all these series were retrospective, the true frequency is probably higher. Males and females seem equally affected, the condition tends to develop in the young, with three quarters of Gastaut's cases developing before the age of 20 years. Adult onset cases also occur and from a distinctive subcategory discussed on pp. 135–7). Patients can suffer repeated attacks. In over half the status lasts 12 hours or less, but it can persist for days, weeks or even months.

Lennox (1960) pointed out that the episodes of status differ from isolated petit mal seizures, not only in length but also in the state of consciousness. He was the first to emphasise that awareness may be only partially impaired and not totally lost, a remarkable phenomenon, the physiology of which is quite unexplained. The clinical features recorded by Lennox (1960) in his 'small series' of cases included the unseeing stare ('The physics of the optical apparatus has been altered. The light of consciousness generated in the brain stem has gone out'), and he noted that clonic movements were less evident than in isolated petit mal.

ALTERATION OF CONSCIOUSNESS: Roger *et al.* (1974) gave a detailed clinical and EEG description of the series of 148 patients compiled for the Xth Marseilles Colloquium (Gastaut *et al.* 1967). Of these, 84 had a history of primary generalised epilepsy, and 11 of Lennox–Gastaut syndrome. The cardinal clinical feature of absence status recorded by Roger, and all prior and subsequent commentators, is clouding of consciousness, which Roger and his colleagues categorised into four degrees (in reality a clinical spectrum), and in a few additional patients consciousness is clear.

1. *Slight clouding* (19% of the 148 patients); slowing of ideation and expression, and psychological effects noted particularly on activities requiring sustained attention, sequential organisation, or spatial structuring. Amnesia may be slight or even absent (Andermann & Robb 1972). There is a very striking contradiction between the severe EEG disturbance in such cases and the slight behavioural change. Indeed, occasional patients are encountered whose behaviour is entirely normal, and who are aware only of a 'lack of efficiency' (Andermann & Robb 1972) in spite of continuous spike–wave electrographic activity (Fincham *et al.* 1979; Gökyiğit, Apal & Çalişkan 1986). In such cases psychometric testing may be necessary to uncover impairment of auditory or verbal responses, and dichotic listening tests may be particularly sensitive in demonstrating attentional defects (Fincham *et al.* 1979). Geier (1978) documented atypical cases with specific isolated psychometric impairments during spike–wave status in three patients, including temporal and spatial disorien-

tation, disturbance of mathematical ability, disturbance of praxis, and delayed motor responses. A notable feature in generalised absence status is the relative preservation of verbal functioning, in marked contrast to in complex partial status.

2. *Marked clouding* (64% of the 148 patients); at its most severe immobility and mutism, simple voluntary actions performed only after repeated requests, long delays in verbal responses, monosyllabic and hesitant speech. Confusion and marked disorientation are present, and a widespread impairment of intellectual functioning. The expression may be expressionless or puzzled, the eyes may be partially closed, and the patient appears groggy or in a trance-like state. Food tends to be kept in the mouth without chewing. The pseudoataxic gait is hesitant and stumbling. Automatisms can occur and even ambulatory epileptic fugues (absence status may be the commonest cause of ictal fugue; Vizioli & Magliocco 1953). Amnesia is usual but variable and may be punctuated by short patches of recall. One patient, for instance, described islands of memory of occasional objects (e.g. a building, a park) encountered during a prolonged ambulatory fugue. The severity of the amnesia usually correlates with the degree of altered consciousness, but Geier (1978) reported patients with marked clouding and complete recall. Widespread deficits can be demonstrated during attacks on psychometric assessment, and include difficulties in sustained attention, visual spatial skills, sequential planning, lack of initiative, memory disturbance, and perseveration; the measured IQ may fall (Andermann & Robb 1972; Geier 1978; Niedermeyer *et al.* 1979; Nightingale and Welch 1982; Guberman *et al.* 1986). Such intellectual deficiencies may lead the unwary to a misdiagnosis of dementia.

3. *Somnolence* (7% of the 148 patients); patients are obtundated, immobile, their eyes usually closed and eyeballs turned upwards. Spontaneous motor response is rare, and the patient staggers when forced to stand. Incontinence of urine, pseudoataxia, pseudodementia and bradyphrenia occur.

4. *Lethargy* (8% of the 148 patients); this is the state previously defined as 'epileptic stupor'. All psychic functions are suspended, the patient is inert and motionless, reacting only to strong painful stimuli, is unable to eat, and is incontinent.

OTHER CLINICAL FEATURES: In addition to clouding of consciousness, about half of the patients show motor features, including myoclonus of variable distribution and frequency, atonia, hippus, rhythmical blinking of the eyelids and quivering of the lips, facial grimacing and smiling. Facial, especially eyelid, myoclonus is a common feature of absence status, but rare in complex partial status, an important feature in differential diagnosis.

The termination of an episode of absence status (especially typical absence status) by a grand mal seizure is highly characteristic. The physiological basis of this pattern is unclear, but presumably related to the powerful inhibitory processes which follow a grand mal seizure. Less often, the grand mal seizure initiates nonconvulsive status, and occasionally grand mal seizures intervene in the middle of an episode without affecting the course.

Psychotic and behavioural changes during nonconvulsive spike–wave status have been emphasised by several authorities, usually in atypical patients, but these are neither as frequent nor as severe as those encountered in complex partial status. How many of the reported cases are truly generalised absence status is not clear. Goldensohn & Gold (1960) report a series of cases in which the spike–wave confusional state was associated with hostility, negativism, aggressivity, and withdrawal. In his intensive study of psychotic features in epilepsy, Dongier (1959/60) similarly describes a variety of psychotic features in patients with 'centrencephalic spike–wave' status, including hebephrenia, catatonia, paranoid and hallucinatory states. Lugaresi *et al.* (1971) recalled a patient with polyspike and wave, in which episodic quarrelsome, irrascible and impulsive behaviour progressed to agitation, a dreamy state and sometimes to stupor, as the EEG discharges became more frequent. Mild confusion may lead to inappropriate behaviour in day-to-day activities. Regressive behaviours may be manifest. Rohr-Le Floch, Gauthier & Beaumanoir (1988) compared petit mal and focal nonconvulsive status, and found that, whilst indifference and perplexity were more common in absence than in psychomotor status, other psychological symptoms (anxiety, aggressivity, negativity, fear, irritability) were not (table 3.11).

Episodes of status can last for hours or days, and occasionally much longer (e.g. the patient of Gökyiğit *et al.* 1986). A surprising periodicity of attacks is observed in some patients. The onset and offset of the confusional state may be abrupt or relatively gradual.

Precipitating features can be identified in some cases and are more common in typical absence status than in complex partial status. They include menstruation, withdrawal of medication, hypoglycaemia, hyperventilation, flashing or bright lights, sleep deprivation, fatigue, stress or grief. Often, though, the status is apparently spontaneous. Most patients have known petit mal (some with myoclonus and/or grand mal also), but occasionally petit mal status is the first manifestation of epilepsy (especially in adults, see pp. 135–6). Episodes of petit mal status can punctuate the course of petit mal epilepsy at any stage, and its occurrence does not seem to prejudice outcome.

Only Rohr-Le Floch *et al.* (1988) have directly compared the symptomatology of typical absence and complex partial status (60 episodes in 52 patients). The most characteristic presentation of petit mal status was a fluctuating confusional state with myoclonus; in contrast, confusion with affective or psychotic states was typical of psychomotor status, and confusion with euphoria or difficulties of programming were seen, mainly in the frontal status group (see table 3.11).

The clinical features of typical and atypical absence status overlap, although obvious differences in emphasis exist. As mentioned above, most case series reviewed here have included examples of both, and the degree to which these syndromes differ is unknown; a large modern comparative investigation would be of the greatest interest.

Table 3.11. *Comparison of the clinical features of petit mal, psychomotor and frontal polar status epilepticus (from the series of Rohr-Le Floch et al. (1988))*

	Petit mal status ($n = 32$)	Psychomotor status ($n = 9$)	Frontal polar status ($n = 19$)
Intellectual features			
Altered consciousness (%)	100	66	58
Fluctuating consciousness	29 (91%)	3 (33%)	6 (32%)
Poverty of speech	8 (25%)	0	4 (22%)
Slowness of speech	3 (9%)	0	3 (16%)
Feeble voice	3	0	1
Slowness of gesture	4	1	3
Confabulation	0	0	4 (22%)
Ideas of persecution	0	3 (33%)	0
Myoclonus (facial/global)	18 (56%)	0	0
Psychiatric misdiagnosis	3	2	4
Attitude			
Indifferent, peevish	7 (22%)	0	4 (22%)
Perplexed/mute	7 (22%)	1	7 (37%)
Sly, ironic	0	0	6 (32%)
Smiling/hilarious	0	0	8 (42%)
Sad	1	0	1
Anxious, frightened	3	4 (44%)	1
Negativistic	1	2 (22%)	2
Irritable, aggressive	1	5 (56%)	2
Agitated	4	1	1
Automatism			
Simple gestural	7 (22%)	1	3
Complex gestural	2	4 (44%)	2
Stereotyped gestural	0	1	3
Ambulatory	1	2 (22%)	0
Verbal	1	2 (22%)	0
Echolalia	0	0	3
Jargon aphasia	0	1	0
Defect in programming	0	0	2

Percentages are of the number of cases in which it was possible to test the patient.

The numbers investigated were small, and the cases selected. This is, however, the only direct published comparison of the clinical appearance of status in the three patient groups.

Electroencephalography

The EEG features of absence status have been extensively described. The diagnostic electrographic pattern is, of course, continuous or almost continuous bilaterally synchronous and symmetrical spike–wave activity, with little or no reactivity to sensory stimuli. The classical EEG appearance with 3 Hz spike–wave is usually seen in the setting of primary generalised epilepsy, and the closer the EEG is to this classic pattern the more typical the clinical features. Other heterogeneous forms have been described, including irregular and slow spike–wave (1.5–4 Hz), prolonged bursts of spike activity, generalised periodic triphasic sharp waves, and polyspike and wave at frequencies of from 2 to 6 Hz. Whether to include such cases within the category of typical absence status and quite where to draw the nosological line is uncertain. The cycling of EEG changes seen in complex partial status is not usual in spike–wave status but does occur, and in some patients the spike–wave is not continuous but rather broken into frequent bursts (see, for instance, the patient of Schwab (1953)). The most comprehensive EEG description was the detailed analysis of 148 patients by Gastaut & Tassinari (1975) for the Xth Marseilles Colloquium. In about 40% of these patients, the spike–wave rhythm was continuous and in about 30% broken up into frequent bursts. In about 15% of patients, arrhythmic spike–wave bursts were repeated and in 10% the EEG showed underlying slow activity with bursts of spikes or spike–wave. In rare cases (fewer than 2%), an isolated rhythm of generalised or anterior spikes at 10–20 per second or slow waves, or very slow complex rhythms mixed with occasional bursts of more rapid activity were observed, although whether these latter forms are true absence status is debatable. The type or degree of clouding of consciousness does not in general correlate strongly with the form of the EEG.

Cause

In the past decade or so, there has been a tendency to subdivide the generalised absence epilepsies into more or less well-defined syndromes, a classification which cuts across the 'seizure type' classification. These syndromes include childhood absence, juvenile absence, juvenile myoclonic, Lennox–Gastaut, myoclonic–astatic, and myoclonic–absence. This subclassification is based on clinical phenomenology, without clear pathophysiological justification and so has been rightly criticised. An alternative approach, recently revived, is to view absence seizures simply as a spectrum (Berkovic *et al.* 1987). This emphasises the multifactorial origin of the generalised absence epilepsies, and makes no distinction between the primary and secondary types. The patients with generalised absence, it is suggested, show a spectrum of inherited epileptic propensity, congenital and acquired (usually prenatal) cerebral damage, and a range of clinical and EEG findings. Absence status is more easily dealt with viewed in this way, as a broad neurobiological continuum, than in either a seizure type or epilepsy syndrome classification, and this approach allows the easy incorporation of atypical or transitional cases. The main case against the 'neurobiological continuum' is the very great difference between the core syndromes exhibiting typical absence (i.e. petit mal) and atypical absence (i.e. Lennox–Gastaut), conditions which have almost nothing else in common. Furthermore, the lumping together of absence epilepsies, whilst avoiding problems of subcategorisation on clinical grounds and allowing the incorporation of transitional cases, does not, however, necessarily provide new insight into physiological or clinical features. Until the basic pathophysiology is better understood, all subclassifications (or none!) are unsatisfactory.

By definition, focal aetiologies should not result in 'typical absence status', a term which is restricted to the generalised epilepsies. The incidence of absence status in the subdivisions of primary generalised epilepsy is not known, and presumably status can occur in any category. The secondarily generalised atypical absence status of the Lennox–Gastaut type may be due to a variety of diffuse and focal cerebral disorders (see pp. 102–3). To what extent generalised absence status can occur outside the primary generalised or Lennox–Gastaut categories is unclear, as discussed above. However, since fairly typical 3 Hz spike–wave discharges are observed on EEG in epilepsies with mesial frontal lobe foci (Bancaud *et al.* 1974), or other frontal regions, with clinical correlations indistinguisable from petit mal, it would be surprising if small focal frontal lesions did not underlie some 'generalised' absence status. Only the application of careful MRI studies to classical absence status cases will resolve this point. In my own experience, minor degrees of frontal cortical dysplasia (especially neuronal migrational disorders, see pp. 72–5) revealed by MRI, are common in cases of apparently generalised absence status. The suggestion that microdysgenesis actually underlies primary generalised epilepsy may provide the conceptual link between the lesional and 'idiopathic' absence epilepsies (see pp. 74–5).

The treatment and prognosis of absence status are described on pp. 290 and 308.

Epilepsia partialis continua

In 1880, Hughlings Jackson first described in detail the focal motor seizure, which henceforward has carried his name (the *Jacksonian seizure*) (see Taylor 1931). He correctly attributed the attacks to epileptic discharges in the contralateral motor cortex, and predicted localised structural pathology. Although such simple partial motor seizures are usually shortlived, occasionally localised clonic jerks can persist, sometimes for hours, weeks, or even years. The status syndrome has come to be known as epilepsia partialis continua (or EPC); a useful definition is that of Obeso, Rothwell & Marsden (1985):

> Spontaneous regular or irregular clonic twitching of cerebral cortical origin,
> sometimes aggravated by action or sensory stimuli, confined to one part
> of the body, and continuing for hours, days or weeks.

Although uncommon, the condition is full of interest. Controversy has been engaged over three particular issues:

1. The site of origin of the clonic jerks (i.e. cortical versus subcortical).
2. The neurophysiological distinction between EPC, myoclonus and other jerks.
3. The aetiology of the syndrome.

Taxonomic confusion abounds (again!), partly because the condition has been investigated from the viewpoint of both epilepsy and also movement disorder research, each arriving at the condition from rather different perspectives. Nosologically, this form of status is best considered first by a geographical–historical approach.

Russian descriptions (Russian spring–summer encephalitis)

Kojewnikoff (1895 *a,b*) described in four patients 'a particular type of cortical epilepsy', which he named *epilepsia corticalis sive partialis continua*. The seizure disorder consisted of frequent jerks continuing for years (3.5–5 years in his four cases) in the same part of the body, uninfluenced by treatment. Kojewnikoff, with remarkable prescience, recognised that these jerks were epileptic discharges in a localised region of the brain, close to, but not coexistent with, the motor strip, and might be due to chronic inflammation. In an excellent early review, Omorokov (1927) found only 42 cases of Kojewnikoff's disease in the literature (mostly Russian), and then described a further 52 examined clinically and pathologically from his own clinic in Siberia. He suggested that the condition was due to an encephalitis afflicting the peasant population of forested areas, confirmed Kojewnikoff's view that the pathology was highly localised, and reported the effectiveness of surgical intervention. In these Russian patients, the epilepsy usually developed 3–4 months after a febrile illness, associated in 30% of cases with a hemiplegia or monoplegia. The jerks typically affect agonist and antagonist muscles, with a rhythmic quality, in short bursts of 1–2 seconds' duration alternating with quiescent phases 2–4 seconds long, persisting in sleep and worsened by action or stress. Jacksonian or generalised epileptic seizures are almost invariable accompaniments, although with a strong tendency to improve with time. The jerking, which is often highly focal, continues relentlessly for years. Sensory symptoms occur in about one fifth of cases, and 80% of cases have a persisting hemiparesis. Brain biopsy reveals highly localised encephalitis with cortical and meningeal inflammatory changes, damage to the ganglion cells of the cortex, with ring-like inclusion bodies; Omorokov postulated that the infectious agent enters the cortical motor cells via the blood vessels. Of his 52 patients, 30 underwent Horsley's operation, with a 30% cure rate (Omorokov 1927). This condition is thus a well-established epidemic form of epilepsy, of cortical origin, due to Russian spring–summer tick-borne encephalitis.

Canadian descriptions (Rasmussen's chronic encephalitis)

Rasmussen, Olszweski & Lloyd-Smith described, in 1958, three cases of persisting focal epilepsy due to a chronic focal encephalitis; a condition henceforward known as Rasmussen's chronic encephalitis. The condition has been the subject of a definitive symposium held in 1988 in Montreal (the excellent proceedings, to which this text is heavily indebted, were published in 1991: Andermann 1991). In Montreal, a total of 48 patients had been identified and described by 1988 (Oguni, Andermann & Rasmussen 1991), and these cases differ in many ways from those of Russian spring–summer tick-borne encephalitis. Only about 50% of cases have a preceding infectious illness (within 6 months). The great majority are children (mean age 6.8 years, with 85% being under the age of 10 years), and all present with epilepsy, usually but not always focal. About half exhibit episodes of EPC, usually within 2 years of the onset of epilepsy. These episodes last hours in some patients, and years in others, and are often discontinuous. The condition is progressive, and after a highly variable period, fixed focal deficits develop, notably hemiplegia, hemianopia or aphasia (see fig. 3.5). The patients have other forms of epilepsy, and EPC may be a minor part of the overall clinical picture. Pathological examination shows a chronic inflammatory process, involving predominantly and sometimes entirely one hemisphere; this has the appearance of a chronic encephalitis, but no infective agent has been identified. The condition obviously differs, both clinically and pathologically, from Kojewnikoff's disease, although both may result in continuous focal motor seizures (EPC).

Evidence for a cortical or subcortical origin, and the differentiation from myoclonus

Both the Russian and the Canadian conditions are well-established entities, with obvious cortical pathology, and EPC coexisting with other forms of epilepsy. Taxonomic confusion began with the publication, from Denny-Brown's laboratory, of the electrophysiological and pathological details of nine patients, who had acute (usually large) cerebral lesions (Juul-Jensen & Denny-Brown 1966). Denny-Brown suggested that the jerks of EPC arose, not from the cortex but from subcortical structures. This view was supported by pathological examination

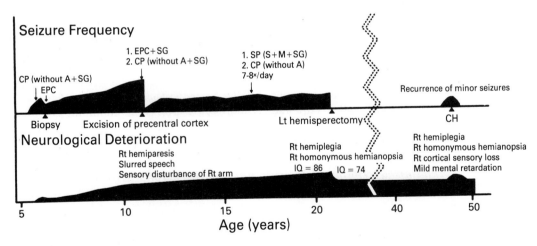

Fig. 3.5. Diagram showing the case history of a 50 year old man with Rasmussen's encephalitis and epilepsia partialis continua (EPC). The patient had EPC from the age of 6–11 years, at which time a cortical excision resulted in temporary relief from seizures. His signs progressed and seizures (without EPC) returned, and at age of 21 he was treated with a left hemispherectomy. The progression of the disease was halted, although hydrocephalus and haemosiderosis developed as late complications of surgery. SP, simple partial seizure; CP, complex partial seizure; S, somatosensory; M, motor; SG, secondary generalisation; A, automatism; CH, cerebral haemosiderosis; Lt, left; Rt, right. (From Oguni *et al.* 1991, with kind permission.)

which showed subcortical damage in all cases (albeit in most cases with coexisting damage in the cortical motor areas), and EEG findings of large blunt waves, often polyphasic, with a large field; characteristics which were taken to point to a subcortical origin. The clonic jerks were thought to be due to release of extra-pyramidal mechanisms from cortical control, and the EPC therefore seen as a *disequilibrium in subcortical reflex activity, of the same type which determines myoclonus.* The bilaterality of the lesion and coincident extrapyramidal signs were seen as confirmatory evidence (Juul-Jensen & Denny-Brown 1966). This theory, backed by the authority of Denny-Brown, spawned a highly confused subsequent litera-ture, notable contributions to which include those of Halliday (1967), Bancaud (1967), and Bancaud *et al.* (1970).

If EPC is viewed as a subcortical phenomenon, the occurrence of other forms of epilepsy is difficult to explain. Indeed, some definitions of EPC excluded patients with other seizures (for a discussion, see Chauvel *et al.* 1992). Another view taken was that the Jacksonian seizures were cortical and the jerks (myoclonus) subcortical. Kuzniecky *et al.* (1988), probably wrongly, further confuse the issue by differentiating focal cortical myoclonus from other cortical myoclonus. Much of the debate revolves around the semantic issues of definition, but classification became highly confused.

From the viewpoint of epileptology, the situation has been greatly clarified by stereoencephalographic (SEEG) studies. Wieser *et al.* (1977) first reported SEEG findings in a 14 year old with EPC associated with tonic–clonic seizures and a progressive hemiplegia (the aetiology was not known, although the clinical features were similar to those that Rasmussen described). The jerks were stimulus sensi-tive, increased on action, and typically involved agonist and antagonist muscles. SEEG recording very clearly demonstrated a neocortical origin and defined its extent. Chauvel *et al.* (1992) presented detailed SEEG findings in four patients, all with coexistent epilepsy. These recordings showed that epileptic seizures and the EPC originated from the same neuronal pool. In some instances, the two seizure types merged clinically and electrophysiologically, and it was concluded that the epileptogenic motor cortex discharge can generate different ictal patterns depending on the speed and extent of propagation. These SEEG findings demon-strate beyond doubt a cortical epileptic origin for the jerks, and demonstrate neurophysiological characteristics of the jerks that are identical with those of cortical myoclonus. All these cases had coexisting epilepsy (as indeed did the Russian and Canadian cases).

Approaching the question of myoclonus from the perspective of movement dis-order research, rather different physiological methods are employed, including back-averaging of recordings of reflex or spontaneous jerks, the study of evoked potentials, and electromyographic recordings of the sequence of recruitment of muscle groups in a myoclonic jerk. These recently developed methods have greatly clarified the taxonomy and physiology of myoclonus, and its relationship to EPC. Here is not the place to describe the myoclonic research in detail (and the reader is referred to excellent reviews by Marsden, Hallett & Fahn 1982; Obeso *et al.* 1985; Menini & Naquet 1986). Current views can, however, be summarised as follows:

1. *Myoclonus:* Myoclonus is a brief muscle jerk, which can be classified physiologically according to whether it is of cortical, brain stem or spinal origin. Typically (but not invariably) in cortical myoclonus, back averaged time-locked EEG cortical potentials precede the jerks, sensory evoked potentials (SEPs) are enlarged, and the myoclonus may be spontaneous, action or stimulus sensitive with a rostrocaudal pattern of muscle recruitment and antagonist and agonist co-contraction. In stimulus-sensitive myoclonus, the reflex timings are compatible with a cortical loop. Neither *brain stem* nor *spinal myoclonus* have this constellation of features. Cortical myoclonus can be viewed as a hyper-synchronous discharge from a group of cortical cells, and in this sense is truly fragmentary epilepsy. Obeso *et al.* (1985) report patients showing a spectrum

(*a*)

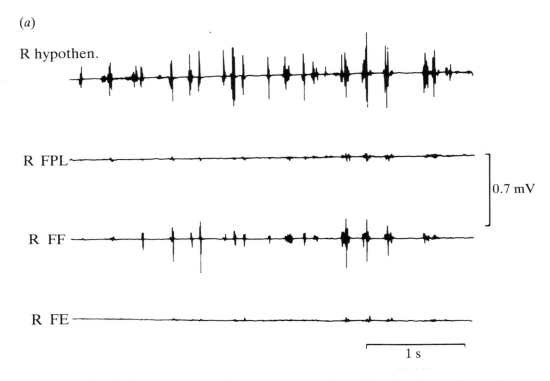

Fig. 3.6. Neurophysiological studies from a patient with epilepsia partialis continua (EPC). Recording from a 33 year old woman with a 3 year history of right-sided upper limb EPC, of uncertain cause. The onset of the condition began with two grand mal seizures which did not recur. Over the subsequent 8 years, the EPC has continued without change, despite therapy, and with no progression. This illustrates the co-contraction of agonist and antagonist muscles, and the cortical origin of the jerk. (*a*) Electromyograph showing jerks in the right hypothenar muscles (R hypothen.), flexor pollicis longus (R FPL), and flexor (R FF) and extensor muscles (R FE) of the forearm.

of spontaneous and stimulus-sensitive myoclonus, EPC, Jacksonian and generalised seizures, with similar physiology, variations which were taken to represent subtle differences in the site of abnormality in sensorimotor cortical
neuronal mechanisms.

2. *Epilepsia partialis continua:* The physiological characteristics of the jerks in
   most cases of EPC are identical to those of cortical myoclonus. This is almost
   always true where the EPC is associated with other forms of epilepsy, and in
   such cases it is now hard to escape the view that the EPC is simply repetitive
   cortical myoclonus (or a very close relation; see fig. 3.6). However, other

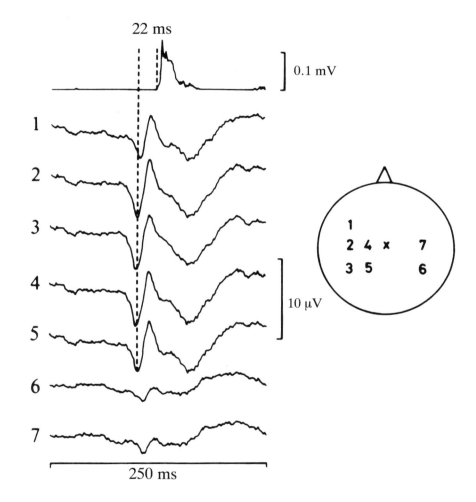

Caption for fig. 3.6 (*cont.*). (*b*) 120 back-averaged EEG records showing a
contralateral positive potential preceding the onset of the spontaneous jerk by 22
milliseconds. Numbers 1–7 denote EEG channels.

(c)

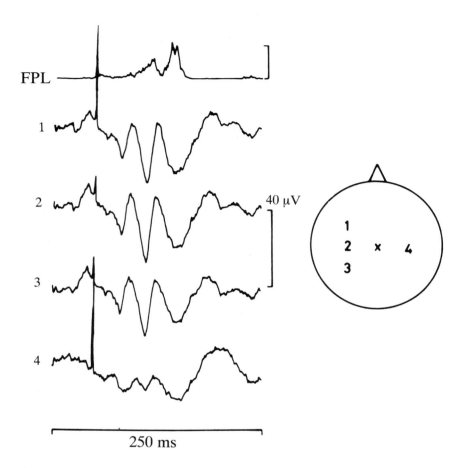

FPL

1

2   40 μV

3

4

250 ms

Caption for fig. 3.6 (*cont.*). (*c*) Sensory evoked potential (SEP) (average of 32 responses) and muscle jerks in flexor pollicis longus (FPL), following electrical stimulation of the thumb. This shows the *giant SEP* seen in some cases of cortical myoclonus. Numbers 1–4 are EEG channels used in (*b*). (With thanks to Dr Philip Thompson, Institute of Neurology, for debating this case; recordings from Obeso *et al.* 1985. The spectrum of cortical myoclonus, *Brain*, **108**, 193–224, with permission from Oxford University Press.)

patients are encountered without a history of other forms of epilepsy whose jerks resemble EPC clinically but not neurophysiologically. In these cases the site of origin of the jerks may not be cortical. Menini & Naquet (1986) suggested that these are of brain stem origin (their type C myoclonus). This variety of EPC (if indeed it exists, which is contentious) is not as common nor as well studied as the cortical variety, nor is its exact nosological position clear.

3. *Myoclonic dystonia:* Dystonic syndromes of subcortical origin may also be

associated with jerks (myoclonic dystonia), which do not have the characteristics of myoclonus of either cortical or brain stem origin. Such myoclonus is often bilateral and multifocal; it is caused by long duration bursts of electromyographical activity, SEPs are normal and the jerks do not have the orderly recruitment of muscles seen in brain stem myoclonus. Since subcortical pathology was especially prominent, some of Denny-Brown's cases might be fitted into this category. Neither these patients nor those with spinal or brain stem myoclonus should be considered examples of EPC.

All of the Russian and Canadian patients would probably be considered examples of cortical myoclonus, and the few reported detailed neurophysiological examinations (all in cases with coexistent epilepsy) essentially confirm this view, although the physiology may be complex (Obeso *et al.* 1985; Chauvel *et al.* 1986, 1992; Cowan *et al.* 1986). Some of the cases reported by Juul-Jensen & Denny-Brown (1966) and Thomas, Reagan & Klass (1977) would probably now be categorised as jerky dystonia or brain stem myoclonus.

The above scheme, tidy and logical as it is, does not account for all cases. Some patients exist, without dystonia or other evidence of severe extrapyramidal disease, or coexisting epilepsy, in whom positive evidence of a cortical origin is also lacking. Detailed studies are few but a subcortical origin is probable in some such cases (see fig. 3.7). At least some of Juul-Jensen & Denny-Brown's patients might be so described, although modern neurophysiology was not carried out. Colamaria *et al.* (1988) reported two patients with EPC, which, it was postulated, was due to striatal necrosis. Widespread cerebral disease was present in addition, and no physiological studies were performed.

EPC as focal motor epilepsy

Since the early 1970s, amongst epileptologists at least, it has become customary to view EPC simply as the status equivalent of the simple partial motor seizures (really as Kojewnikoff had done years earlier). One advantage of this oversimplistic view is that it allows the inclusion of cases with widely varying aetiologies, although admittedly avoiding the thorny questions of physiology or differentiation from other conditions with clonic features. An example of this approach is the retrospective record review of 32 patients presenting over a 23 year period to the Mayo Clinic, Rochester, MI, with EPC defined as: 'regular or irregular clonic muscular twitching affecting a limited part of the body, occurring for a minimum of one hour, and recurring at intervals of no more than 10 seconds' (Thomas *et al.* 1977). This was a very heterogeneous group. Some patients were in deep coma from an acute cerebral insult, and some were fully conscious with EPC for up to 20 years; the latter were considered to have either no obvious pathology or postinflammatory brain disease. The topology of the jerks varied, some were highly focal, and some widespread; most were asynchronous irregular and low amplitude twitches, varying in intensity and rhythm. Eight autopsies were performed (six with stroke, one with tumour and one with meningitis), showing cerebral damage which included motor cortical regions in each case. This was a highly disparate group of cases in terms

91

(a)

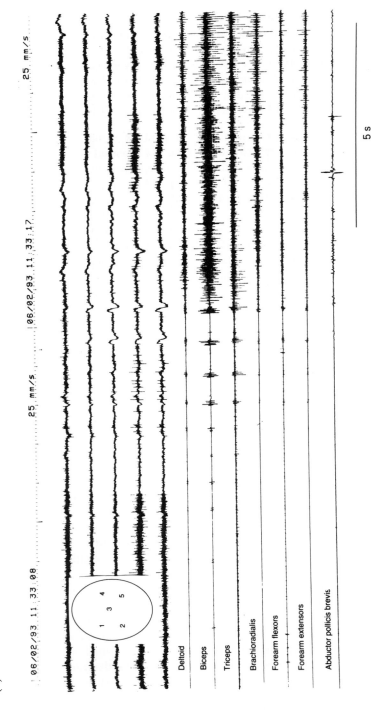

06/02/93 11:33:08   25 mm/s   06/02/93 11:33:17   25 mm/s

25 mm/s

5 s

1 4
3
2 5

Deltoid

Biceps

Triceps

Brachioradialis

Forearm flexors

Forearm extensors

Abductor pollicis brevis

(b)

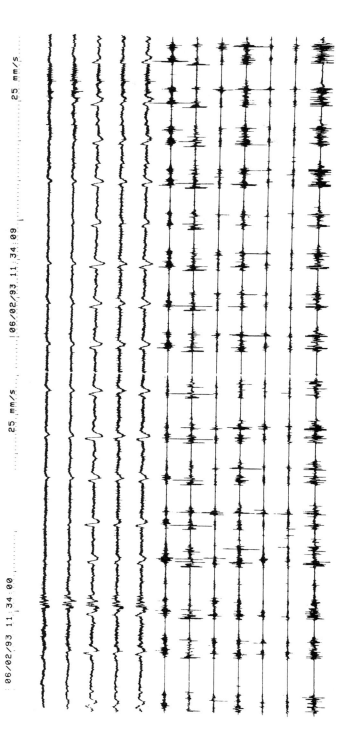

Fig. 3.7. Simultaneous EEG and electromyograph recording from a 56 year old male with a nonprogressive 10 year history of jerking of the right arm and trunk, for which no underlying cause has been identified. There are often discrete intermittent episodes starting with jerking in the shoulder muscles spreading to the forearm and after a few moments tonic flexion of the arm (a). At other times relentless jerking of proximal and distal muscles occurs for hours or days at a time (b), sometimes frequently interrupted by the discrete episodes. The EEG shows no epileptic activity either during the jerking or interictally, and detailed volumetric magnetic resonance imaging is normal. The diagnosis of epilepsia partialis continua has been made, but the site of origin of the convulsive movements is uncertain and may be subcortical. (With thanks to Dr Philip Thompson, the Institute of Neurology, London, for preparing this illustration.)

of aetiology, presentation, duration, clinical and EEG findings, accompanying signs (including coma), and outcome. Some cases would now be best categorised as *myoclonic status in coma*, some as myoclonic dystonia and some possibly as nonepileptic myoclonus of noncortical origin. Bancaud (1985) reported 22 cases of a more obviously epileptic nature. He divided these into two categories. The first had an epileptic focus in the rolandic area, with focal EEG disturbances, the absence of mental disturbance and often an identifed fixed lesion. The epilepsy is not progressive, and surgical resection may be helpful. The second group had a progressive disorder, with epilepsy, an evolving focal deficit, mental deterioration, and diffuse EEG abnormalities, and surgical intervention was of limited value. At least some of the latter cases were likely to be due to Rasmussen's chronic encephalitis, although pathological findings were not published.

Clinical and electroencephalographic features of EPC

The myoclonic jerks in EPC can affect any muscle group. In some individuals, the jerks are confined to a single muscle or muscle group, but in others the distribution is more widespread, and the distribution of the jerks can vary over time. Agonists and antagonists are affected together, and distal muscles are more commonly involved than is proximal musculature (see fig. 3.5). When widespread, the jerking is usually synchronous. The clonic jerks most commonly affect the face, trunk or upper limb, and are unilateral (whether cases with multifocal bilateral myoclonus should be embraced within the rubric of EPC is debatable, although some were included by Löhler & Peters (1974) and Thomas *et al.* (1977). Palatal myoclonus is occasionally seen. By definition, in EPC (in contrast to nonepileptic myoclonus) the jerks are spontaneous, although they may be exacerbated on action (a well-recognised feature of the Russian variety, for instance), or by stimuli (e.g. startle or sensory stimuli: startle-induced seizures are well documented in the SEEG-documented cases of Chauvel and colleagues). The jerks can be single or can cluster, and may have a rhythmic quality and a wide range of frequencies. Some jerks recur only every few minutes and others are more frequent. Rapid myoclonus may display a continuous 'shivering' quality. The intensity of the clonic jerks also varies, without obvious reason. In most patients the jerks continue in sleep (a constant feature of the Russian patients, apparently), although this was not the case in ten of the patients described by Thomas *et al.* (1977). In chronic cases the myoclonus may have continued relentlessly for months or years. In some individuals with long-lasting myoclonus, periods of freedom from jerking are experienced, without obvious cause.

Other neurological signs are common, and depend on the aetiology. In the encephalitic varieties of EPC, hemiparesis or hemiplegia are common, and are associated with other cortical signs such as aphasia, hemionopia or sensory disturbance. In Rasmussen's chronic encephalitis, hemiparesis gradually develops within months or years of the onset of seizures (mean about 3 years), and is progressive to become complete or almost complete (at a mean of 4 years). The typical time course of a patient with Rasmussen's encephalitis is shown in fig. 3.5. Mental deterioration occurs in over four fifths of patients, hemianopia in about one half, and sensory loss, dysarthria, dysphasia, and behavioural disturbance less frequently. In other conditions, cortical, extrapyramidal, sensory, brain stem or cerebellar signs depend on the underlying aetiology.

In the Russian and Canadian encephalitides, seizures other than EPC are common, and take the form of Jacksonian, complex partial or generalised attacks. In Rasmussen's condition, such seizures are at times frequent or severe, and episodes of generalised status occurred in 21% of the 48 cases reported from Montreal (Oguni *et al.* 1991). In Russian spring–summer encephalitis, the seizures are initially severe then tend to improve. In other cases, the occurrence of other seizures depends on the underlying pathology; seizures are common in cases in the epileptological literature and less common in that of the movement disorders (e.g. only 5 of the 11 patients of Obeso *et al.* (1985)).

The EEG findings again depend on the underlying pathology. In Rasmussen's encephalitis, there are epileptiform and nonepileptiform changes, usually lateralised but not exclusively unilateral. The background activity is typically slow, in a focal or generalised distribution, and the interictal epileptic spike or spike–wave discharges also more widespread than the clinical seizure phenomenology might lead one to expect. Ictal recordings are often disappointing, and scalp EEG recordings often apparently unchanging during EPC. SEEG, EcoG or back-averaged EEG will, however, demonstrate a spike focus. In other conditions, the EEG reflects the cause. Of the 245 EEGs carried out in the 32 patients of Thomas *et al.* (1977) all but 7 were abnormal. This was a selected group and a normal or almost normal scalp EEG is more common than this study suggests. Focal spiking was the commonest finding, but other changes included sharp and spike–wave paroxysms, generalised and lateralised slow activity, and PLEDs; Löhler & Peters (1974) reported similar findings.

Causes

The Russian and Canadian cases of EPC, described above, are due to encephalitic conditions. The Russian spring–summer tick-borne virus has been isolated from monkey brain after several months of incubation, which supports the concept of a slow virus disease, and the pathological appearances of inclusion body encephalitis are well established. In contrast, the organism underlying Rasmussen's encephalitis has not been identified. Viral inclusions are not seen on light or electron microscopic studies, immunocytological and ultrastructual electron microscopic studies have been negative, as has *in situ* hybridisation for herpes simplex and papovavirus, and polymerase chain reaction studies, although there is a single recent report of cytomegalovirus in biopsy specimens examined by *in situ* hybridisation (Power *et al.* 1990). Viral transmission either in humans or to other animal species has not been reported (Robitaille 1991; Asher & Gajdusek 1991). Curiously, pathological examination of brain biopsy and resective tissue in many patients with typical EPC, whether conforming to the picture of a chronic encephalitis or not, is often unhelpful, with degenerative or inflammatory lesions found which cannot be characterised; quite how such cases will be resolved eventually is uncertain (see Cowan *et al.* 1986; Verhagen *et al.* 1988; and fig. 3.8).

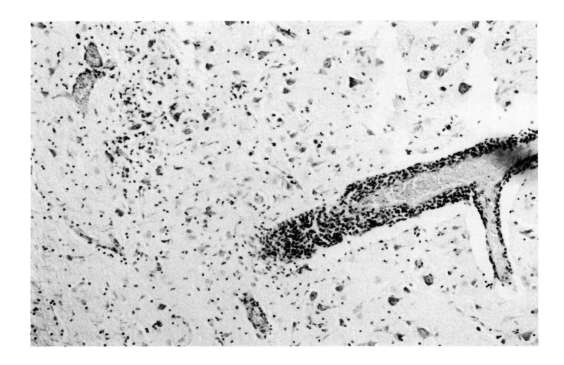

Fig. 3.8. A post-mortem slide of cerebral cortex from the frontal lobe, stained with haematoxylin-eosin. The patient was female, with a strong family history of epilepsy and of mental retardation, who developed severe thyrotoxicosis requiring partial thyroidectomy at age 24 years. At the same time she developed behavioural disturbance and intellectual deterioration, which over a 5 year period progressed to profound dementia and mutism. At the age of 20 she had developed epilepsy, taking the form of complex partial seizures, generalised tonic–clonic seizures and in the last 2 years of her life long periods of epilepsia partialis continua affecting her face. Intensive investigations were normal, except for oligoclonal bands on immunoelectrophoretic analysis of the cerebrospinal fluid. She died aged 29 years, and pathological examination of her brain revealed scattered perivascular lymphocytic cuffs, and small clusters of microglia in the cerebral cortex. These changes were seen scattered through the cerebral cortex bilaterally, and have the appearance of chronic encephalitis. The cause of the encephalitic illness was not established, and a diagnosis of atypical Rasmussen's encephalitis was made. (With thanks to Dr B.N. Harding, Institute of Neurology, for preparing this illustration.)

The aetiological profile of other cases clearly depends on how wide a definition of EPC is accepted. Löhler & Peters (1974) reviewed 162 patients in the literature of whom 85 had pathological confirmation (see table 3.12). Thomas *et al.* (1977) included patients in myoclonic coma and acute lesions; of the 32 patients, cerebral

Table 3.12. *Causes of epilepsia partialis continua in a series of 85 pathologically verified cases (Löhler & Peters 1974ª)*

Causes	*n*	(%)
Cerebral neoplasia (1)	13	(15)
Infective mass lesion (2)	10	(12)
Encephalitis (3)	26	(31)
Vascular lesions (4)	15	(18)
Traumatic lesions (5)	15	(18)
Miscellaneous (6)	6	(7)

(1): metastasis, astrocytoma, oligodendroglioma, carcinomatosis.
(2): abscess, tuberculoma, gumma.
(3): viral encephalitis, meningitis, cysticercosis, granulomatous tissue, encephalitis of unknown aetiology.
(4): arteriosclerosis, embolus, cortical venous thrombosis, cerebral haemorrhage, other cerebral vascular disorders.
(5): postraumatic cyst, subdural haematoma, epidural haematoma, haemorrhagic meningitis, intracerebral haematoma.
(6): focal gliosis, no pathological changes, pathological changes of uncertain nature.
ª With modern neuropathology, the spectrum of identified causes would be rather different. For further explanation, see the text.

infarction or haemorrhage accounted for 8, cerebral tumour and presumed encephalitis for 5 each, hepatic encephalopathy and trauma for 2 each, and subarachnoid haemorrhage for 1, and 9 had no obvious cause. In all eight cases coming to autopsy, the motor cortex was affected by the pathogenic process, with variable damage to other cortical and subcortical areas. Focal motor status can also be precipitated by exposure to drugs, including metrizamide (in myelography) and treatment with penicillin, azlocilin and cefotaxime (Wroe *et al.* 1987). More recently, newer investigatory methods have demonstrated other causes of EPC, including mitochondrial disease, subacute measles encephalopathy in immunosuppressed children, nonketotic hyperglycinaemia and Alper's disease. Recently, a patient with EPC and the pathological findings of Alper's disease was found to have a cytochrome *c* deficiency (Bourgeois & Aicardi 1992). SPECT and positron emission tomography (PET) scanning has been carried out in children with Rasmussen's chronic encephalitis, showing an (unsurprising) interictal decrease and ictal increase in blood flow in the epileptogenic region (Hwang *et al.* 1991), and magnetic resonance spectroscopy has demonstrated focal lactate accumulation in the cortical epileptogenic regions (Matthews, Andermann & Arnold 1991).

The 'subcortical' cases reported in the literature are also often of uncertain aetiology, even if post mortem or biopsy specimens are examined. Two patients with striatal necrosis due to measles encephalitis in an immunosuppressed patient and acute hyponatraemia were reported by Colamaria *et al.* (1988). The eight cases of Juul-Jensen & Denny Brown (1966) considered to be subcortical in origin were mostly of vascular or infective origin, but again damage was widespread.

The treatment and prognosis of EPC are described on pp. 290 and 308–9.

Myoclonic status epilepticus in coma

Status epilepticus is not uncommon in coma. Acute anoxic brain damage is the cause encountered most frequently, for instance after cardiopulmonary resuscitation (17% incidence of status; Krumholz, Stern & Weiss 1988), cardiopulmonary surgery or failed suicide. A similar clinical picture can also be seen in toxic or metabolic encephalopathies, the terminal stages of degenerative cerebral disorders such as Jakob–Creutzfeldt disease, and in acute cerebral injury (e.g. after cerebral haemorrhage) or trauma (see table 3.13)

Several seizure types occur, including tonic–clonic, tonic, simple and complex partial seizures, but much the most characteristic is continuous myoclonia, which has a distinctive clinical and EEG appearance. This is best named *myoclonic status epilepticus in coma*. Other terms which have been used include: myoclonic status epilepticus, status myoclonus, and generalised status myoclonicus, and generalised myoclonic status epilepticus, but these are best avoided, failing as they do to differentiate the myoclonic status in coma from myoclonic status in other syndromes (e.g. Lennox–Gastaut syndrome (pp. 101–3), the other myoclonic epilepsies (pp. 109–10) and primary generalised epilepsies (p. 149)) which have very different pathophysiology, clinical and EEG features, and prognosis. Myoclonic status in coma should also be differentiated from *subtle status epilepticus*, which is an end-stage of tonic–clonic status (see p. 54).

In acute anoxia, the status usually develops within a day or two of the onset of acute coma, occasionally later, and lasts for hours, days or even weeks. Seizures comprise irregular, asynchronous, typically small amplitude, repetitive myoclonic jerking of the facial musculature, and less consistently of the limbs (Celesia, Grigg & Ross 1988; Jumao-as & Brenner 1990; Lowenstein & Aminoff 1992). These jerks may be slight and observed only on careful scrutiny. Tonic–clonic, clonic or tonic seizures commonly interrupt the ongoing myoclonic status. In about 50% of cases, the myoclonus may be stimulus sensitive. In some patients motor activity is restricted to slight jerking of the mouth or eyelids. The patients are usually comatose, with flaccid paralysis, and absent oculocephalic reflexes. Rhythmic, small amplitude, vertical or horizontal eye movements have also been described in electrographic status (continuous spike–wave or repetitive organised rhythmic stereotyped discharges), in the absence of other motor manifestations. Alternating myoclonus has been observed, similar to 'erratic' neonatal seizures (Bortone *et al.* 1992). There is usually no prior history of epilepsy and myoclonic status epilepticus in coma is a sign of profound cerebral injury.

Table 3.13. *Some causes of myoclonic status epilepticus in coma*

Acute anoxic–ischaemic cerebral damage
Cardiopulmonary surgery
Coronary resuscitation
Other surgical procedures
Acute intracerebral vascular events
Carbon monoxide poisoning
Carbon dioxide narcosis
Subarachnoid haemorrhage

Metabolic/toxic encephalopathies
Hepatic failure
Renal failure
Hypoglycaemia
Hyponatraemia
Dialysis syndrome
Toxins (e.g. bismuth and heavy metal poisoning)
Drug overdose (including lithium, L-dopa, tricyclics, anticonvulsants, penicillin, sedatives, opiates)
Neonatal metabolic disorders (see table 3.2)
Nonketotic hyperglycaemia
Thiamine and other cofactor deficiencies

Physical encephalopathies
Post-traumatic
Heat stroke
Electrocution
Decompression injury

Degenerative cerebral disorders (terminal stages)
Jakob–Creutzfeldt disease
Alzheimer's disease
Other dementias

Acute viral or inflammatory encephalopathy
Herpes simplex encephalitis
Other viral and bacterial encephalitides
Subacute sclerosing panencephalitis
Disseminated postinfectious encephalomyelitis
Infections in immunosuppressed subjects (including HIV infection)
Progressive multifocal leucoencephalopathy

HIV, human immunodeficiency virus.

The EEG appearances vary. In a series of 23 cases, defined by the presence of EEG abnormality, 11 (48%) showed generalised periodic complexes of spike or polyspikes, with intervals varying from 0.5–5 seconds but which were relatively consistent within individuals, 4 (17%) showed burst suppression with interburst intervals of 1–10 seconds, and others exhibited continuous rhythmic activity consisting of spikes or slow waves, or irregular bursts of spike or polyspike discharges (Jumao-as & Brenner 1990). Periodic bursting and burst suppression are rather characteristic features of the EEG in this condition (Giorgi *et al.* 1991), and carry a very dismal prognosis, most patients dying or remaining in a persistent vegetative state.

In some patients, identical motor manifestations occur without EEG correlates, and it may become difficult to define what is and what is not 'epileptic'. In a series of 47 patients in coma usually due to anoxic, infective or metabolic causes, small clonic movements of the eyes, face or upper extremities were seen in 33 (in only 5 of whom were limb movements involved) with EEG epileptic discharges, in 9 without EEG correlate, and in 5 EEG discharges were present without clinical signs (Lowenstein & Aminoff 1992). To categorise patients on the basis of EEG seems futile, and the differences are probably based on a spectrum of cerebral damage. Nonepileptic reticular and segmental myoclonus can also occur if cerebral damage is diffuse.

Pathological examination of the brains of patients dying in status myoclonicus in coma shows widespread damage in structures concerned with the propagation and generalisation of epileptic activity. It has been suggested that the unique clinical appearances of the status are due to: profound disruption of the neocortical architecture, preventing the intracortical spread required in normal epilepsy; disruption of thalamic function, preventing normal seizure generalisation; or basal ganglia or cerebellar disturbance, preventing normal tonic inhibitory phenomena (Celesia *et al.* 1988). Another possibility is that the anoxic or biochemical changes in the efferent pathways interrupt the transmission of impulses, especially if brain stem structures are destroyed. Whatever the mechanism, the fragmentary nature of the clinical seizures is highly characteristic and a reflection of diffuse cerebral damage.

The treatment and prognosis of myoclonic status in coma are described on pp. 290 and 309.

Specific forms of status epilepticus in mental retardation

Nowhere are the nosological problems of status more apparent than in children and adults with mental retardation (the term used here to denote those with impairment of cerebral functioning, most commmonly due to prenatal congenital or developmental cerebral damage, resulting in low intelligence). In the mentally retarded, the clinical and electrographic forms of severe epilepsy (and status) seem to be determined as much by the incompleteness of cerebral development as by the specific aetiology, or indeed even by age. The classic types of status do occur, but, more characteristically, both epilepsy and status take unusual forms. Classification, though, is very confused, and this is a most ill understood and poorly investigated subject. Four clinical types of status occur almost exclusively in the mentally retarded, and are best grouped together: atypical absence status, subclinical status, tonic status and minor motor status. In many patients, these seizure types coexist, and often overlap, with converging clinical features. Similar seizure disorders are seen in mental retardation of widely varying aetiology and clinical presentation, with few if any distinguishing features; at least as far as is known.

100

These types of seizure disorder are best therefore viewed together as nonspecific epileptic manifestations of diffuse cerebral damage and impaired (compromised) cerebral development. Little is understood about the epileptic mechanisms of these forms of status, which ∴ .. fertile area of further research.

The frequency of status in the mentally retarded is unknown. Between 1% and 2% of the population are mentally retarded (IQ below 70) and about 0.5% severely retarded (IQ below 50). Epilepsy occurs in about one third of the severely mentally impaired and about 12% of those with mild mental retardation. In table 3.9 are shown the underlying causes of epilepsy in a mentally handicapped population in which there was a history of convulsive status in 19% of cases. No details of the frequency of nonconvulsive or atypical forms were given, forms which are probably more common.

The best-studied epilepsy 'syndrome' amongst the mentally handicapped is the *Lennox–Gastaut syndrome*. Here again is a nosological jungle, with opinion divided as to whether this is a distinct entity or simply an inclusive term which incorporates disparate cases with mental handicap and severe epilepsy. Certainly, the dividing line between the syndrome and other secondarily generalised epilepsies in the mentally retarded is vague. The Lennox–Gastaut syndrome is defined by the EEG appearance of slow spike–wave, yet this can also be seen in other epilepsies, not conforming to the clinical descriptions of the syndrome. The reliance on such an EEG pattern for classification is quite unsatisfactory. Status in the Lennox–Gastaut syndrome resembles status in other mentally retarded persons with epilepsy (especially those with myoclonic epilepsies), and the clinical forms will therefore be considered together.

Lennox–Gastaut syndrome

When Lennox first noted the particular electroencephalographic pattern of diffuse slow spike–wave, he considered it to be a variant of petit mal (Gibbs *et al.* 1937). By 1950, however, these cases had been distinguished from true petit mal by Lennox and his colleagues (Lennox & Davis 1950; Lennox 1960), who compared 200 cases with slow spike–wave and 200 cases of 3 Hz generalised spike–wave, and found, in the first group, earlier age of onset, a high incidence of mental retardation and signs of other brain damage, the existence of frequent atypical absence, tonic and myoclonic seizures, and a poor response to anticonvulsant drugs. Dravet in 1965 completed a thesis on the petit mal variant under the tutelage of Gastaut, and in 1966 Gastaut *et al.* published a definitive paper on the syndrome, which was henceforth termed the Lennox–Gastaut syndrome (see Niedermeyer & Degen 1988). A substantial body of literature from the Marseilles school and others has formed subsequently (Neidermeyer 1968; Ohtahara *et al.* 1970; Doose *et al.* 1970; Chevrie & Aicardi 1972; Blume, David & Gomez 1973; Aicardi 1973; Markand 1977; Gastaut 1982; Dravet *et al.* 1985*b*; Tassinari *et al.* 1985; Beaumanoir 1985; Doose 1985; Roger *et al.* 1987), and the condition has been the subject of a conference with published proceedings (Niedermeyer and Degen 1988).

As originally defined by Gastaut *et al.* (1966), the syndrome is a severe variety

Table 3.14. *The underlying pathologies in 265 cases of Lennox–Gastaut syndrome*

Disease	Number
Cryptogenic	68
Pathological mental defect	32
Cerebral palsy	74
Postencephalitic	33
Sequelae of West syndrome	21
Tuberose sclerosis	10
Hydrocephalus	5
Porencephaly	4
Others[a]	18

[a] Includes multiple anomalies (2), microencephaly (3), cavum vergae or cavum septi pelucidi (2), agenesis of the corpus callosum (2), hemiconvulsion-hemiplegia-epilepsy syndrome (2), Down's syndrome (1), Sjøgren-Larsson syndrome (1), Von Recklinghausen syndrome (1), dyssynergia cerebellaris myoclonica (1), Alper's disease (1), Louis Bar syndrome (1), Lowe syndrome (1).
From Ohtahara *et al.* 1988.

of childhood epilepsy, refractory to treatment, characterised by frequent tonic and atypical absence seizures, progressive mental retardation, and interictal EEG records showing diffuse slow spike–wave patterns. Other seizure types occur including tonic–clonic seizures, clonic seizures, unilateral seizures and partial seizures. This clinical and EEG syndrome can be produced by many different cerebral pathologies (table 3.14), although often no cause is uncovered.

Its nosological position has been the subject of considerable debate. The same clinical and EEG picture can occur in mild and severe forms, can evolve from other types of epilepsy, and can be caused by a great number of different pathological disorders. Furthermore, Oller-Daurella (1973) noted that only 184 patients of 250 with slow spike–wave on the EEG met the clinical criteria of Gastaut *et al.* (1966), and approximately similar proportions are reported by Aicardi (1973); Osawa *et al.* (1977) and Beaumanoir (1982). Many doubt whether this condition fully earns the sobriquet of a true 'syndrome', and others view it as a relatively nonspecific developmental response of damaged brain. Whether the Lennox–Gastaut syndrome is a true entity or not, there is no doubt that patients with this clinical and EEG pattern have a profound epileptic encephalopathy, and the term has acquired wide clinical usage.

The clinical description given by Gastaut *et al.* (1966) has not been bettered. The cardinal features are a severe epileptic disorder with mental deterioration. The epilepsy is characterised by frequent atypical absence, tonic, myoclonic and tonic–clonic seizures (usually in combination); other seizure types may also occur. The patients fall frequently, and are prone to injury. Associated with the severe epilepsy is progressive mental retardation, and neither the epilepsy nor the mental impairment are easily controlled by medical means. Overt and covert status are common. The outcome is generally poor, few children acquire normal intellectual functioning and most continue to have epilepsy. Many require institutionalisation.

The age of onset is generally between 1 and 7 years. In a series of 265 patients (Ohtahara *et al.* 1988), all cases developed epilepsy between the ages of 4 months and 14 years, the great majority being between 11 months and 6 years. However, apparently adult-onset patients are also encountered, as are adult patients, with static clinical features, who developed the condition in childhood. There is some heterogeneity within this clinical picture, and specific subgroups have been defined including the 'myoclonic variant' and the 'intermediate petit mal' type. The condition can evolve in children initially exhibiting infantile spasm or West syndrome, or from partial epilepsy, and in some cases there is overlap (from the clinical or electrographic points of view) with the severe myoclonic epilepsies, post-traumatic partial epilepsies, myoclonic–astatic epilepsy, ESES (electrical status epilepticus during slow wave sleep), Landau–Kleffner syndrome and other progressive cerebral degenerations.

The signature of the Lennox–Gastaut syndrome is, of course, the repetitive 1–2.5 Hz spike–wave complex, spread widely in both hemispheres with varying asymmetries, roughly bilaterally synchronous and with a bifrontal predominance. These discharges can persist for long periods of time, occupying over two thirds of the EEG record, for hours or days at a time. The complexes are rarely induced by hyperventilation or by photic stimulation, in this respect differing from the 3 Hz spike–wave of petit mal, and are enhanced in non-REM sleep. The background activity is slow during wakefulness, and normal arousal and sleep potentials are diminished or absent. Variable EEG patterns are seen in clinical events, and variable clinical events for the same EEG pattern (Blume 1988). During a clinically evident atypical absence attack, the EEG may at times show little change and at others a distinct slow spike–wave paroxysm. Other seizure types are usually but not always accompanied by EEG change; nevertheless in many cases, the distinction between ictal and interictal state on EEG grounds may be difficult.

Forms of status epilepticus in the Lennox–Gastaut syndrome and other types of mental retardation

There is a high incidence of clinically evident status in patients with the Lennox–Gastaut syndrome. Of 184 reported cases (Aicardi & Gomes 1988; Beaumanoir *et al.* 1988; Weiermann & Jacobi 1988) 63% had a history of discrete episodes of both nonconvulsive and convulsive status, often lasting hours to weeks or more, and in other syndromes of mental retardation status is also common. Generalised tonic–clonic, simple and complex partial status occur, not unlike the episodes of status seen in any symptomatic epilepsy, although often highly refractory to treatment; these are described elsewhere. Four distinctive clinical patterns of status, though, are both common in, and relatively specific to, the Lennox–Gastaut

103

syndrome and other forms of mental retardation: atypical absence status, sub-clinical status, tonic status, and minor motor status.

ATYPICAL ABSENCE STATUS EPILEPTICUS: This type of status is very common in the Lennox–Gastaut syndrome. The phenomenology of absence status is described in detail on pp. 76–8, and the reader is also referred to pp. 79–81 for a discussion of the nosological confusion that surrounds the differentiation of typical and that of atypical forms. Suffice to say here that the clinical phenomenology of typical and that of atypical absence status overlap greatly, although to exactly what extent is not known. Nevertheless, there are dissimilarities. First, of course, is the clinical context; typical absence status occurs in normally intelligent patients with primary generalised epilepsy, which is very different from the clinical picture of the Lennox–Gastaut syndrome. The tempo and the temporal course of the status also differ; in atypical absence status the episodes are generally longer and more frequent, with a gradual onset and offset of the status. Atypical absence status is often preceded by an alteration in the general physical and mental state of the patient, with changes in motor activity, mood or intellectual attainment, persisting for hours or days before the overt seizures develop ('bad days'; possibly due to subclinical nonconvulsive status, see below). Atypical absence status tends to fluctuate, and minor motor, myoclonic or more typically tonic seizures interrupt, but do not terminate an episode. In some patients, the mental state fluctuates gradually in and out of this ill-defined epileptic state over long periods (some attacks last weeks or even months), with little distinction possible between ictal and interictal phases. The initiation or termination of the status with a tonic–clonic seizure, a common pattern in petit mal (typical absence) status, is unusual in atypical absence. Beaumanoir *et al.* (1988) distinguish five varieties of tonic and atypical absence status in their 34 cases of Lennox–Gastaut, emphasising the evolution from one type to another during the episode, but whether these categories are distinctive is debatable. Unlike typical absence status, the atypical absence status often responds poorly to benzodiazepine injection. Indeed anticonvulsant therapy may be futile, and the condition waxes and wanes in its own time, uninfluenced by external force. One has a strong impression that absence status in Lennox–Gastaut is more likely if the child or adult is understimulated, or is drowsy, another reason not to overmedicate. Some cases have a striking and unexplained periodicity (fig. 3.9).

The EEG during absence status may show continuous irregular slow (2–2.5 Hz) spike–wave or more discrete ictal patterns (Beaumanoir *et al.* 1988).

The occurrence of overt status in the Lennox–Gastaut syndrome is not clearly related to outcome (Dravet *et al.* 1985; Beaumanoir *et al.* 1988; Weiermann & Jacobi 1988), nor are clear-cut mental sequelae common after even prolonged epiosdes of overt nonconvulsive or tonic status. Neverthless, it is tempting to posulate that the inexorable intellectual decline in the Lennox–Gastaut syndrome might be related to the electrographic status which is universal in the syndrome, though this proposition is untestable whilst therapy is so ineffective.

SUBCLINICAL STATUS EPILEPTICUS: The mental state of some retarded children, especially those with the Lennox–Gastaut phenotype, is rather similar in kind, if not in degree, to that in atypical absence status. This raises the possibility that the 'interictal' condition is in fact a form of subclinical status epilepticus, a view supported by the clinical and EEG similarity of ictal and interictal phases and the lack of clear onset and offset of ictal phases. It is possible to view the overt status as a 'decompensation' (Beaumanoir's (1982) excellent term) of the chronic epileptic encephalopathy, thus emphasising the close relationship between the interictal and ictal states (see fig. 3.10).

These are conundrums which raise philosophical as well as practical questions about the nature of epilepsy which are outside the scope of this book. Nevertheless, it would be of great interest to know whether or not the interictal state with electrographic status is equivalent to overt status in physiological terms, for therapeutic as well as prognostic reasons. The issue is further compounded by the fact that subtle changes in awareness, alterations in tone, and occasional jerks are also frequently seen in patients in an apparently interictal phase without electrographic status.

TONIC STATUS EPILEPTICUS: This form was first clearly delineated by Gastaut *et al.* in 1963, and the clinical and EEG features were comprehensively documented in a series of 28 cases for the Xth Marseilles Colloquium by Roger *et al.* (1974). Almost all episodes of tonic status occur in children or adults, with the clinical features of the Lennox–Gastaut syndrome. Ohtahara *et al.* (1979) reported that about half of cases of childhood status are tonic status, but most authorities record a much lower incidence.

The status comprises severe and frequent tonic seizures. The clinical symptomatology may be similar to that of isolated tonic attacks, or modified particularly as the status progresses. Gastaut, in his seminal work on this topic (Gastaut *et al.* 1963), divided individual tonic seizures into three types: the axial tonic seizure, the axial-rhizomelic tonic seizure, and the global tonic seizure. In the Marseilles series, each type is represented in status (Roger *et al.* 1974). As the status progresses, motor phenomena tend to lessen, at times to a stage where clinical manifestations are confined to slight eyelid blinking, eye deviation or pupillary or respiratory changes only. Such seizures can occur with extraordinary frequency. Autonomic features may be prominent, with tachycardia, hypertension and pronounced tracheobronchial secretion. In a significant proportion (14%) of the cases reported by Roger *et al.* (1974), seizure manifestations were slight from the onset of status, and in 17% the status comprised of electrographic tonic seizures without any motor features at all. The condition may present as a confusional state (Somerville & Bruni 1983), and may also evolve from or into atypical absence status. In Roger's series, the duration of individual tonic seizures in status was 70 seconds, longer than that of individual isolated tonic seizures (mean 15 seconds). In established status in the tonic seizures recurred at a frequency of 2–45 per hour in wakefulness, and up to 100 per hour during sleep. The duration of an episode of status was very variable, the average being 9 days, but cases with status continuing

(*a*)

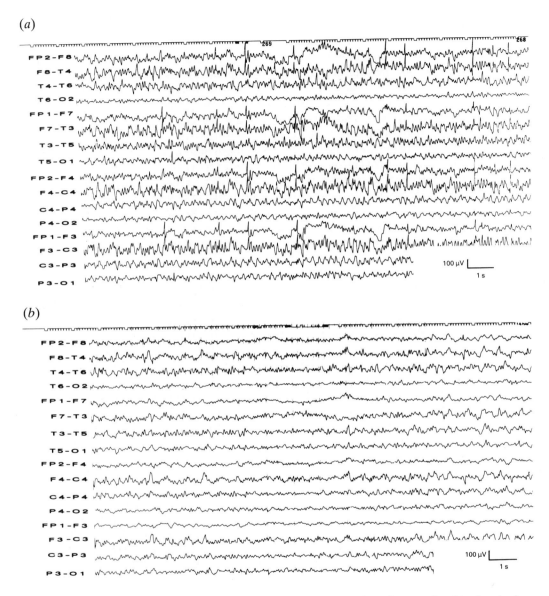

(*b*)

Fig. 3.9. Scalp EEG of a 25 year old male who developed generalised tonic–clonic seizures in the first year of life, which continued at a frequency of about one every 3 months. His development was slow from this time, and he is mentally retarded. At the age of 11 years, following drug changes, he experienced recurrent episodes of severe tonic–clonic status epilepticus over a 4 month period. Since then, he has had generalised seizures every few months, and also episodes of atypical absence status at a regular frequency of one every 5 days, for several years.

for up to 4 months were observed. The mental state between attacks varies from full consciousness to deep coma. Tonic status responds poorly, if at all, to anti-convulsant therapy, and occasionally ends fatally. Variants occur, and the condition very occasionally develops in patients without mental retardation or the Lennox–Gastaut phenotype. Tanganelli & Regesta (1991) reported a remarkable patient in which status persisted for 5 months, with up to 130 seizures an hour at times. There was no response to therapy (which included pentobarbitone anaesthesia), but after 5 months the status subsided, and the patient remained subsequently seizure free. Usually, on recovery, no long term deficit is evident, although at least one reported patient showed intellectual deterioration (Somerville & Bruni 1983).

The EEG is very important diagnostically, especially in patients with few motor features, and demonstrates one of three patterns: desynchronisation, a rapid (20 Hz) initially low amplitude rhythm increasing gradually to 100 µV, and a 10 Hz recruiting rhythm of high amplitude from its onset. Occasionally, however, tonic seizures occur without EEG correlate, or with atypical forms.

MINOR MOTOR STATUS (MYOCLONIC ENCEPHALOPATHY): In 1966, Brett published an influential report describing 22 cases of minor epileptic status in which frequent myoclonus and akinetic attacks occurred to a suffcent degree to simulate severe ataxia and dementia (pseudoataxia and pseudodementia) (Brett 1966). Many cases would now be included within the rubric of the Lennox–Gastaut syndrome but not all and various other syndromic diagnoses were subsequently made. The minor motor status may last for hours, days or even weeks. The child is obtunded, drooling, speech is absent or slurred, and the head may tend to fall forward. Variable symmetric and assymetric myoclonic jerks are seen in the limbs, trunk, and eyes. Sudden atonia may occur, resulting in head nodding, flexion of the trunk, or falls. Walking is unsteady, the gait lurching and unsteady (pseudoataxia). Fine movements may be interrupted by the myoclonus, and in severe cases even

Caption for fig. 3.9 (*cont.*).
These attacks are initiated with a generalised seizure, followed by absence lasting an entire day, with motor retardation, confusion, and a pseudo-ataxic gait. The recurrent status at the age of 11 was precipitated by sulthiame withdrawal, and continued despite intensive therapy. Remarkably, on restarting sulthiame, all epileptic activity ceased (for 8 months at the time of writing). The illustrated EEG (*a*) was recorded during the atypical absence status and shows persisting rhythmic activity over both hemispheres, with bilateral anterior predominance, and spikes showing shifting localisation. The second trace (*b*) was recorded 10 minutes after the intramuscular injection of 10 mg of midazolam. There is a marked improvement in the EEG, with the virtual abolition of spikes, although the EEG is not normalised. The clinical state did not change markedly; such an incomplete response of absence to acute benzodiazepine administration is not uncommon, and can be contrasted with the classic response shown in fig. 5.7. (With thanks to Dr David Fish, National Hospital for Neurology and Neurosurgery, for preparing this illustration.)

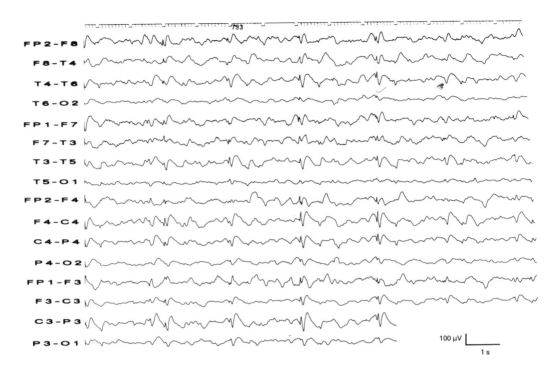

Fig. 3.10. Scalp EEG from a 26 year old male with Lennox–Gastaut syndrome,
following a left frontal lobe abscess at the age of 1 year. He experiences frequent
tonic–clonic, atypical absence, tonic and myoclonic seizures, mild mental
retardation (full scale IQ 66) which is static and without focal neurological signs. The
EEG shows slow spike–wave (2–3 Hz) on a slow background without focal
features. At times, he is much slower and more obtunded than at others ('bad
days'), thought to be due to continuous subclinical activity (the form of status
common in Lennox–Gastaut syndrome) but during these periods, there is little
change in the scalp EEG, which fluctuates largely independently of the clinical state.
The illustrated EEG shows ongoing epileptic activity which in this example is taken
during a 'bad day' when he was obtunded and exhibited marked motor retardation.
(With thanks to Dr David Fish, National Hospital for Neurology and Neurosurgery,
for preparing this illustration.)

simple activities are impossible. The EEG shows multifocal continuous spikes
and spike–wave discharges, in most cases of the Lennox–Gastaut type. The
response to treatment is poor, as is the prognosis, which relies ultimately upon
the underlying pathology. In a few cases the condition largely resolved (E.H. Brett,
personal communication).

The treatment and prognosis of the various specific forms of status in mental
retardation are described on pp. 291 and 309–10.

Other syndromes of myoclonic status epilepticus

As discussed above, the myoclonic encephalopathies of childhood and the myoclonic epilepsies in the differing forms of mental retardation are hopelessly entangled nosologically. There are, however, three other situations with myoclonic status which are highly distinctive. First, is myoclonic status in coma, discussed on pp. 98–100; second, the myoclonic status in patients with primary generalised epilepsy; and finally, myoclonic status in the progressive myoclonic epilepsies.

Myoclonic status epilepticus in primary generalised epilepsy

The spectrum of the primary generalised epilepsies comprises a series of subgroups, which include childhood absence epilepsy, juvenile absence epilepsy, juvenile myoclonic epilepsy, epilepsy with generalised tonic–clonic seizures on awakening, epilepsy with myoclonic absences, and childhood grand mal epilepsy. To what extent these form separate syndromes is a source of tangled controversy, without the scope of this book; suffice to say here, that the clinical features often overlap, and some if not all of the syndromes can, from a clinical perspective, be considered part of a broad spectrum. Status takes three forms in these conditions: tonic–clonic, absence and myoclonic (or myoclonic-absence) status. Tonic clonic status is described on pp. 53–76, and occurs in primary and secondarily generalised epilepsies. Absence status (petit mal status) is discussed on pp. 76–84, and in its pure form occurs only in patients with primary generalised absence epilepsy. Myoclonic (or myoclonic–absence) status is probably less common than the other status types, being only occasionally encountered, particularly in children. The status will usually take the form of the *myoclonic storm* in which myoclonus builds up in a fulminating manner to reach the intensity of status. At its height, awareness is altered, and the myoclonic status may be succeeded and terminated by a tonic–clonic seizure. A specific syndrome of *epilepsy with myoclonic absences* has been delineated by Tassinari *et al.* (1992), and seems particularly to be associated with myoclonic status. This syndrome developes in older children (mean age 7 years) with a male preponderance. Generalised absences are accompanied by severe bilateral rhythmical myoclonias. The seizures are frequent and about 50% of cases show pre-existing mental retardation. The interictal EEG is normal, and the ictal EEG shows 3 Hz spike–wave discharges, similar to those of childhood absence epilepsy. In about one third of cases, absence or myoclonic status develops. In some cases, the clinical picture evolves to resemble that of the Lennox–Gastaut syndrome, raising some questions as to the nosological position of the syndrome.

Status epilepticus in the progressive myoclonic epilepsies

In older children and adults, the syndrome of *progressive myoclonic epilepsy* is fairly well defined and can be differentiated from the other myoclonic encephalopathies (Berkovic *et al.* 1986, 1989*b*; So *et al.* 1989). It is characterised by progressive myoclonus, dementia and epilepsy. Other signs may also occur, depending on the underlying cause. Tonic–clonic, partial and absence seizures accompany the myoclonus, but are seldom the central clinical problem; tonic–clonic or nonconvulsive status are rare. As the condition proceeds, myoclonus may become more and more persistent, and frequently reaches status proportions. The myoclonus is erratic, asymmetrical, affects limbs and trunk, and facial musculature, is often continuous for long periods of time, and can be exacerbated by action or startle. It is of cortical origin, and is usually accompanied by time-locked EEG potentials. Even when the myoclonus is continuous and severe, consciousness is usually preserved, the syndrome thus differing from the myoclonic encephalopathies described above. Sometimes a massive increase in the frequency and amplitude of the myoclonus is produced by movement, which may be misinterpreted as a tonic–clonic seizure (the preservation of consciousness should help to differentiate the two seizure types). Progressive myoclonic epilepsy has a number of underlying causes, of which the most common in my own practice are mitochondrial cytopathy (MERRF), Lafora body disease, Unverricht–Lundborg disease, and dentato-rubro-pallido-luysian degeneration. Less common causes include sialidosis (types I and II), juvenile neuroaxonal dystrophy, Gaucher's disease, neuronal ceroid-lipofuscinosis (Batten's and Kuf's diseases), GM_2 gangliosidosis, poliodystrophy and biotin-responsive progressive myoclonus. The clinical course and prognosis of the myoclonic epilepsy is determined largely by the underlying cause, but in over half of the patients encountered in adult neurological practice, no specific cause can be found.

Myoclonus without epilepsy rarely if ever reaches the proportions of status, and has a rather different aetiological spectrum (e.g. the myoclonus in Wilson's disease, torsion dystonia, Huntington's disease, ataxia telangiectasia, the spinocerebellar degenerations, progressive supranuclear palsy, and multi-system atrophy, Hallervorden–Spatz syndrome).

The treatment and prognosis of myoclonus status in the primary generalised and progressive myoclonic epilepsies are outlined on pp. 291 and 310.

Nonconvulsive simple partial status epilepticus

The subdivision of partial seizures into simple and complex categories was a most important revision of the second International League Against Epilepsy classification of seizure type (Commission on Classification and Terminology of the International League Against Epilepsy 1981). Simple partial seizures are defined as focal seizures occurring without, and complex partial seizures those with, altered consciousness. Consciousness is difficult to assess clinically (or indeed to define), and the classification has thus been heavily and justifiably criticised. It is also now clear that a subdivision of partial seizures on the basis of consciousness is not meaningful in either physiological or anatomical terms. The widely held view that altered consciousness in epilepsy implies bilateral limbic involvement, although generally true is not reliably so, and altered awareness has been demonstrated in strictly unilateral temporal as well as extratemporal epilepsy

(Wieser *et al.* 1985). Presumably the physiological disturbance in simple partial status is very similar to that in complex partial status, albeit restricted in distribution, and their differentiation on the basis of 'consciousness' is rather futile.

Simple partial status can be defined as a prolonged simple partial seizure. It is possible that simple partial nonconvulsive status is more common in neocortical than in limbic epilepsy, but convincing evidence on this point is lacking. Convulsive simple partial status is usually classified as *epilepsia partialis continua* (see pp. 86–98), and is more common than nonconvulsive simple partial status. Oculoclonic status epilepticus (nystagmoid status) is a rare form of adversive status of occipital origin (see the interesting case of Kanazawa, Sengoku & Kawai (1989)). Prolonged ictal paralysis (somato-inhibitory status) is another occasional form of nonconvulsive simple partial status (Tinuper *et al.* 1987) that can be difficult to distinguish from a postictal (Todd's) paresis. There is also substantial overlap between simple partial status with psychic symptomatology and the boundary syndromes discussed below, and conceptual difficulties arise when the correlation between electrographic and clinical symptoms is loose (as is often the case).

Prominent psychic symptomatology is much commoner in complex partial than in simple partial epilepsy, but can occur in the latter. The most common symptom is ictal fear. Williams (1956) found, from 2000 personal cases, 100 who showed affective symptoms. Sixty-one exhibited fear, often associated with visceral sensation, and always associated with anterior temporal epileptic discharges. One patient was described who had episodes lasting for 24–48 hours during which time he was frightened ('an unnatural sense of fright about nothing'), bad tempered, obstinate, mildly confused and depressed; the depression was severe enough to engender suicidal thoughts. Henriksen (1973) described in great detail a patient with prolonged periods of fear often followed by epigastric sensations lasting for days, and associated with spiking in the right anterior temporal region and at the right sphenoidal electrode. The fear was maximal when spiking was most frequent, and subsequent corticography confirmed the presence of spiking over the anterior temporal isocortex. Zappoli *et al.* (1983) reported another patient with prolonged episodes of fear (motiveless anxiety and vague alarm) associated with frequent bursts of left anterior temporal epileptic activity.

Geier (1978) and Sacquegna *et al.* (1981) reported cases of electrographic partial status, in which, at times, the only clinical manifestations were disturbances of spatial data organisation and other cognitive impairments, which were barely appreciable on clinical examination and which were detected reliably only on neuropsychological testing. Such phenomena, although rare in partial status, are relatively common in atypical absence status.

The specific syndrome of acquired aphasia in association with electrographic status in children (the Landau–Kleffner syndrome) is described on pp. 51–2. In adults, too, isolated motor and sensory aphasias have been reported, with few other signs, during episodes of electrographic status (Boudouresques, Roger & Gastaut 1962; De Pasquet *et al.* 1976; Gastaut 1979; Hamilton & Matthews 1979; Dinner *et al.* 1981; Knight & Cooper 1986; Rosenbaum *et al.* 1986; Primavera,

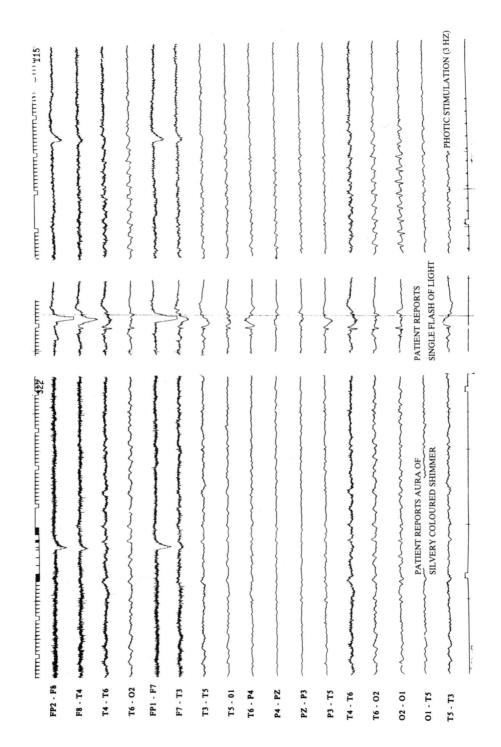

PHOTIC STIMULATION (3 HZ)

PATIENT REPORTS
SINGLE FLASH OF LIGHT

PATIENT REPORTS AURA OF
SILVERY COLOURED SHIMMER

FP2 - F8
F8 - T4
T4 - T6
T6 - O2
FP1 - F7
F7 - T3
T3 - T5
T5 - O1
T6 - P4
P4 - PZ
PZ - P3
P3 - T5
T4 - T6
T6 - O2
O2 - O1
O1 - T5
T5 - T3

Bo & Venturi 1988; Blatt, Jackson & Dasheiff 1992; Wells, Labar & Solomon 1992; fig. 3.12). The temporal course differs from the Landau–Kleffner syndrome in that language reverts to normal at the end of each electrographic episode (often after days or weeks), and neither intellectual nor behavioural regression occur. Cases in the elderly without a prior history of epilepsy have also been described, and the evidence of a true epileptic basis in some is doubtful (Racy *et al.* 1980). The speech disturbance may be associated with other psychometric abnormalities, including alexia, agraphia, word deafness, and ideomotor or constructional apraxia (Boudouresques *et al.* 1962; De Pasquet *et al.* 1976), but the language disturbance predominates. As in other status syndromes, language functions seem particularly affected, but the physiological basis of this sensitivity is unknown. The status may be the first epileptic manifestation (Wells *et al.* 1992).

Simple and complex visual hallucinations have also been reported as an isolated prolonged epileptic phenomenon (Sowa & Pituck 1989). These include flashes of light, patterns of colour and light, misperception of size or orientation, and hallucinations of objects and animals (see fig. 3.11). Ictal blindness is also a relatively common symptom in occipital focal status (status epilepticus amauroticus) and was originally reported by Ayala (1929) in a patient with attacks of cortical blindness culminating in an episode of persisting blindness lasting 15 days, punctuated by focal motor and grand mal seizures. Engel, Ludwig & Fetell (1978) reported a meticulously studied case of complex partial status, in which blindness occurred when seizure activity spread into the temporal-occipital region. More recently Barry *et al.* (1985) detailed four cases of blindness occurring in the context of nonconvulsive status, variably associated with confusion, forced eye

Fig. 3.11. Three sections of EEG from a 29 year old male with a history of occasional secondarily generalised seizures since the age of 3 years. From age 13, he experienced recurrent prolonged attacks of simple partial status. The attacks evolve slowly, initially he experiences single momentary flashes of light, and episodes of shimmering silver light lasting a second (like a flashlight of a camera) followed by a headache. These visual phenomena recur at increasing frequencies, from one an hour to one every 2 minutes, over a period of 2 days, during which his headache also progressively worsens. Then, over a 3 minute period, the shimmering lights become continuous in the left visual field, grow in size and intensity, he experiences a dark blob in the middle of his visual field, which increases in size to obscure his vision, totally. He is still conscious at this stage, but experiences hallucinations of faces, a dreamy feeling and a rising epigastric feeling, his eyes flicker, he repeatedly swallows and he loses consciousness, and a tonic–clonic seizure occurs. This seizure disorder is classified as a simple partial status, evolving into a complex partial and then a secondarily generalised seizure. No cause for his epilepsy was found despite detailed magnetic resonance imaging studies and other intensive investigation. The first EEG segment shows a posterior ictal discharge during the aura, the middle section shows a spike–wave complex recorded during the experience of a flash, and the segment on the right shows a following response at 3 Hz photic stimulation. (With thanks to Dr Shelagh Smith, National Hospital for Neurology and Neurosurgery, for preparing this illustration.)

deviation, and focal hemisensory and motor signs, where the EEG showed occipital or bi-occipital discharges.

Prolonged 'auras' are another enduring epileptic phenomenon, best categorised as simple partial status. Four of my cases have exhibited prolonged episodes of a 'butterfly' sensation in the stomach, rising epigastric sensations (fig. 3.13), and persisting olfactory sensations. The latter sensations lasted for weeks on end, fluctuating in intensity. The focal onset was temporal or frontal in the four cases,

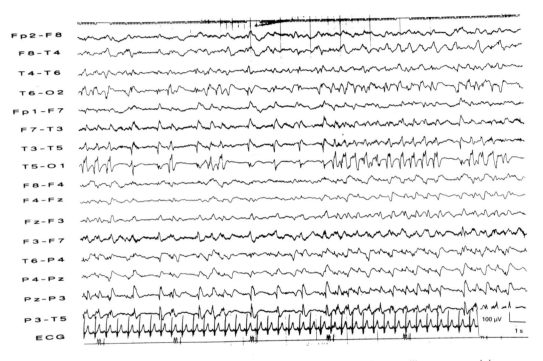

Fig. 3.12. Scalp EEG from a 44 year old male with a subacute illness comprising headaches, diplopia, confusion and bilateral papilloedema. Findings on investigation included a high cerebrospinal fluid protein and cell count, meningeal thickening on MRI, and persisting raised intracranial pressure. A presumptive diagnosis of neuro-sarcoidosis was made. His treatment included steroid therapy, optic nerve sheaf fenestration, and insertion of a ventriculo-atrial shunt complicated by an extradural haemorrhage requiring surgical evacuation. Three months later he developed tonic–clonic seizures, then an episode of tonic–clonic status epilepticus, and then repeated episodes of simple partial status epilepticus. These episodes, which lasted hours or days, took the form of a marked dysphasia with expressive and receptive components. The EEG recorded during an episode shows repetitive bursts of left temporal spike and spike–wave activity, highly characteristic of both simple and complex partial status epilepticus. (With thanks to Dr David Fish, National Hospital for Neurology and Neurosurgery, for preparing this illustration.)

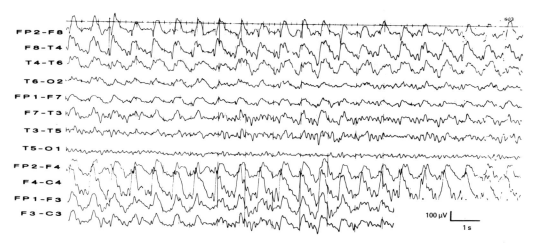

FP2-F8
F8-T4
T4-T6
T6-O2
FP1-F7
F7-T3
T3-T5
T5-O1
FP2-F4
F4-C4
FP1-F3
F3-C3

100 µV
1 s

Fig. 3.13. Scalp EEG from a 25 year old male with a history of complex partial seizures of frontal lobe origin since the age of 10 months. The seizures comprise a strange sensation of 'butterflies' in his stomach, sometimes rising to the neck, followed by loss of awareness and often a loud cry and manual automatisms, jerking movements of the limbs and bizarre speech. These seizures tend to cluster. At times, the butterfly sensation (long aura) persists for hours on end, without any other manifestation. The illustrated EEG was recorded during a long aura, and shows right frontal spiking which persisted during the period of the aura. A right frontal lobectomy was carried out, and the histological specimen demonstrated small areas of focal cortical dysplasia, in the region of the ictal discharges. This case illustrates the clinical and EEG semiology of a case of simple partial status, with histological evidence of dysplasia and resolution following surgical resection. (With thanks to Dr David Fish, National Hospital for Neurology and Neurosurgery, for preparing this illustration.)

and the prolonged auras were often followed by an overt seizure or cluster of seizures (Manford & Shorvon 1992). Three similar cases of 'continuous symptoms' (numbness in a hand, repeated blankness of mind, causeless terror) often terminating in a seizure undoubtedly due to enduring seizure activity were reported by Scott & Masland (1952).

In the reported cases of simple partial status, EEG has always been abnormal (by necessity to confirm the diagnosis), and ictal changes have shown spikes and spike–wave paroxysms in varying neocortical or mesial temporal sites. The EEG abnormalities are usually frequent and are restricted or widely distributed. The case of Sacquegna *et al.* (1981), for instance, showed focal and generalised spike–wave discharges lasting many hours, unresponsive to eye opening or closure and unaffected by intravenous diazepam. Ictal and scalp depth EEG (carried out by Dr David Fish, fig. 3.12; case 1 of Manford & Shorvon (1992)) in a patient with recurrent auras showed frequent widespread spikes and spike–wave activity

115

initially in medial frontal, but spreading to other frontal, temporal neocortical and hippocampal regions.

The aetiological basis of simple partial status has not been fully explored. Most reports have concentrated upon EEG or clinical manifestations to the exclusion of aetiology. Recorded cases have included cerebrovascular disease, mesial temporal sclerosis and cortical dysplasia (Dinner *et al.* 1981; Primavera *et al.* 1988; Manford & Shorvon 1992). Whether the range of causes differs from other forms of focal epilepsy is not known.

The treatment and prognosis of the nonconvulsive simple partial status are described on pp. 291 and 310–11.

Complex partial status epilepticus

Cases of what were undoubtedly complex partial status were recounted sporadically as 'interesting freaks' in the nineteenth century. Perhaps Hughlings Jackson was the first clearly to report a fugue state in temporal lobe epilepsy. One fascinating case was of a physician, who, during prolonged temporal lobe attacks with total loss of awareness and amnesia, was able to carry out normal activities, on one occasion actually ascultating a patient's chest and correctly diagnosing left basal pneumonia, and on another travelling by train on the Metropolitan line, negotiating the ticket collection, and walking straight home (see Taylor 1931). The first case authenticated by EEG was that reported by Gastaut *et al.* (1956), and until very recently this was thought to be a rare form of epilepsy (see, for instance Roger *et al.* 1974). With the conceptual advances of the last two decades, however, it has become clear that episodes of possible complex partial status are common events in the course of many focal epilepsies. No published statistics exist, but in my own adult practice, at least, this form of status is indubitably more common than other types of nonconvulsive or indeed tonic–clonic status. A history of possible complex partial status can be obtained from over 15% of patients encountered with chronic active partial epilepsy.

Definition and subclassification of complex partial status epilepticus

Since its first identification in 1956, there have been numerous attempts to define and subclassify complex partial status, and the result has been obscuration and confusion. Heintel's (1969) early example used convulsive status as a model, and defined complex partial status as an epileptic state in temporal lobe epilepsy in which serial complex partial seizures occur without intervening recovery of full consciousness, and with an EEG showing ictal changes. Gastaut & Tassinari (1975) and Lugaresi *et al.* (1971) refined this, dividing complex partial status into two types: (a) frequently recurring complex partial seizures with full or almost full recovery of consciousness in between (discontinuous form) and (b) a long-lasting episode of mental confusion and/or psychotic behaviour (continuous form). Most cases fall into one or other pattern, although transitional cases are seen, cases which exhibit both forms and cases in which one form evolves into the other (the celebrated case detailed by Wieser (1980), for instance). This was the first of what was to become a series of dichotomous (or at least oligotomous) classifications, none of them entirely satisfactory. Celesia (1976), for instance, recognised two types of complex partial status: the first of recurrent complex partial seizures with intervening confusion, and the second a prolonged confusional state indistinguishable clinically from absence seizures. Modifying the earlier categorisation, Mayeux & Lüders (1978) proposed that case definition should meet one of the following criteria: (a) continuous complex symptoms accompanied by a continous EEG seizure pattern which is either focal (usually in the temporal lobe) or secondarily generalised from a focal pacemaker; (b) repetitive episodes of complex symptoms with an EEG seizure pattern of focal origin (usually temporal), with continuous postictal focal or generalised EEG abnormalities between clinical seizures.

Escueta *et al.* (1974) postulated, on the basis of a single patient, that complex partial status comprises two electroclinical phases: (a) a continuous twilight state with reactive automatisms 'in which the lateral temporo-parietal cortex and/or the frontocentral regions of both cerebral hemispheres do not have to be involved continuously', and (b) staring and stereotyped automatisms in which 'the right and left medial anterior temporal lobes are engaged simultaneously'. This was the first 'physiological' definition of status (of any sort), but unfortunately these electrographic patterns are not observed in most patients, and the explanation has proved too simplified. Treiman & Delgado-Escueta (1980, 1983) expanded on this theme, and suggested (probably correctly) that continuous and noncontinuous forms in fact represent a clinical spectrum. They proposed (on the basis of 11 cases) that the essential difference between complex partial status and other forms of twilight state is the *cyclical* nature of clinical behaviour between unresponsive and partially responsive phases in complex partial status. It was suggested that episodes of complex partial status were made up of continuously recurring complex partial seizures, each comprising three phases (stare, stereotyped automatism and reactive automatism; this three-phase explanation of a complex partial seizure was then, but is not now, fashionable). The view that all episodes are thus constituted has not been supported by subsequent clinical observation (either personal or published), at least in most cases, and yet has had a woeful effect on subsequent discussion. Furthermore, even in cases in which cycling is observed, this may be present only for a part of the episode (see for instance the case of Roberts & Humphreys (1988)). The same authors also proposed four criteria for the diagnosis of complex partial status (Treiman & Delgado-Escueta 1983): (a) recurrent complex partial seizures, without full recovery of consciousness between seizures, or a continuous 'epileptic twilight state' with cycling between unresponsive and partially responsive phases; (b) ictal EEG with recurrent epileptiform patterns like those seen in complex partial seizures; (c) prompt observable effects of intravenous antiepileptic drugs on both ictal EEG and clinical manifestations of the status; (d) interictal EEG with a consistent epileptiform focus, usually in one or both temporal lobes. None of these criteria is consistently present in either personally observed or published cases. In 1988, Rohr-Le Floch *et al.* proposed that nonconvulsive status be classified on anatomical not physiological or clinicoelectrographic criteria. They recognised three varieties of nonconvulsive status: petit mal status,

117

psychomotor status and frontal polar status, the latter two sometimes taking the form of simple or complex partial status (table 3.11). This emphasis on the anatomical basis of the seizures, although simplistic, has the advantage of avoiding a mechanistic reliance on seizure type. The importance of the frontal lobe in complex partial epilepsy was further demonstrated by Williamson *et al.* (1985), who described the clinical and intracerebral EEG findings in eight cases of complex partial status, in seven of whom the seizures were found to arise in the frontal cortex. It is also clear that other neocortical sites can be involved. Delgado-Escueta & Treiman (1987) then modified their previous electrographic schemes, perhaps in the face of the evident importance of extratemporal epilepsy, and divided cyclic complex partial status into two further subcategories. The first (psychomotor status of hippocampal, amygdalohippocampal or amygdala origin) is defined as a continuous twilight state with partial responsiveness and reactive automatisms, frequently interrupted by an arrest reaction with staring, total unresponsiveness and stereotyped automatism. During the twilight state, bilateral slow activity is seen diffusely, and during the arrest reaction a mesial seizure discharge occurs. This status tends to develop from serial complex partial mesial temporal seizures, increasing in frequency. The second type of cyclic status epilepticus (entitled secondary involvement of the amygdalohippocampal region by lateral posterior temporal neocortical epilepsy, opercular epilepsy, occipital–hippocampal epilepsy, and frontal epilepsy) has cycling clinical features which, it is postulated, are due to extratemporal seizures spreading to amygdalohippocampal regions. The presence of noncyclic forms is also acknowledged, and thought to be of frontal origin. Whether this categorisation will stand the test of time remains to be seen.

It seems obvious that a more synoptic definition of complex partial status is needed, one less specific physiologically or anatomically, but able to encompass all clinical forms encountered. The following definition is proposed:

> a prolonged epileptic episode in which fluctuating or frequently recurring
> focal electrographic epileptic discharges, arising in temporal or
> extratemporal regions, result in a confusional state with variable clinical
> symptoms.

This definition stresses the importance of anatomical subdivision, avoids specifying EEG detail and emphasises the diversity of clinical features.

Clinical features

At least 150 cases of complex partial status have now been recorded (e.g. Passouant *et al.* 1957, 1967; Goldensohn & Gold 1960; Janz 1960; Bonduelle *et al.* 1964; Dreyer 1965; Dongier 1967; Gastaut *et al.* 1967; Kroth 1967; Rennick, Perez-Borja & Rodin 1969; Wolf 1970; Hess *et al.* 1971; Celesia, Messert & Murphy 1972; Henriksen 1973; Escueta *et al.* 1974; Roger *et al.* 1974; De Pasquet *et al.* 1976; Adebimpe 1977; Kugoh & Hosokawa 1977; Belafsky *et al.* 1978; Engel *et al.* 1978; Grier 1978; Markand, Wheeler & Pollack 1978; Mayeux & Lüders 1978; Fincham *et al.* 1979; Kitagawa *et al.* 1979; Mayeux *et al.* 1979; Behrens 1980; Karbowski 1980; Racy *et al.* 1980; Wieser 1980; Dinner *et al.* 1981;

McBride, Dooling & Oppenheimer 1981; Sacquegna *et al.* 1981; Treiman, Delgado-Escueta & Clark 1981; Bauer, Aichner & Mayr 1982; Aguglia, Tinuper & Farnarier 1983; Ballenger, King & Gallagher 1983; Drake & Coffey 1983; Silverberg Shalev & Amir 1983; Treiman & Delgado-Escueta 1983; Zappoli *et al.* 1983; Aguglia *et al.* 1984; Mikati, Lee & DeLong 1985; Munari *et al.* 1985; Van Rossum, Groeneveld-Ockhuysen & Arts 1985; Willliamson *et al.* 1985; Lim *et al.* 1986; Rosenbaum *et al.* 1986; Tomson, Svanborg & Wedlund 1986; Delgado-Escueta & Treiman 1987; Dunne, Summers & Stewart-Wynne 1987; Kramer *et al.* 1987; Manning & Rosenbloom 1987; Murasaki & Takahashi 1988; Roberts & Humphreys 1988; Rohr-Le-Floch *et al.* 1988; Béquet *et al.* 1990; El-Ad & Neufeld 1990; Varma & Lee 1992). The clinical phenomenology of complex partial status is highly variable, and the manifestations are not simply prolonged or iterated versions of isolated complex partial seizures. This clinical heterogeneity undoubtedly reflects the very varied underlying pathophysiology, the nature of which has been greatly illuminated by recent SEEG work.

PATTERNS: Episodes of complex partial status typically last for a period of hours, although both shorter and much longer examples are encountered (in my own practice are several patients with presumptive histories of months, and one with intractable frontal lobe status lasting continuously, or almost continuously, for 2 years). The condition is unusual in children (McBride *et al.* 1981; Silverberg Shalev & Amir 1983), and most common in early adult life. The youngest reported case is in the first year of life, and the oldest an octogenarian. There is a preponderance of female patients in the published literature, and most but not all cases have a pre-existing history of epilepsy (see Van Rossum *et al.* 1985). Precipitating factors include menstruation, alcohol and drug withdrawal (but not usually photic stimulation or overbreathing as in typical absence status). The onset and offset are usually less well defined than in absence status, and the response to intravenous therapy more gradual. Complex partial status may typically follow a grand mal seizure (or cluster of seizures), but is rarely terminated by a grand mal fit, as is often the case in typical absence status. Complex partial status is usually recurrent, indeed it is rare in my experience for patients to experience single attacks (see figs. 3.14–3.17). Occasionally there may be a remarkable periodicity (see fig. 3.14).

CONFUSION: Confusion is the cardinal clinical feature of complex partial status, and an essential diagnostic feature. The confusional state may fluctuate or be fairly continuous. The alteration in consciousness is generally more severe than that in absence status. Extremes are encountered, varying from profound stupor with little response to external stimuli in some patients (Mikati *et al.* 1985), to occasional patients without overt confusion in whom cognitive testing may show subtle abnormalities (Sacquegna *et al.* 1981). The patient is usually but not always amnesic for the whole episode. Patients with extratemporal status are said to show less alteration of consciousness and amnesia than those with status arising in mesial temporal (limbic) structures, an inviting concept for which there is little convincing supporting evidence.

119

(*a*)

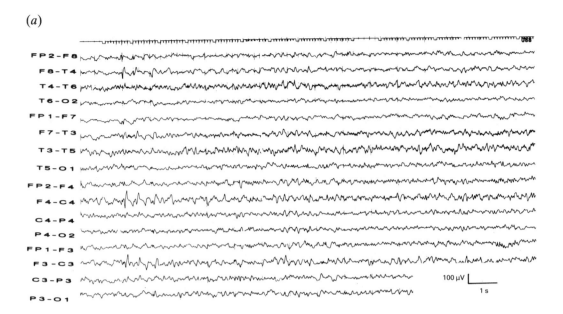

Fig. 3.14. (*a*) Scalp EEG and (*b*) axial proton-density weighted magnetic resonance imaging (MRI) of a 61 year old male with secondarily generalised epilepsy since the age of 14 years, and complex partial seizures since the age of 35 years. From the age of 56, at a frequency which has varied from one attack a week to one a fortnight, he has experienced episodes of complex partial status each lasting 1–2 days. During these episodes he is bedbound, relatively unresponsive, confused, fidgety with a tendency to try to rearrange clothes, able to eat and drink and continent, and does not sleep in the episodes. In between episodes he is quite normal, active and carries out skilled carpentry as a hobby. He is amnesic for the episodes, which have not responded to intensive anticonvulsant therapy. The EEG, recorded during an episode, shows fluctuating sharp and spike–wave activity maximal in the right anterior segment, but seen bilaterally and occurring in short runs, with widespread 2–3 Hz slow activity showing right hemisphere predominance. This activity is eliminated temporarily by 10 mg i.v. midazolam with less clear-cut temporary clinical improvement. The interictal EEG shows infrequent frontotemporal slow activity. Computed tomography was repeatedly normal, but MRI revealed a temporal neocortical mass (arrowed). (With grateful acknowledgement to Drs David Fish and Mark Cook, National Hospital for Neurology and Neurosurgery, for preparing these illustrations.)

MOTOR FEATURES: Alterations in posture, convulsive movements and tonic spasm may all occur intermittently in complex partial status (see fig. 3.15); these are rare in absence status (either typical or atypical). Adversion of the head and eyes is common, and occasionally may persist for hours. The tendency to adversion may

(b)

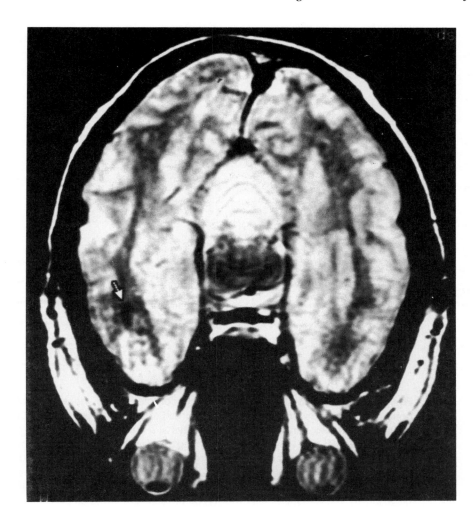

be profound, and some patients walk in circles. Motor features, including adversion, are more common in central or frontal status than in mesial temporal complex partial status. Focal myoclonic jerks are common, but eyelid or bilateral facial myoclonus (if it occurs at all) is much less common than in absence status. Palatal myoclonus has been observed (Emre 1992). Motor automatisms are seldom as dramatic, coordinated or violent as in isolated complex partial seizures. Lip-smacking, orofacial automatism, posturing or gestural automatism are common. Occasionally prolonged ambulatory fugue (poriomania) occurs, the first well-defined example in a case of temporal lobe epilepsy was probably Jackson's, referred to above (p. 116). The distinction between this and psychogenic fugue may be difficult (Mayeux *et al.* 1979), nor it is clear whether poriomania in complex partial status is more or less common than in absence status.

121

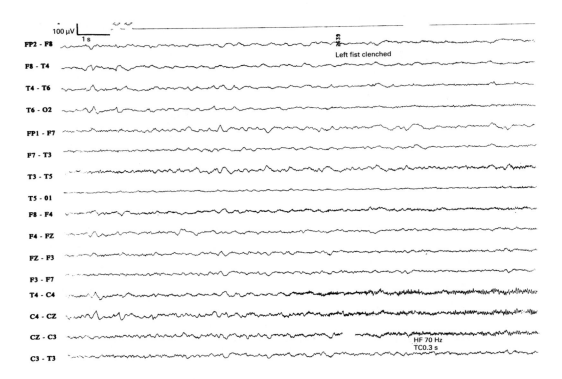

Fig. 3.15. EEG from a 48 year old male with complex partial and secondarily generalised seizures since childhood, with mild retardation. He has a history of attacks of complex partial status, lasting days at a time. During an attack, his left fist clenches, his left arm elevates as if 'pointing', stiffens, flexes and abducts with some clonus of head and left arm. The motor attack lasts 20 seconds, and recurs every 2 minutes or so, for 24–48 hours. During an episode of status epilepticus, in between motor attacks he is drowsy, able to follow simple commands only, and occasionally vocalises. He has other types of recurrent complex partial status comprising confusion and obtundation without focal motor features. Investigation failed to reveal a cause for the status. Magnetic resonance imaging and interictal magnetoencephalography are normal. The EEG during a period of status shows cycling of repeated discrete short-lived ictal episodes, one of which is illustrated here. (With thanks to Dr Shelagh Smith, National Hospital for Neurology and Neurosurgery, for preparing this illustration.)

BEHAVIOURAL AND PSYCHOLOGICAL FEATURES: Behavioural changes range from agitation, excitation or even occasionally mania, through fairly normal motor behaviour to severe psychomotor retardation and stupor. Most commonly, the patient appears alert but rather sluggish, behaves in a restless and apparently questing fashion, and may seem facile or silly. Ideational sluggishness may be evident, with slowness of reactions or gesture, torpor, obtundation, or a true *état crépusculaire*. The patients can usually be guided to sit down or walk about. Aggressive, hostile, negativistic, anxious or irritable behaviour may occur, but less commonly than in the automatisms of isolated complex partial seizures.

Psychotic or autistic symptoms may be prominent, much more so than in typical absence status (although sometimes, differentiating between the two may be difficult, see fig. 3.16). These include inaccessibility, delusions, visual or auditory hallucinations, ideas of reference, paranoia, thought disorder, illogical responses, and often a curious perseverative obsessive insistence on oppositions, such as black/white, good/bad, left/right (see fig. 3.17). Severe catatonia is only occasionally encountered, but mild degrees are quite common. Affective symptoms, typically anxiety but also depression, may be a predominant feature of complex partial status as can be prolonged dreamy states with altered perception of time or space. A psychiatric misdiagnosis is common where psychotic features are prominent and some patients have long histories of repeated psychiatric hospital admissions before the status is recognised. Treatment with antipsychotic drugs may of course make the seizures worse.

In some patients, specific psychological deficits can be detected, such as constructional or spatial apraxias, loss of visual perceptual skills, or even cortical blindness. Simple perceptual alterations such as flashing lights or repetitive noises occasionally occur. Specific cortical deficits are probably commoner in status of parietal–occipital–lateral temporal than frontomesial temporal origin.

SPEECH AND LANGUAGE DISTURBANCE: Even in patients without gross aphasia, speech patterns may be very abnormal, with marked perseveration, confabulation, echolalia, repetitive utterances or stereotyped responses. Characteristically, language may be sparse, and responses to questions, although eventually appropriate, may show a marked delay between question and answer. A motor aphasia, with other psychological functions relatively intact, is a not uncommon feature (De Pasquet *et al.* 1976; Racy *et al.* 1980; Dinner *et al.* 1981; Knight & Cooper 1986; Rosenbaum *et al.* 1986), and frank mutism can also occur (see fig. 3.18). Receptive language problems seem less common. The peculiar susceptibility of language functions to disturbance in status has also been noted in generalised absence status, and in the childhood epilepsy syndromes. Whether or not epileptic discharges 'functionally ablate' specific language areas, or whether the disturbance of speech simply reflects the widespread and complex cortical basis of speech production is not clear. Prolonged affliction of speech can occur after single left temporal complex partial seizures, and it has been suggested that some prolonged postictal 'confusion' is in fact simply dysphasia (Privitera, Morris & Gilliam 1991).

OTHER CLINICAL FEATURES: Autonomic disturbances may occur including belching, borborygmi and flatulence, change in colour, pupillary dilatation, and fever (El-Ad & Neufeld 1990). Sensory symptoms or signs seem less common than psychic or motor signs, but may be encountered.

Sometimes the diagnosis of complex partial status is based on the clinical or

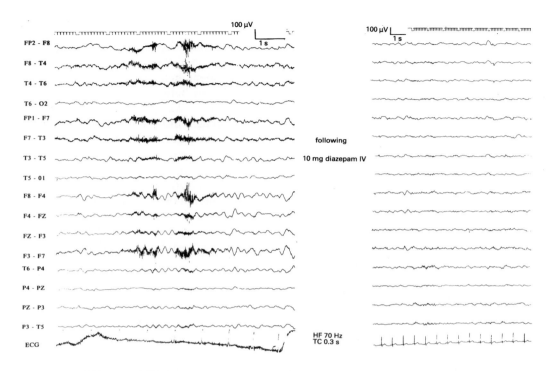

Fig. 3.16. EEG from a 31 year old male with absence, complex partial and secondarily generalised seizures, and morning myoclonus since age 13 years. He is of low average intelligence, but there are no other neurological abnormalities. Interictal EEG shows high voltage 4 Hz generalised polyspike and wave paroxysms, without focal features. Other investigations were normal. For 2 years he experienced episodic psychosis, lasting 4–30 days, during which he experienced hallucinations of hair growing over his body, saw aeroplanes flying over his bed trailing string, believed the voices on the radio were talking about him, and thought that a dragon was blowing wind from his umbilicus. There were no motor features, no retardation, and no change in affect. During the episodes of psychosis, the EEG shows generalised slow wave and at times 3–5 Hz spike and slow wave activity with varying maximal localisation. Diazepam (10 mg) injection resulted in abrupt cessation of the ictal activity. This effect lasts for several minutes and is followed by the recurrence of clusters of polyspike and wave bursts. The injection had no immediate effect on the psychotic delusions. Electroclinical classification of his status is uncertain, and the history has features both of atypical absence and complex partial status. ECG, electrocardiograph. (With thanks to Dr Shelagh Smith, National Hospital for Neurology and Neurosurgery, for preparing the slide.)

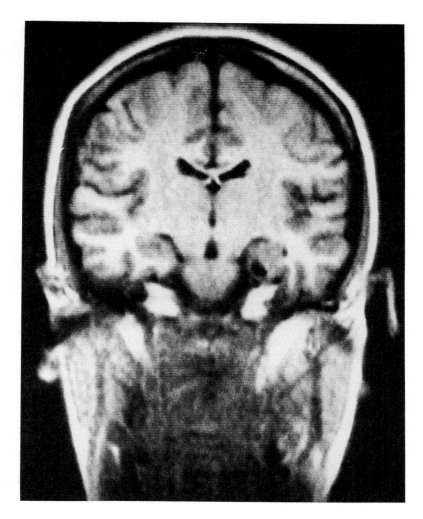

Fig. 3.17. Coronal magnetic resonance imaging (MRI) scan in the temporal region of a 31 year old female of above-average intelligence, with a history of complex partial seizures since age 12 years, and occasional secondarily generalised seizures since age 17. From age 26, generalised seizures were followed by periods of 1–4 days during which she was agitated, panicky, somewhat disinhibited, and experienced auditory hallucinations. During these episodes, she was preoccupied with thoughts that she had multiple sclerosis or was having a heart attack, concerned with physical and philosophical oppositions (black/white, good/bad, etc.), and exhibited pressure of speech. EEG during the attack showed widespread slow activity at 2–4 Hz over both hemispheres, which cleared on diazepam injection and showed clinical improvement. Computed tomography was normal. The MRI shows a small left temporal lobe mass, removed at temporal lobectomy with resolution of the psychotic periods (but still occasional complex partial seizures).

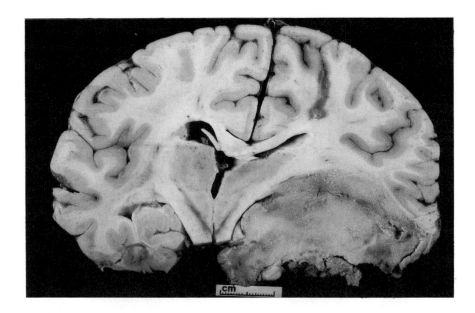

Fig. 3.18. Pathological specimen from a 34 year old right-handed male with complex partial and secondarily generalised seizures since the age of 3 years, and low average intelligence. From the age of 30, he experienced recurrent episodes of complex partial status, characterised by motor retardation and profound mutism. He was able to walk hesitantly but unaided, his eyes were open, there was a coarse tremor of the left hand, a tendency to drool, and he showed slow responses to questions (but after prolonged delay, often an appropriate and correct reply). The episodes lasted days at a time, and recurred every few months. A temporal lobe glioma was diagnosed by magnetic resonance imaging, and confirmed by brain biopsy at age 32. There was a rapid neurological deterioration in the last 6 months of life, and he died aged 34. The figure shows an extensive malignant glioma infiltrating the region of the right temporal lobe. (With thanks to Dr Alsanjari, National Hospital for Neurology and Neurosurgery, for preparing this illustration.)

EEG response to the acute administration of intravenous benzodiazepine. Whilst there is no doubt that this manoeuvre improves the EEG and clinical signs in status, the response is relatively nonspecific, and similar changes occur in a wide variety of degenerative cerebral conditions (a recent example in my own practice was in Jakob–Creutzfeldt disease), psychiatric states, and other epileptic and nonepileptic neurological conditions. It is an unreliable diagnostic feature in this situation, as indeed it is in nonacute epileptic states.

FLUCTUATION AND CYCLING OF SIGNS: The distinction between continuous and discontinuous forms of status was made in the earliest descriptions. In some cases, the confusional state and other signs are continuous or virtually continuous over long periods of time and, in others, fluctuations or cycling of signs are a prominent feature. The recognition that a discontinuous form can be due to rapidly repeated discrete complex partial seizures has certainly clarified the clinical picture in some patients in whom separate seizures are discernible within the confusional state. These may be clear cut and facilitate diagnosis, although it is rare for the automatisms or motor activity to be as marked in status as in individual seizures. In some cases, individual seizures are subtle in form and difficult to detect, manifest only by brief motor automatisms, intermittent pallor or changes in colour, pupillary dilatation, myoclonus, or sometimes nothing more than the cessation of ongoing activity. Treiman & Delgado-Escueta (1983) suggested that cycling between unresponsive and partially responsive phases is an essential diagnostic feature, but in practice clear-cut cycling is not clinically observable in all cases (see figs. 3.14, 3.16 and 3.18). Furthermore, cycling of signs can occur in atypical absence status (Tomson *et al.* 1986). It is therefore not a reliable diagnostic sign, nor does it reliably indicate a temporal as opposed to a frontal focus.

Electroencephalography

Ballenger *et al.* (1983) could find only 17 case reports of complex partial status in which EEG findings were documented. Since then there have been further detailed studies and from these and personal cases, it is apparent that complex partial status has widely varying scalp EEG patterns. Indeed, scalp EEG findings may be very disappointing. Although seldom normal, the interictal and ictal recordings in complex partial status are often very similar, and a whole range of EEG patterns are seen. Different ictal patterns include continuous or frequent spike or spike–slow wave, or spike–wave paroxysms which can be widespread or focal, and also episodes of desynchronisation. Treiman & Delgado-Escueta (1983) contend that the EEG changes are more specific, at least in patients with cycling clinical activity, comprising bimedial temporal or lateralised temporal 8–20 Hz spikes alternating with one of three patterns: low voltage fast activity with bursts of diffuse slow activity, or rhythmical bilateral diffuse spikes or slow waves, or anterior temporal spikes on a normal background. It is claimed that the specific EEG pattern is determined by the frequency in which individual cycles occur. The cases reported by Heintel (1969) and Ballenger *et al.* (1983) more or less conform to this submission; nevertheless, intermediate or transitional cases are just as common, as are cases without any of these electrographic features. Tomson *et al.* (1986) reported cases without clinical or EEG cycling, and also EEG cycling in some cases of atypical absence status. The longer the status proceeds, the less likely discrete ictal activity is to be noticeable (see for instance the case of Roberts & Humphreys (1988)). The focal abnormalities can be maximal in temporal or extratemporal sites. Engel *et al.* (1978) describe a case of parietotemporal complex partial status in which fluctuating focal EEG patterns cycled from one hemisphere to the other, independent of clinical changes.

SEEG has been much more informative than scalp EEG in the understanding of the physiology of complex partial status. The first SEEG case reported was by

Wieser (1980), in which EEG and clinical phenomena were meticulously correlated. It was noticeable in this case that the scalp EEG was 'uncharacteristic',
although at times desynchronisation was noted. In contrast, the depth EEG
showed impressive changes. Frequent focal seizures within the right hippocampal
formation were first seen, later to be replaced by continuous increasingly monotonous discharges. Spread of the discharges to lateral temporal neocortex was
associated with dream-like states, that to Herschl's gyrus with musical hallucinations, and that bitemporally with severe alteration in consciousness. Wieser (1980)
suggested that the continuous phase might be the equivalent of a prolonged afterdischarge. Wieser *et al.* (1985) have subsequently reported three further SEEG
cases in unilateral limbic status. Williamson *et al.* (1985) then reported EEG
findings in eight intensively studied patients. During the status epilepticus, discrete
seizure discharges were seen on the scalp EEG in only one case and in the others
diffuse slow activity was seen (without the sequence of changes stressed by
Treiman & Delgado-Escueta (1983)). The SEEG, however, showed recurrent
seizure activity in all patients. Ictal EEG discharges were often preceded by diffuse
or localised high amplitude sharp and/or slow complexes with disorganised slow
activity between seizures. A focal frontal onset was firmly estalished in four cases,
and was felt probable in one other. The onset typically varied within a wide area
of frontal cortex, and appeared diffusely in two cases. The EEG seizure frequency,
duration, intensity and spread diminished as episodes of complex partial status
progressed, and seizures which were initially poorly localised became more localised. Recurrent seizure activity at the end of some episodes simply showed EEG
desynchronisation or flattening. Delgado-Escueta & Treiman (1987) published
three further cases each demonstrating cycling, with EEG findings essentially
similar to the individual complex partial seizures.

All cases of complex partial status recorded with SEEG have shown a mixture
of discrete and continuous focal ictal activity. EEG activity fluctuates over time,
and the poor correlation of scalp and depth EEG is striking. Both discontinous
and continuous behavioural changes can be associated with frequent ictal events
recorded by depth studies. In three of the eight cases of Williamson *et al.* (1985),
subtle behavioural changes only could be detected each time an EEG seizure
discharge occurred (e.g. changes in pupillary size, stare, squirming or changing
position); in one patient no behavioural change was noticeable even on meticulous
scrutiny, despite electrical seizures each lasting 30–45 seconds, occurring every
minute or so.

Anatomical site

Until relatively recently, it was assumed that almost all cases of complex partial
status were temporal lobe in origin; indeed, the terms temporal lobe and complex
partial status were used synonymously in early case reports. Whilst there is no
doubt that patients with temporal lobe epilepsy may develop complex partial status,
a proportion – perhaps even the majority – of cases are extratemporal in origin.
Williamson *et al.* (1985) reported 8 patients with complex partial status, investigated with SEEG (the 8 were from 87 patients with complex partial seizures, of

whom 60 had temporal and 27 extratemporal epilepsy). Seizures arose extratemporally in all 8 patients, and the authors concluded that temporal lobe complex partial status is rare. Similarly, in a series from Zurich of 25 patients with frontal lobe epilepsy examined by SEEG, all had a history of episodic complex partial status (Wieser *et al.* 1992). I have observed cases of complex partial status with temporal, frontal, parietal and occipital foci, and many of the cases reported since 1985 have had extratemporal foci (e.g. Tomson *et al.* 1986; Murasaki & Takahashi 1988; Fujiwara *et al.* 1991). It is a clinical impression that there is a higher than expected incidence of parieto-occipital as well as frontal cases.

Three-hertz spike—wave discharges, indistinguishable from petit mal, are a relatively common finding in frontal lobe epilepsy, and some reported cases of 'petit mal status' may in fact be frontal complex partial seizures. This is particularly likely in atypical cases, or where a syndromic diagnosis of primary generalised epilepsy cannot be made. This diagnostic trap may account for some of the earlier nosological confusion evident in the literature. New MRI techniques demonstrate focal abnormalities in a high proportion of frontal lobe epilepsies, and it is to be hoped that the application of imaging to these cases will elucidate underlying mechanisms in a way that EEG can not.

Causes

Remarkably, aetiology is often ignored in published reports (especially earlier accounts), which have concentrated upon EEG patterns and clinical phenomenology. The impression that complex partial status usually occurs in cryptogenic epilepsy is probably false, and certainly in my practice a high incidence of focal cerebral abnormalities is encountered. The spectrum of reported causes are similar in range to those seen in focal epilepsy in general, and although there is inadequate documentation in published cases there is no conclusive evidence to suggest that status has a different causal emphasis. Published aetiologies include trauma, tumour, cerebrovascular disease, haematoma, infections, atrophy, dysplasia, infantile hemiplegia, perinatal injury, mental retardation, alcohol and metabolic disturbances (Gall, Scollo-Lavizzari & Becker 1978; Markand *et al.* 1978; Ballenger *et al.* 1983; Silverberg Shalev & Amir 1983; Zappoli *et al.* 1983; Van Rossum *et al.* 1985; Williamson *et al.* 1985; Tomson *et al.* 1986; Murasaki & Takahashi 1988; Roberts & Humphreys 1988; Rohr-Le Floch *et al.* 1988; Takeda 1988; Fujiwara *et al.* 1991). In patients with epileptic confusional states due to acute precipitants, it is often not possible to decide whether this is due to complex partial or late onset absence status (e.g. cases of Callahan & Noetzel 1992; Gilliam, Simonian & Chiappa (1992).

A small number of pathological reports from patients with complex partial status are reported, but series giving surgical pathology will inevitably be biased towards structural lesions. Transient focal abnormalities suggestive of oedema and hypervascularisation have been reported with CT, MRI and SPECT during focal status (Kramer *et al.* 1987; Bauer *et al.* 1989; Fujiwara *et al.* 1991), and I have observed similar findings after prolonged focal seizures. One case of apparently generalised absence status has also been reported with transient mesial frontal and anterior temporal MRI changes (Callahan & Noetzel 1992). Neither CT nor MRI changes (particularly the latter) should therefore be assumed invariably to indicate the presence of a permanent structual lesion.

The treatment and prognosis of complex partial status are described on pp. 291–2 and 311.

Boundary conditions

The definition of status epilepticus arrived at in chapter 2 permits the inclusion not only of the conventionally accepted syndromes of status described above, but also other fascinating yet ill-understood conditions; these can be termed boundary syndromes. A debate about classification is fruitless (epilepsy has had far too many such debates), but brief consideration of the boundary symptoms might stimulate thought about the nature of epilepsy and of status. The conditions are overlapping, and distinctions between them (or indeed the more conventional syndromes of nonconvulsive status) are somewhat arbitrary.

Electrographic status epilepticus with subtle clinical signs

Seemingly subclinical electrographic status may happen in both partial and generalised epilepsies. In patients with complex partial epilepsy, EEG (usually depth EEG) recordings not uncommonly show continuous or frequent seizure discharges, occurring at times when consciousness is normal and there is no confusion. Changes in affect may be observed during the discharges, especially anxiety or tension, obsessional neurotic thoughts, or fragmentary somatic symptoms such as vertigo, epigastric sensations, nausea and headache. Subtle psychometric changes can occur, and sometimes no symptoms at all can be elicited. The contrast between the severity of the electrographic status and the absence of clinical symptoms is intriguing. The clinical distinction between complex partial status, simple partial status and these 'subclinical' attacks may be only one of degree. A parallel spectrum of EEG also seems to exist from, at one extreme, continuous focal spike–wave paroxysms to, at the other, only occasional spikes. At what point these can be defined as 'seizures' or even 'status' is quite unclear. Generalised epileptic discharges without clinical signs or with slight disturbance again are not uncommon. Gökyiğit *et al.* (1986) presented a well-documented case of electrographic status that had lasted 17 months without clinical or psychiatric disturbance. This followed an episode of mumps in which a single overt seizure had occurred. The EEGs showed continuous bilaterally synchronised and symmetrical 2.5–3.5 Hz spike–wave, suppressed by eye opening. The pattern persisted during daytime sleep. Similarly, patients with the Lennox–Gastaut syndrome commonly have electrographic slow spike–wave without overt seizures (see p. 105); whether these patterns should be considered as 'seizures' (and thus status) or simply a nonepileptic response of damaged cerebral tissue is contentious. This is a taxonomic jungle.

Prolonged postictal confusional states

Prolonged confusion, bizarre behaviours and amnesia are not uncommon following discrete epileptic seizures. These symptoms can resemble complex partial status, and it is possible that many such 'postictal' events are physiologically identical with nonconvulsive status. A diagnosis of complex partial or generalised absence status is straightforward, when the EEG shows continuing or repetitive ictal bursts, as shown in the case illustrated in fig. 3.19, the eight cases reported by Fagan & Lee (1990), and in the ten patients of Bauer *et al.* (1982). Typically these prolonged confusional states follow a tonic–clonic seizure (or a cluster of seizures). The confusional state lasted 8–36 hours amongst the eight patients recorded by Fagan & Lee (1990), there were various motor signs and psychotic features, and consciousness was usually impaired. The EEG showed a spectrum of epileptic patterns.

When focal or secondarily generalised paroxystic EEG discharges occur, diagnosis is straightforward. The now commonplace demonstration that seizures recorded by SEEG (including prolonged or frequent seizures) can occur without scalp EEG correlates, however, widens the scope of the argument. It is probable that many more 'postictal' confusional states, with unremarkable scalp EEG or with diffuse slow activity, are due to underlying focal status, though to what extent is quite unknown. The cases reported by Levin (1952) from a psychiatric institution may have such occult status, and one encounters large numbers of patients with prolonged confusional states after seizures with nonspecific EEG changes; how many such cases might in fact be due to nonconvulsive status is unknown (the patient whose EEG is illustrated in fig. 3.20 is a particularly striking, but by no means unique, example of this diagnostic conundrum). Similar clinical states occur in other epileptic situations (e.g. after tonic status epilepticus; Somerville & Bruni 1983). This of course is not simply of nosological significance, but may have therapeutic or prognostic implications also. This is a fascinating and ill-understood boundary of status, which is surely to be greatly clarified by the application of modern imaging and electrophysiological methods.

Epileptic behavioural disturbances and psychosis

Perhaps even more intriguing is the possibility that some abnormal mental states in epilepsy are due to prolonged nonconvulsive seizure activity.

The most extreme and best-studied epileptic behavioural disturbance is psychosis. Epileptic psychosis can be divided broadly into postictal and interictal categories, each with distinctive features (see Trimble 1991). The ictal psychosis in complex partial and absence status is described earlier (and see fig. 3.16). Both patterns of psychosis are characterised by delusions often of a paranoid kind, visual and auditory hallucinations, and mood disturbances. Other psychotic features include paranoid ideation, ideas of influence, thought disorder, a preoccupation with religious or mystical thoughts, feelings of passivity and catatonic states. The postictal psychosis is usually associated with delirium, altered consciousness and amnesia, and the interictal psychosis with clear consciousness, retained memory and less severe behavioural disturbances.

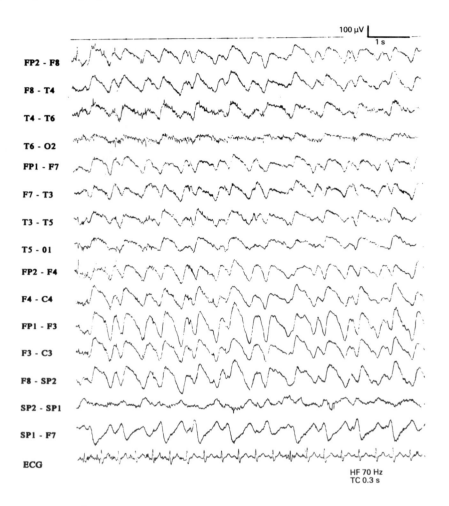

Fig. 3.19. EEG during a period of prolonged postictal confusion in a 41 year old female with a history of tonic–clonic seizures from age 12 years, of unknown aetiology. The epilepsy was initially mild. The seizures worsened at age 36, with each convulsion being followed by a phase lasting up to 3 hours of prolonged postictal confusion during which she is agitated, irritable, complains of headache, and is unable to concentrate. The EEG during this postictal confusional state shows recurring generalised epileptic bursts, without a clear focus, taking the form of nonconvulsive status. (With thanks to Dr Shelagh Smith, National Hospital for Neurology and Neurosurgery, for preparing this illustration.)

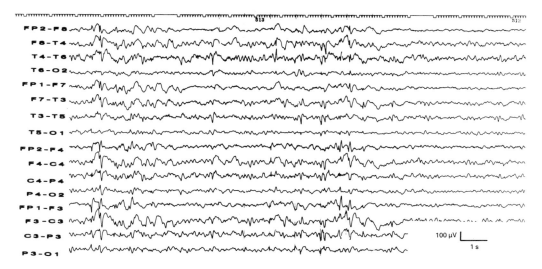

Fig. 3.20. Scalp EEG from a 42 year old male with a history of secondarily generalised seizures, intellectual dulling (full scale IQ 61), and intermittent psychotic episodes since age 10 years, with no obvious cause. At age 23, bilateral Field of Forel stereotactic lesions were made in an unsuccessful attempt to control his seizures. He continued to have frequent and severe seizures over the years. At the age of 42, he developed tonic–clonic status epilepticus, lasting about 12 hours. Following this, he developed an encephalopathy comprising a state of profound mutism and motor retardation. During this period, he lay stuporous, without any movement of the limbs even on stimulation, made no attempts at communication nor displayed any evidence of awareness. This state persisted for several days, to be followed by fluctuating awareness and variable paralysis with slow improvement over 2 weeks to normal. During this time, tube feeding was necessary, and he was incontinent. The EEG during this period showed frequent spike activity with marked background slowing, without focal features (this EEG is an example, taken 1 week after the onset of the encephalopathy). The spiking and the slow activity were loosely correlated with his fluctuating neurological deficit. Other intensive investigation, including examination of the cerebrospinal fluid, magnetic resonance imaging of the head and spine, and biochemical and pharmacological screening failed to demonstrate any other abnormality. This encephalopathy was attributed to persisting 'subclinical' epileptic activity, an extreme example of ictally driven 'postictal' confusion. (With thanks to Dr David Fish, National Hospital for Neurology and Neurosurgery, for preparing this illustration.)

In many apparently postictal psychotic states, repetitive EEG abnormalities can be recorded on scalp and depth EEG, and there is little doubt that some cases, at least, are due to nonconvulsive status (resembling the ictal psychosis of complex partial status, see fig. 3.17); these merge clinically with cases of prolonged postictal confusion on the one hand and functional psychosis on the other; where a semantic

133

line should be drawn is unclear. The response to anticonvulsant (especially benzo-diazepine) therapy and the self-limiting course provide some support for the contention that the psychoses are ictally driven, as does the observation that postictal psychosis typically happens after severe seizures or clusters of seizures, and may recur periodically. Some postictal psychosis occurs with normal scalp EEG, often more normal than either the ictal or the asymptomatic interictal record. See Trimble (1991) for a discussion of the concept of this *forced normalisation*. It seems possible at least that limbic ictal activity is continuing during this phase, but evidence is lacking. The temporal relationship of psychosis and overt seizures often becomes less clear cut as time passes, and the episodic postictal psychoses begin to merge with interictal psychotic behaviour. The interictal psychosis in epilepsy tends to be chronic and persisting; in its fully developed form it is unaffected by the occurrence of overt seizures.

The scalp EEG in cases of interictal psychosis often shows nonspecific changes. Depth EEG (SEEG) recording from mesial temporal and limbic structures has been more informative, albeit in small numbers of highly selected patients. Intense hippocampal or amygdaloid epileptic activity can occur without any disturbance of the scalp EEG; this is a frequent observation in patients with partial seizures undergoing pre-surgical evaluation. It is a small conceptual step to attribute other epileptic behavioural phenomenon to ongoing ictal activity. Although human SEEG studies are limited, their results are intriguing and challenge our concepts of behavioural disturbance in epilepsy. The first (and controversial) use of SEEG to study human behavioural changes was in prisoners suffering from mental illnesses and sometimes overt epilepsy. Psychotic behaviour was consistently correlated with spike–wave activity in the rostral septal region and amygdala, without obvious changes on scalp EEG. Control epileptic patients without psychosis showed no such rostral septal spiking (see review by Heath 1986). Wieser *et al.* (1985) described four cases with unilateral limbic status undergoing bitemporal depth recording. During episodes of unilateral status, prolonged pleomorphic psychological symptoms were experienced including headache, behavioural disturbances with episodic aggressivity, stickiness, sexual exhibitionism and disinhibition. During the periods of status, although confusion was absent clinically, tachistoscopic psychometric testing showed impaired cognitive performance only in tests presented to the affected side (indeed tests presented to the unaffected side were sometimes better performed during episodes of contralateral status). Both the postical and interictal psychotic disorders are more common in patients with severe uncontrolled epilepsy, in partial seizures and cerebral damage.

It is difficult to escape the conclusion that at least some of the interictal psychotic behaviour in patients with epilepsy is driven by limbic status epilepticus. This is of course a controversial area, and the deterministic flavour of this evidence has philosophical as well as physiological implications that cannot be addressed here. How far one can extrapolate from the very small number of highly selected reported cases studied with SEEG is quite unclear. Nevertheless, there is indisputable evidence that prolonged EEG discharges, characteristic of status, in hippocampal and amygdaloid regions can be associated with behavioural abnormalities.

These can occur without scalp EEG changes, and to what extent the generality of interictal behaviour is due to such 'subclinical status' in deep structures is quite unknown. Clearly, though, a re-evaluation is due of all neurophysiological research on persisting psychotic and behavioural changes. Noninvasive and structural functional imaging may throw light on this murky subject.

Status epilepticus confined to adult life

De novo absence status epilepticus of late onset

A curious feature of absence status is its onset in adult, especially late adult, life. In some patients, this is typical absence status occurring in patients with pre-existing primary generalised epilepsy (e.g. cases of Niedermeyer & Khalifeh 1965; Lob *et al.* 1967; Thompson & Greenhouse 1968; Böhm 1969; Andermann & Robb 1972; Heathfield 1972; Roger *et al.* 1974; Gall *et al.* 1978; Nightingale & Welch 1982). In a series of 18 adults with absence status (20% of all cases of status in adults) admitted to a general hospital over a 28 month period, 10 had primary generalised epilepsy (Dunne *et al.* 1987). The status developed between the ages of 18 and 81, and 5 patients were over 50. A remarkable feature is that the epilepsy has often been in long remission prior to onset of status (Niedermeyer & Khalifeh 1965; Lob *et al.* 1967; Andermann & Robb 1972; Gall *et al.* 1978; Nightingale & Welch 1982). Seizure-free intervals of between 2 and 40 years in 4 of the 10 patients were reported by Dunne *et al.* (1987). Quite why status suddenly recurs after long seizure-free periods is not known, and in only a minority of patients are precipitating factors obvious. Myoclonic or clonic movements of the face, eye or jaw are usual, and simple or complex automatisms may occur. Tonic–clonic seizures are also common, often initiating a period of status. The onset is usually acute, and the duration of status varies from hours to days.

In the majority of reported cases there is no past history of epilepsy (over 80 in the published literature: Goldie & Green 1961; Lob *et al.* 1967; Amand 1971; Schwartz & Scott 1971; Wells 1975; Vignaendra, Loh & Lim 1976; Ellis & Lee 1978; Terzano, Gemignani & Mancia 1978; Richard & Brenner 1980; Weiner *et al.* 1980*b*; Goldmann, Glastein & Adams 1981; Rumpl & Hinterhuber 1981; Vercelletto & Gastaut 1981; Berkovic & Bladin 1982; Bateman *et al.* 1983; Pritchard & O'Neal 1984; Lee 1985; Van Sweden 1985; Bourrat *et al.* 1986; Guberman *et al.* 1986; Dunne *et al.* 1987; Van Sweden & Mellerio 1988; Hersch & Billings 1988; Thomas *et al.* 1992). The EEG changes, although showing spike–wave activity, are atypical, and the clinical precipitation, the course, the response to treatment and the prognosis differ from typical absence status. In a review of 64 such cases from the literature (Thomas *et al.* 1992), 66% were female, with a mean age of 62 years (range 42–88). This form of late-onset absence status presents, like ordinary absence status, as an acute confusional state, with variable alteration of consciousness ranging from profound stupor with catatonia and loss of sphincteric control at one extreme, through mental dullness and abulia, to mild

135

motor retardation and specific intellect disturbances (e.g. apraxia, amnesia) at the other. Amnesia may be total, patchy or occasionally inapparent. Moderate confusion is usual, with the ability to obey simple commands but not to follow complex or sequential tasks. Psychometric assessments during absence status have shown good retention of language function in some patients, in the presence of other widespread psychological deficit (Guberman *et al.* 1986). Changes in affect are common, including irritability, euphoria, agitation or depression. Motor retardation or perseveration are common, the gait is often pseudoataxic and slow, and other motor features include myoclonic jerking, posturing, repetitive movements and automatisms. Catatonia may be a prominent feature (Lim *et al.* 1986) as may myoclonus (Terzano *et al.* 1978). Verbal responses are frequently slow and delayed, speech is monosyllabic, monotonous and dysprosodic. Although the condition fluctuates, there is usually no cycling of signs as in complex partial status. Generalised tonic–clonic seizures are reported in about 50% of cases, but not initiating nor terminating the status, as in typical absence status. Psychotic features with paranoid ideation, hallucinations, and delusion may occur, also bizarre or inappropriate behaviour (Ivanainen *et al.* 1984). Almost invariably, a primary psychiatric misdiagnosis is made. The EEG confirms the organic nature of the confusional state, and is usually diagnostic, showing continuous or frequent spike–wave activity at frequencies of between 1 and 4 Hz, sometimes irregular, and usually diffuse or generalised. Other EEG patterns described include bursts of spikes, triphasic waves, and irregular slow activity; but how such cases should be classified is a conundrum. EEG cycling does not usually occur.

In a remarkably high proportion of patients precipitating factors can be identified. Benzodiazepine (or other drug or alcohol) withdrawal is the commonest cause, and identifed in 16 of 29 cases in three series (Dunne *et al.* 1987; Van Sweden & Mellerio 1988; Thomas *et al.* 1992). As there is a high incidence of pre-exisiting psychiatric disorder in adult-onset nonconvulsive status, psychotropic drug withdrawal may have passed unrecognised in other reported cases. Nonconvulsive status of the absence type (and other prolonged epileptic states) may be precipitated by electro-convulsive therapy (Weiner *et al.* 1980*a,b*; Varma & Lee 1992), by metrizamide myelography (a particularly common cause; Pritchard & O'Neal 1984; Vollmer *et al.* 1985), cerebral angiography, lithium therapy, acute metabolic disturbances, toxic or other pharmacological agents (Schwartz & Scott 1971; Vignaendra *et al.* 1976; Ellis & Lee 1977; Beaumanoir, Jenny & Jekiel 1980; Richard & Brenner 1980; Rumpl & Hinterhuber 1981; Lee 1985; Van Sweden 1985; Bourrat *et al.* 1986; Dunne *et al.* 1987; Hersch & Billings 1988; Gilliam *et al.* 1992; Thomas *et al.* 1992). Such status often occurs in the context of other medical or surgical disturbances; sometimes several potential precipitating causes exist. The rapid response of the clinical condition to intravenous diazepam has been universally reported, and the EEG changes are immediately reversed.

The nosological position of such cases is (like that of other nonconvulsive status syndromes) controversial, but a relatively homogeneous and distinctive core syndrome exists. It would seem reasonable to distinguish these cases from primary generalised absence status (typical absence status), other forms of secondarily generalised epileptic encephalopathies (e.g. Lennox–Gastaut), or complex partial status. In view of the fact that the condition is often precipitated by drug withdrawal, metabolic or toxic factors, Thomas *et al.* (1992) suggested the designation 'situational related nonconvulsive generalised status epilepticus', and included these cases amongst the category of 'Special Syndromes – situation-related seizures' in the 1985 ILAE *Classification of the epilepsies and epileptic syndromes*.

The treatment and prognosis of the *de novo* absence status of late onset are described on pp. 290 and 311–12.

Pseudostatus epilepticus

Of all the curiosities of medicine, pseudostatus must be one of the most bizarre. If status epilepticus is the *maximum expression* of epilepsy, pseudostatus is its psychogenic equivalent, and is indubitably an extreme form of aberrant human behaviour.

The term refers to repeated or continuous seizures which are psychogenic in origin, and which resemble (at least superficially) convulsive status epilepticus (Toone & Roberts 1979; Howell, Owen & Chadwick 1989; Shorvon 1989). To the experienced observer, the 'seizures' are not convincing, and differentiation from true status is usually easy. The motor movements do not have the classic features of convulsive seizures, but fluctuate in intensity, frequency or distribution as the status proceeds, often influenced by emotional external factors. Vocalisation is common, as is bizarre behaviour, explosive emotional expression, and resistance to examination. Preservation of consciousness can often be deduced in spite of the continuing convulsions. Incontinence, tongue biting and cyanosis do occur but are less common than in true status. Opisthotonus was first depicted by Charcot, and is a dramatic motor manifestation, sometimes accompanying flapping and twisting of the limbs (Bateman 1989). The previous medical history is important in diagnosis. Inquiry usually reveals a long history of psychiatric or personality disorder, often with hysterical features, and previous episodes of pseudostatus. The epilepsy history is usually atypical, showing an odd pattern of seizures over time, an inconsistent response to treatment and repeatedly normal EEG. The more dramatic the presentation of status, the more likely is it pseudostatus (a recent patient of mine was flown in by helicopter, so dire appeared her predicament, from a distant hospital). EEG during the episode will definitively confirm or refute the diagnosis, if there is clinical doubt.

The frequency of pseudostatus is unclear. Amongst 110 of my patients with pseudoseizures diagnosed on videotelemetry, 7.5% had recorded attacks lasting longer than 30 minutes (Meierkord *et al.* 1991), and many more a history of prolonged attacks . In my neurological practice, full-blown convulsive pseudostatus is more frequently encountered than true status; and this is probably common experience (Howell *et al.* 1989). The condition is, however, insufficiently

137

recognised in routine hospital practice, and for instance about 80% of all emergency out-of-hours EEG requests for new status at the National Hospital reveal pseudostatus (D. Fish, personal communication). The danger of the condition is that misdiagnosis results in mistreatment. A disastrous therapeutic cycle is all too commonly embarked upon. Status epilepticus is misdiagnosed, and intravenous anticonvulsants are given. Seizures persist, and more drugs are administered to the point of unconsciousness. These have a temporary effect but as consciousness is regained, seizures recur, and more intravenous anticonvulsants are given, often including intravenous anaesthetics, and full ITU care and assisted ventilation are then required. Seizures recur whenever the patient recovers consciousness, and further treatment is given, and the cycle can persist even to the stage of tracheostomy.

This is all the more unfortunate, as once the true diagnosis is made, treatment is straightforward. All anticonvulsant and sedative therapy should be withdrawn immediately, and sympathetic but firm verbal encouragement given. This will rapidly terminate the episode. Diagnosis may be complicated in a minority of patients who suffer from both seizures and pseudoseizures, and occasionally a period of pseudostatus can be preceded by a genuine tonic–clonic seizure.

Patients will often have a history of previous status-like episodes, and one reported case had had 80 emergency admissions to 9 different hospitals in 3 health regions; 21 episodes were diagnosed and treated as status, and she was admitted to intensive care on 5 occasions (Howell *et al.* 1989). A recent patient of mine, with a history of over 40 previous episodes, was treated and returned to the referring district by train, only to gain admission with recurring pseudostatus to another hospital at the first intermediate station.

The psychological mechanisms, in many cases, are obscure. A few patients malinger, some have a psychopathic disposition, some a history of sexual abuse, but most have no formal psychiatric diagnosis other than personality disorder. In some the seizures seem to occur simply in the context of unhappiness or loneliness. The behaviour is potentially dangerous, as the large doses of sedative drugs given carry a high risk of iatrogenic morbidity and mortality. Long-term treatment should attempt to prevent repeated episodes of this hazardous maladaptive behaviour. Recidivism is more common if there is a lack of family support, in chronic cases, and in the absence of a clear psychogenic mechanism (Meierkord *et al.* 1991; Pakalnis, Drake & Phillips 1991).

CHAPTER 4

Neurophysiology, neuropathology and neurochemistry of status epilepticus

Scientific investigation of the mechanisms of status focused upon first neuropathology, then electroencephalography and neurophysiology, and in the past two decades also neurochemistry and neuropharmacology. In the future, molecular genetic studies in epilepsy seem likely to flourish, although as yet these are scarcely begun. In this chapter, I consider the basic human and experimental research concerned with status in the fields of neurophysiology, neuropathology and neurochemistry in an attempt to provide a synthesis and overview of current ideas.

Although Bourneville had described Ammon's horn sclerosis in 1876, Pfleger (1880) is generally credited with the earliest detailed pathological study of a patient dying in status. He identified abnormalities, especially in the hippocampus, which have been confirmed many times since. The lesions, both macroscopic and microscopic, were patently slight, and contemporary thought was summed up by Gowers (1888) in his usual prescient manner: 'the changes in the nerve centres are probably of that fine kind which is revealed only by altered function and eludes the most minute research'. Pathology has made erratic progress since Pfleger's early report, as is reviewed later in this chapter, but Gower's statement still applies largely today. The contrast between the spectacular clinical appearances of status and the minor findings of morbid anatomy is quite disconcerting. With the introduction of EEG as a method of measuring altered function, the direction of basic research in epilepsy altered, and structural and histological inquiry diminished. The new electrographic studies concentrated mainly upon the physiological mechanisms of epilepsy, both at a cellular and a systems level, and status, viewed merely as iterative seizures of little instrinsic interest, was largely neglected. In the past two decades, though, neurochemical research (Gower's 'most minute' level?) has again focused on status, using newly developed animal models of epilepsy. This has, in turn, stimulated new types of neurophysiological and pathological study, and essential differences between isolated seizures and status in neurochemical, physiological and pathological terms have been recognised. The work on status has addressed two particular questions:

1. What are the mechanisms of status as distinct from those underlying normal epilepsy?
2. What are the features and mechanisms of the cerebral damage caused by status?

In this chapter, both questions are reviewed. I consider the experimental neurophysiological, pathological and neurochemical investigations of tonic–clonic and partial status. What little work there is on other clinical forms of status is discussed in the relevant sections of chapter 3. I confine this review where possible to specific studies of status rather than of the larger topic of epilepsy, and emphasise aspects which concern status specifically. A critical difference between status and epilepsy, of course, lies in the dimension of time, and many of the physiological and chemical mechanisms of status and pathological changes evolve as the duration of seizure activity lengthens.

Experimental neurophysiology of status epilepticus

This is not the place to describe the basic neurophysiology of epilepsy or of the epileptic discharge. This vast topic is beyond the scope of this book, and is reviewed excellently elsewhere (see, for instance, the following recent reviews: Jasper & van Gelder 1983; Schwartzkroin & Wheal 1984; Prince 1985; Delgado-Escueta *et al.* 1986*a,b*; Heinemann 1987; Jefferys & Roberts 1987; Meldrum, Ferendelli & Wieser 1988; Heinemann & Jones 1990; Jefferys 1990, 1993). Since the advent of EEG, an understanding has been gathered of such topics as the cellular events associated with epilepsy, the mechanisms of synchronisation, the patterns of spread, and the anatomico-physiological correlations of both focal and generalised seizures. The neurophysiological exploration of status, though, is still at an early stage, and largely animal based. Physiological changes at a systems (in contrast to cellular) level show marked species differences, and caution is needed before extrapolating the animal experimental findings to the human condition. The EEG features of the various forms of clinical status are described in chapter 3.

Initiation of seizure activity in status epilepticus

The neurophysiological processes which initiate status are, by common agreement, very similar to those producing isolated seizures. Evidence for this can be garnered from the close resemblence, clinically and electrophysiologically, between seizures at the onset of status and isolated attacks. In human tonic–clonic status, for instance, the condition is often preceded by increasing isolated seizures, and the initial seizures in status are identical in clinical and electrographic form with isolated attacks (see pp. 53–4, 61–6). Similar conclusions have been reached in almost every animal model studied. Although the electroclinical forms of the seizures are similar, the precipitants of status and isolated seizures are not. In animal experimentation, the intensity of the epileptic stimulus can define whether or not isolated seizures or status occur (examples are the duration of electrical stimulation in animal models of epilepsy produced by hippocampal or amygdaloid stimulation, or the dose of convulsant applied in chemically induced seizures). In human status, too, the factors which precipitate status differ, in relative terms, from those precipitating ordinary seizures; for instance, the relatively stronger propensity for status to occur following drug withdrawal, fever, or metabolic disturbance. What defines 'intensity' is not known, but this is likely to be related to the persistence of the precipitating influences on the pacemaker systems initiating seizures, rather than some more fundamental difference in type or mechanism; however, this question requires further research.

Most work has been carried out on focal epilepsy, facilitated by the large number of animal and brain slice models. Seizure initiation requires the presence of cells with intrinsic burst-generating properties (pacemaker cells), loss of postsynaptic inhibitory control around these cells, and synchronisation of the epileptic discharges (Schwartzkroin 1986). The mechanisms of intrinsic burst generation have been the subject of intensive study, concentrating on ion flux across membranes (the reader is referred to large reviews, e.g. Jasper & van Gelder 1983; Prince 1985; Delgado-Escueta *et al.* 1986*b*; Wong, Traub & Miles 1986; Heinemann 1987; Heinemann & Jones 1990). Cells with burst potential are particularly evident in the hippocampal pyramidal cells in the CA1 and CA3 layers, and in neocortical cells, especially in layers IV and V. How far defects in cellular membrane function underlie status is unclear, although the disturbances of ion flux are well documented. Inhibition, at a cellular level, is mediated largely by γ-aminobutyric acid (GABA) at interneurone level, in feedback and feedforward circuits, producing inhibitory postsynaptic potentials (IPSPs) that raise membrane potentials and inhibit depolorisation (see discussion of GABA$_A$ and GABA$_B$ inhibitory function by Thompson & Gähwiler (1989)). Synchrony may be due to excitatory transmission, largely glutamate mediated (for review see Wong *et al.* 1986), although nonsynaptic mechanisms may also be involved (Dudek, Snow & Taylor 1986). The synchronous generation of depolarisation shifts at a cellular level sum to produce extracellular field potential changes, culminating in the epileptic spike. Prince (1985) suggested that epileptogenesis may be due to such processes as selective impairment of inhibitory processes, alterations in membrane properties causing hyperexcitability, establishment of new synaptic connectivity, gliosis leading to accumulation of ionic potassium, and disturbed metabolic control of membrane excitability. Wong *et al.* (1986) described the mechanisms by which neuronal synchrony develops, relating the activity of individual cells to the synchronised discharges of a large population of neurones. A detailed discussion of these is beyond the scope of this book, but this complicated process can be described neurophysiologically at a cellular or systems level; the key differences in status seem likely to reside mainly in the latter.

Spread and maintenance of seizure activity in status epilepticus

Propagation of the epileptic discharges is largely along existing pathways (for a review, see Meldrum *et al.* 1988), but potentially also by nonsynaptic mechanisms including direct electrical field effects and electrotonic junctions, and changes in extracellular ionic (potassium) and possibly other neurochemical concentrations. The relative importance of these may change over time as seizure activity continues. The mechanisms of spread of focal and generalised status are quite distinct, and furthermore, very obvious species differences exist; extrapolation of experimental results to human status must be highly circumspect. It is now quite clear that, as status progresses, specific physiological and chemical changes occur which act to perpetuate seizure activity; the mechanism underlying these changes is a key feature of status physiology. In the rodent tetanus-toxoid model of focal epilepsy, prolonged seizure activity always involves both hippocampi, and it may be that widespread neural systems are necessary to sustain seizure activity. In slice preparations, low magnesium concentrations also cause prolonged activity, suggesting that the activitation of ionic channels may potentially affect the maintenance of seizure discharges.

The experimental neurophysiological model of focal status most completely studied is that of limbic status in the rat (Lothman 1990; Lothman *et al.* 1989; VanLandingham & Lothman 1991*a,b*; Lothman & Bertram 1993). Limbic status is induced by continuous hippocampal stimulation, and a sequence of neurophysiological changes occurs over time as the status develops. Initially stimulation produces discrete seizure activity; the seizures lengthen and become more frequent, and then become continuous (fig. 4.1). After stimulation has stopped, seizures persist, initially continuously and then evolve into a pattern of recurrent short seizures and finally simply periodic epileptic discharges without clinical seizures, a sequence reminiscent of the stages in seizure activity in human tonic–

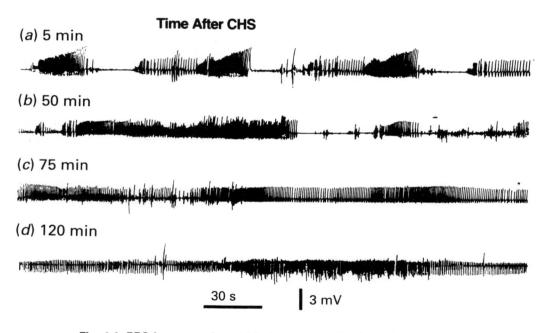

Fig. 4.1. EEG from experimental limbic status epilepticus. Evolution of limbic status induced by continuous hippocampal stimulation (CHS), in the rat (the *self-sustaining limbic status epilepticus* model of Lothman and colleagues). The recordings are by bipolar electrodes positioned in the hippocampus. Discrete seizures are noted 5 minutes after stimulation, evolving to longer seizures at 50 minutes, and then continuous seizure activity with periodic epileptiform discharges at 75 and 120 minutes. (From Lothman 1990, with kind permission.)

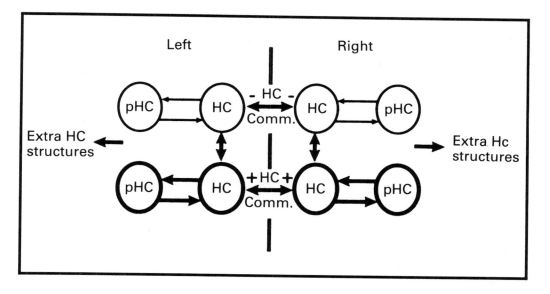

Fig. 4.2. Self-sustaining limbic status epilepticus: anatomical circuits. This is a diagram of the anatomical circuits underlying self-sustaining limbic status epilepticus (in the rat model reported by VanLandingham & Lothman 1991*a*). The left and right hippocampi (HC) are connected by the hippocampal commissure (HC Comm). On each side, the dorsal and ventral hippocampi are connected via longitudinal associational pathways. The hippocampi and parahippocampus (pHC) sustain a reverberating self-sustaining circuit (the hippocampal–parahippocampal loop). Transection of the hippocampal commissures does not block the status epilepticus, but the dorsal commissure appears to exert a relatively inhibitory influence, and the ventral commissure a relatively excitatory influence. The ventral hippocampal–parahippocampal loop is more important than the dorsal loop in the maintenance of status epilepticus in this model. (From VanLandingham & Lothman 1991*a*, with kind permission.)

clonic status. In this model, by measuring regional cerebral glucose utilisation during status, a feedback loop has been identified between the hippocampal and the parahippocampal structures (subiculum and entorhinal cortex), and, it is postulated, seizure activity reverberates in this loop, thus maintaining the status for many hours (fig. 4.2). Included in this loop, interestingly, is the dentate gyrus, which normally serves to retard seizures, a controlling mechanism that seems to break down in status. The status also spreads outside the ipsilateral limbic structures, both contralaterally to limbic structures and also to other cortical areas; again parallels with human status are obvious. In the rat, but probably not in the human, spread from one hippocampal region to the other is through the hippocampal commissures. These structures are not, however, crucial in maintaining seizures or status, because unilateral status still occurs in commissurotomised animals.

143

This model of status has provided the most detailed experimental analysis of seizure spread in status to date, but similar changes in the EEG over time have been observed in other rodent models (Treiman *et al.* 1990). The recognition of reverberating circuits in status has been noted before, and herein may be the crucial neurophysiological mechanism for maintaining recurrent seizures, especially of the nonconvulsive type in humans. Circuits could be maintained by the breakdown of inhibitory mechanisms or the enhancement of excitation, the neurochemistry of which is discussed below. Whichever is more important, it is apparent that as time passes, the recurring seizure activity induces physiological changes which act to perpetuate seizure discharges; it is this temporal dimension which above all others differentiates the physiology of status from that of isolated seizures. In human status, cycling of electrographic activity is a common feature of complex partial status, and may be due to reverberating circuits (see pp. 126–8). If these mechanisms can be identified in human status, therapy specifically directed towards interrupting reverberating circuits might prove possible. The limbic status epilepticus model is of interest for other reasons also. Chronic epilepsy and interictal spiking are a common sequel to an episode of status, with hippocampal pathological changes which have a parallel in chronic human temporal lobe epilepsy. Furthermore, studies from hippocampal slices from the same animals show a decrease in GABA-mediated inhibition and an altered sensitivity to extracellular ions, suggesting that these are the biochemical changes that might underlie chronic focal epilepsy (Lothman *et al.* 1990).

In another recent study of limbic status produced in rats by continuous amygdaloid stimulation, the changes in clinical and electrographic activity over time were also scrutinised. The temporal evolution of the seizure activity in this animal model has echoes in human status. Stimulation produced limbic seizures which evolved in some animals to convulsive, and in others to nonconvulsive, status (Handforth & Ackermann 1992), and the following salient observations were made:

1. The initial physiological changes in the limbic status seem identical with those in individual seizures, morphologically and anatomically, and clinical correlates were also similar. This is confirmation that seizures and status have a common substrate and mode of initiation. Presumably, the distinction between seizures and status has more to do with failure to contain or terminate the epileptic processes in status than with any differences in origin.
2. In many rats, the limbic seizures evolved into convulsive status. The electrographic and clinical findings initially were similar to isolated convulsive seizures, but as status progressed, the initially discrete seizures merge into continuous ictal activity, and later still the motor activity becomes progressively less and less marked (very similar to human status). Electrographically, the evolution from seizure to status in this model resembles an enhancement of the afterdischarge. A very similar observation was made by Wieser (1980), in human complex partial status, and this is an analogy which deserves further study.

The similarities between convulsive status in the rodent and human have also been stressed by Treiman *et al.* (1990), who were able to detect five electrographic stages in human convulsive status (fig. 3.2), and also in the EEG of three different rat models of status (Trieman *et al.* 1990). Such a sequence presumably reflects the evolving neurochemical changes of prolonged status, and may be the physiological signature of status-induced neuronal damage.

In generalised epilepsy, the mechanisms of seizure spread and persistence are almost certainly very different from those in focal seizures. The experiments of Meldrum & Horton (1973) in the adolescent baboon (*Papio papio*), with bicucul-line-induced seizures provide detailed neurophysiological data (fig. 4.3). At the onset of status, myoclonic jerks, associated with irregular widespread cortical spike–wave, are followed by tonic spasm for 10–30 seconds with fast activity, and then rhythmic spikes on the EEG evolving into rhythmic polyspike and waves as the

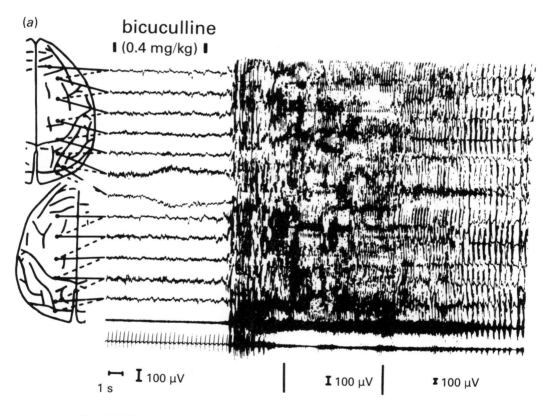

Fig. 4.3. Electroencephalographic (EEG) records showing the progression of seizure activity in status induced by intravenous bicuculline (0.4 mg/kg) in a baboon. Also shown is the electromyograph from the right elbow flexors. The seizure begins with generalised irregular myoclonus, which after 2 seconds evolves into a generalised flexor spasm.

145

(*b*)　　　**+ 10 min**

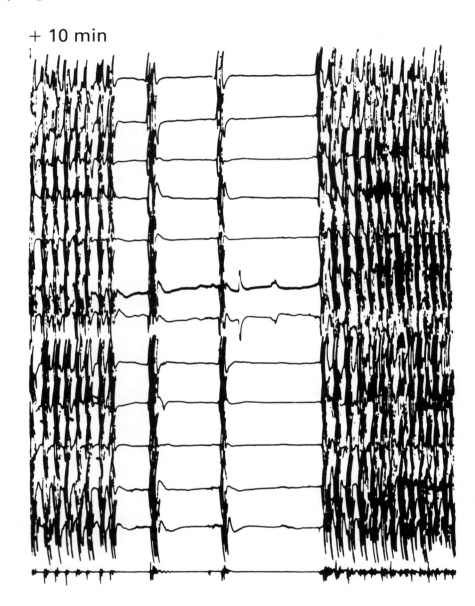

Caption for fig. 4.3 (*cont.*). At 10 minutes, seizure activity is intermittent with transient arrest of seizure activity.

(c) + 161 min

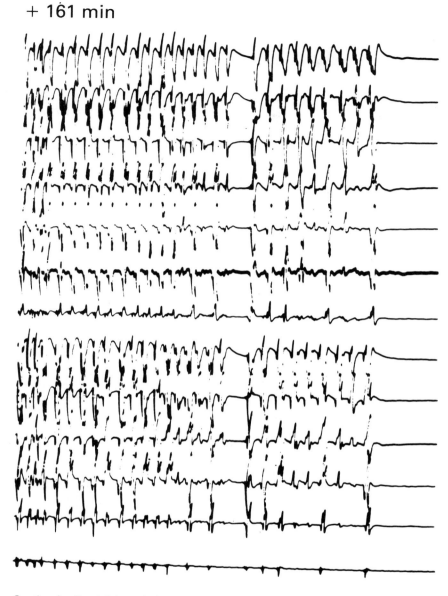

Caption for fig. 4.3 (*cont.*). At 161 minutes, the myoclonus had slowed, and the seizure activity is more continuous. Seizure activity ceases at 168 minutes, and is followed by postictal depression.

(*d*)

+ 173 min	+ 198 min	+ 302 min

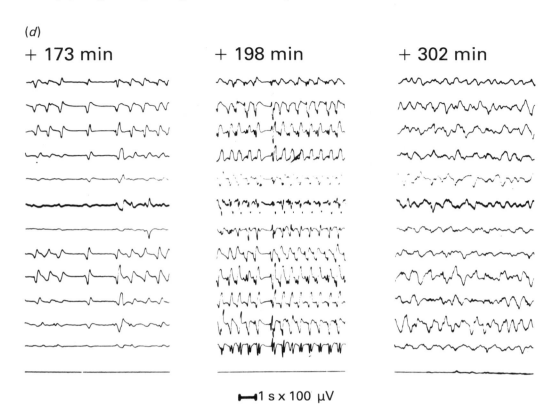

►◄1 s x 100 µV

Caption for fig. 4.3 (*cont.*). Isolated biphasic waves appear by 173 minutes. By 198 minutes, these waves become more rhythmic, generalised and paroxysmal in appearance. At 302 minutes, the EEG pattern evolves into diffuse high-voltage delta activity. (From Meldrum & Horton 1973, Physiology of status epilepticus in primates, *Archives of Neurology*, **28**, 1–9, copyright 1973, American Medical Association, with kind permission.)

clonic phase develops. This clinical and electrographic pattern could be sustained for 40–50 minutes, although often interrupted for a few seconds by electrical silence followed by more fast activity or the resumption of rhythmic spiking. After 1–2 hours, the jerks began to wax and wane, and become asymmetrical, involving only parts of the body, and the EEG activity becomes irregular in rhythm and distribution. Discharges faded away from the occipital cortices whilst continuing in the frontal and parietal regions. At the end of the status, cortical activity ceased synchronously, and the postictal electrographic silence was then followed by delta waves, augmented in amplitude and becoming rhythmic and symmetrical, at times taking on a paroxysmal quality, with sporadic spikes or spike-bursts. Physiological changes were demonstrable in these baboons as they are in humans (see pp. 54–61 and fig. 3.1), and Meldrum & Horton were the first to point out that status results in physiological decompensation, and that two distinct phases can be defined (the shift from phase I to phase II occurring after about 20 or 30 minutes of continuous seizure activity in the baboon). In phase I, arterial and cerebral venous pressure rise and small subarachnoid haemorrhages occur. Arterial oxygen concentrations fall, as do arteriovenous differences for oxygen and carbon dioxide, and glucose and lactate concentrations levels rise. In the second phase, hyperpyrexia becomes severe, arteriovenous oxygen and carbon dioxide differences are enhanced, and although arterial oxygen concentrations fall they are not critically reduced. Blood glucose levels fall, and in the later stages severe hypoglycaemia can develop. Hyperkalaemia occurs late, and the electrolyte and pH disturbances induce cardiovascular malfunction, which is a common cause of death. There have been no more detailed neurophysiological studies of generalised epilepsy in any other animal models, and none in humans (as the inevitable efforts to treat status of course interfere with the neurophysiological study), and this work provides our best available model of generalised status.

In generalised epilepsy, the importance of cortico–subcortical reverberating circuits has been stressed by others, especially in the experiments using the feline penicillin model of generalised epilepsy reported by Gloor and co-workers (see Gloor 1979; Gloor & Fariello 1988). These studies provide one possible theoretical basis for spike-wave seizures and, by extrapolation, status. Modest stimulation of reticular thalamic neurones causes seizure discharges, and the basic defect in generalised status may reside in these reticular thalamic generators, and possibly also in the general hyperexcitability of cortical cells (see Steriade & Llinas 1988). Whilst the neurophysiological experiments in generalised status provide detailed descriptive neurophysiology, several important issues remain unresolved: by what mechanisms do seizures persist, what are the exact pathways of spread in generalised epilepsy, why does seizure activity change over time? These are essential questions to which future research should be addressed.

Termination of status epilepticus

The sudden cessation of epileptic activity at the termination of an ordinary epileptic seizure is remarkable. The physiological processes causing the abrupt end of seizure activity are unclear but could have relevance in status. It is now firmly established that seizures are not usually terminated because of energy failure (this is discussed below), but rather by synaptic and ionic mechanisms. The cessation of seizures or status could be due to the sudden inhibition of pacemaker (generator) cells, the interruption of synchronisation or reverberating circuits, or the activation of a widespread inhibitory system. It is obviously tempting to postulate that defects in these termination mechanisms lie at the centre of status physiology, and there is some evidence to support this. In human and experimental isolated seizures, when the seizures cease, the EEG usually shows either delta activity or attenuation. The changes are usually most pronounced over the site of maximal seizure activity (electrographically), but not always. In the early seizures of human status (and indeed in the baboon), these typical postictal changes are sometimes absent (Roger *et al.* 1974), suggesting that the usual inhibitory mechanisms are impaired in status. The synaptic inhibition is probably mediated at the GABA$_B$ receptor, particularly by the slow IPSPs (not the fast IPSPs of the GABA$_A$ receptor). Changes in synapses induced by chronic seizure activity can also predispose cells to prolonged ictal activity, perhaps by increasing the density of excitatory receptor sites.

The Na$^+$/K$^+$-ATPase system is of central importance in the termination of seizure activity (Heinemann & Jones 1990). Activation of this system during a seizure causes hyperpolarisation, at a presynaptic level, reducing the amount of neurotransmitter release, and at a postsynaptic level, repolarising the cell membrane. In this process, adenosine is released into the extracellular space which also acts to hyperpolarise the postsynaptic membrane. How this system is altered in status is uncertain, but clearly these inhibitory effects of ionic shift are overridden. Extracellular ionic concentration may be important. Recurrent seizure-like activity can be produced in low-calcium or low-magnesium hippocampal slice preparations, in which ion flux across membranes is impaired. The persistence of seizures in status might thus be, to an extent, due to abnormalities in ion movement as a result of membrane defects. Low extracellular calcium and high potassium also facilitate nonsynaptic effects which may circumvent normal inhibitory processes (Dudek *et al.* 1986). It has also been postulated that status arises when excitatory influences are enhanced to the extent that they outlast the normal refractory period of a cell after hyperpolarisation, thus repeatedly retriggering burst activity. The hyperexcited neuronal state could also be due to impairment of GABAergic function, GABA being the most important pre- and postsynaptic inhibitory transmitter; this hypothesis is discussed at more length below. Opioid peptides are also released by seizure activity and have a role in self-limiting seizures (Tortella, Long & Holaday 1985). It is easy to postulate that status is caused by impairment of such inherent negative feedback mechanisms, a proposition that has as yet been incompletely studied.

Cerebral energy in status epilepticus

Cerebral energy metabolism in status has been evaluated using positron emission tomography (PET) and magnetic resonance spectroscopy. Epileptic seizures consume more energy than any other cerebral event, and a study of energy relations in status would seem a promising method of identifying basic neurophysiological or neurochemical abnormalities. Unfortunately, early experiments in this area have rather disappointingly provided few new insights into inherent status mechanisms (for a review see Chapman 1985). Ictal PET scanning during complex partial status (and individual focal seizures) shows an unsurprising increase in cerebral blood flow and oxygen consumption, roughly correlating with the regions of EEG abnormality. In the focus, oxygen extraction is somewhat reduced, suggesting that oxygen utilisation by the mitochondria is impaired. A relative increase in nonoxidative metabolism has been postulated, perhaps reflecting calcium ion influx into cells during status, but changes were not gross. The supply of glucose also seems quite sufficient to support the metabolically active brain (Franck *et al.*

1986*a,b*). This is an important point, and evidence against the theory that cerebral damage in status is due to an impaired ability to meet metabolic demands. If seizures continue long enough, however, hypoxic metabolic changes can be observed, especially in limbic and cortical regions and in the presence of falling blood pressure (Hempel, Kariman & Saltzman 1980; Ingvar & Siesjö 1983; Kriesman, Magee & Brizzee 1991). How important such mechanisms are in human status is unclear. There may also be an age effect, as energy requirements in the neonatal primate brain have been shown to exceed glucose supply (Fujikawa *et al.* 1989*a*). It has also been shown in experimental models that moderate reductions in oxygen or glucose supply lessen seizure activity (Blennow *et al.* 1978), a physiological mechanism that protects cerebral tissue from hypoxic damage. Again, the relevance of this mechanism in human status is unknown. *In vivo* nuclear magnetic resonance phosphorus spectroscopy has proved another new and versatile method for studying, serially, the chemistry of energy systems in status. In paralysed and ventilated rabbits, generalised status, induced by bicuculline, causes a decrease in phosphocreatine levels and in intracellular pH, about 10–20 minutes after the first bicuculline injection. ATP levels are maintained thoughout the status, suggesting that energy failure is not the reason for seizure termination and that the pH fall is due probably to lactic acidosis. Rather similar changes have been noted in the neonatal dog (Young *et al.* 1985). Changes do not correlate closely with seizure activity, nor with the effects of drug action, and their relevance to the maintenance of status is unclear (Petroff *et al.* 1984). The lack of derangement of energy-producing systems and the lack of tissue catabolism, as judged by protein breakdown, in status contrast greatly, for instance, with the massive abnormalities induced by hypoglycaemia or ischaemia (Auer & Siesjö 1988). Anaerobic glycolysis and lactic acid production are increased in status, but, in the well-ventilated subject at least, lactic acid concentrations do not reach damaging levels.

Neuropathology of status epilepticus

As discussed in chapter 1, neuropathological studies have a long pedigree. By 1880, the macroscopic and microscopic appearances of the brain in status had been described, but the hunt for the essential 'lesion' of epilepsy was then, and is still, largely unsuccessful both in focal and generalised status. Furthermore, many pathological changes in status are the result not the cause of the condition, an issue debated at some length below.

In focal status, pathologies are often found which are the immediate cause of the epilepsy. Common examples include cerebral tumours, vascular lesions, developmental anomalies, hippocampal sclerosis, and post-traumatic or infective cerebral damage. Although causal in the sense that they precipitate seizures, at a cellular level such pathologies are not the *intrinsic defect* of epilepsy. The pathological correlate of the neurophysiological and neurochemical changes of status has not been identified, at a macroscopic, light or even electron microscopic level, and this is deeply disappointing. Indeed the normality of pathological appearances

151

is often in remarkable contrast to the severity of the epileptic condition. Progress in the field of developmental pathology, however, may shed light on this problem. Recent evidence, requiring further evaluation, suggests that minor developmental abnormalities (disorders of neuronal migration) are present in many apparently idiopathic epilepsies. To demonstrate clearly that these underlie epileptogenesis, it will be necessary to confirm the observations, and to establish a mechanistic link with the physiological and neurochemical changes of epilepsy; this is an exciting research area of great potential.

Neuropathological changes in status epilepticus: cause or effect?

Assessing neuropathological findings in status is seriously complicated by the fact that status not only results from but can also cause pathological changes. Whilst there is now no doubt that status can induce cerebral damage, the degree to which this occurs in humans, and the nature of these changes, are still highly controversial. In human status, the problems are compounded by differing definitions of status, the treatment employed, and the fact that the propensity for cerebral damage depends on the cortical site, duration and type of status, and the age of the patient. Furthermore, the underlying aetiology of the status may itself result in cerebral damage, as can the secondary systemic effects of status. Perhaps it should not therefore surprise us that much still remains to be learnt, although it is difficult to disagree with Corsellis & Bruton (1983) that future advances lie not within the realm of the morbid anatomist, but rather with the experimental neurochemist and neurophysiologist.

Human pathological studies

Gross postmortem examination of the brains of patients dying in acute status often shows no obvious changes. In some cases the brain is swollen and congested, and there may be scattered small haemorrhages. The hippocampus can be swollen in the acute phase, especially in young children, and later become atrophied, shrunken and scarred. Severe atrophic changes may also be visible in the cerebellum.

HIPPOCAMPAL CHANGES: Particular attention has been paid to damage to the hippocampus (figs. 4.4, 4.5), since the important early description of Sommer (1880). Sommer documented, using Nissl-stained preparations of the brains of chronic epileptics, a pattern of damage which is now referred to as Ammon's horn sclerosis (or hippocampal sclerosis), in which gliosis and pyramidal cell loss occur, predominantly in the CA1 region of the hippocampus (a sector now bearing Sommer's name). Subsequent investigators have confirmed these findings, and also recorded damage in other regions, notably the end folium and CA3 region of the hippocampus, certain regions of the cerebral neocortex, specific nuclei of the thalamus and in the cerebellum. Sommer proposed that the hippocampal lesions were the cause of epilepsy (although generalised not psychomotor seizures), but Pfleger (1880), describing haemorrhagic lesions in mesial temporal regions of a patient with status epilepticus, concluded they were the sequel of status, possibly due to impaired blood flow or nutrition. Controversy on this point has raged ever

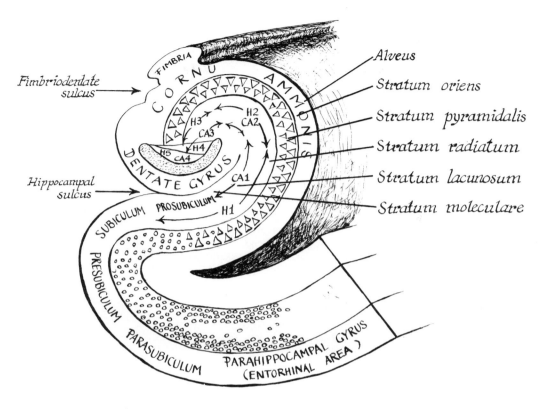

Fig. 4.4 Diagram of the human hippocampus showing the internal anatomy, topography and anatomical relationships. Also shown are two schemes of notation in common use; that of the Ammon's horn fields (CA1–CA4), and that of the hippocampal fields (H1–H5). (Redrawn from Williams *et al.* 1989, by Dr Sveinbjornsdottir, Institute of Neurology.)

since. Although the pathological findings are not in doubt, the relationship of the lesion to epilepsy, causal or consecutive, or both, remains uncertain. Other notable contributions to the description of hippocampal pathology were made by: Bratz (1899), who confirmed Sommer's findings (in 25 of 50 cases of chronic epilepsy examined), noted end plate changes and felt the lesion to be congenital; Spielmeyer (1927), who attributed the changes to ischaemic nerve cell death (*ischamischen ganglienzellenerkrankung*), a descriptive concept still held by many today; and Scholtz (1933) and Oppenheim, who also felt the cerebral changes to be the result, not the cause, of seizures. The link between hippocampal sclerosis and temporal lobe epilepsy was not firmly appreciated until Sano & Malamud (1953) showed that Ammon's horn sclerosis in 29 of 50 institutionalised epileptic patients was associated with anterior temporal spikes or spike–wave discharges.

153

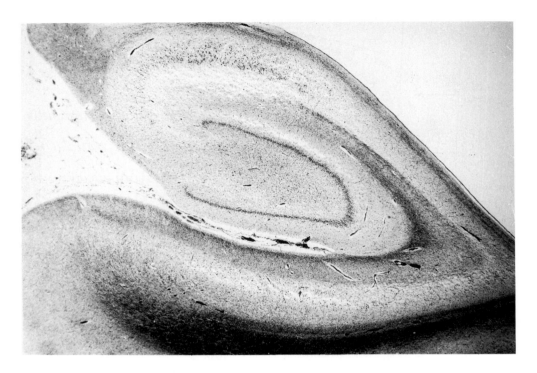

Fig. 4.5. Section through the hippocampus of a male who developed severe multifocal seizures at 28 months. At the age of 36 months he was noted to be ataxic and hypotonic, and his liver was enlarged. The computed tomography scan was normal and electroencephalography showed generalised slow activity and multifocal spikes, maximal in the right anterior region. At the age of 39 months he had an episode of severe status epilepticus requiring intubation, and was noted to have developed liver failure. He died aged 41 months. This specimen shows loss of pyramidal cells from the Sommer sector and end plate, with preservation of H2. Stained with Luxol fast blue-cresyl violet. Examination of the rest of the brain revealed Alper's disease, and this case demonstrates that severe hippocampal cell loss can occur in various pathologies. Alper's disease is a commoner cause of fatal status than is frequently recognised. (With thanks to Dr B.N. Harding, Institute of Neurology who prepared this specimen, which is also published in Harding *et al.* 1986.)

There then followed a series of studies carefully documenting the acute changes in status (Norman 1964; Ounsted, Lindsay & Norman 1966). Recent ischaemic hippocampal lesions were identified in 11 children dying in status epilepticus. The Ammon's horn was the most frequently damaged area (neuronal necrosis being present in 10 of 11 cases, and in the eleventh case old lesions attributed to fits were found), and the Sommer sector and end folium. The preservation of H2 was also noted and it was termed the 'resistant sector'. Amygdaloid and uncal changes were also found and more widespread neuronal damage in the neocortex, striatum, thalamus and cerebellum. The calcerine cortex was usually spared and there was patchy necrosis in other cortical and deep grey matter. Margerison & Corsellis (1966), in a detailed studies of 55 institutionalised patients, found significant damage in the hippocampus in 65%, in the cerebellum in 45%, in the amygdala in 27%, in the thalamus in 25% and in the cortex in 22%. It was concluded that hippocampal sclerosis was due to ischaemic brain damage in early childhood seizures or status epilepticus, and that status-induced ischaemic hippocampal damage was probably the cause of subsequent temporal lobe epilepsy. Corsellis & Bruton (1983) examined the brains of 8 children and 12 adults dying during or shortly after an episode of status epilepticus, and found swelling and almost complete loss of neurones in the Sommer sector in all the children and three of the adults. This acute lesion was recognised as the precursor of Ammon's horn sclerosis, in which the gliosis and atrophy would develop subsequently as the lesion matured. They also noted damage in the cerebellar cortex, the cerebral neocortex and thalamus. The contrast between the vulnerability of the childhood and adult brains is striking, a feature which has been repeatedly confirmed. However, changes can occur *de novo* in adults, as shown by Noel *et al.* (1977), who reported findings similar to those of Pfleger (1880) in a 55 year old woman after 6 days of status epilepticus associated with an acute viral hepatitis. Thus, by the late 1970s there was indisputable evidence that status could induced hippocampal damage, and more controversially that this lesion may also cause subsequent temporal lobe epilepsy. The relative vulnerability of the prosubiculum, CA1 and CA3 regions to damage in human status have been confirmed more recently by quantitative measurements of neuronal densities (DeGiorgio *et al.* 1992).

EXTRAHIPPOCAMPAL CHANGES: Although there is general agreement that the hippocampus is the brain region particularly severely and consistently affected in patients (especially children) with histories of status epilepticus, other brain regions are also clearly affected (fig. 4.6). Chaslin (1889) was the first to note widespread cortical neuronal loss and gliosis, and saw the Ammon's horn changes as simply part of this widespread gliosis, which he considered was the pathological process causing epilepsy; similar changes in the cerebellum in epilepsy were reported by Alzheimer (1898), who considered the gliosis to be a secondary reaction to cell loss. Theories of epileptogenesis at the time favoured the cerebral cortex as the 'primary seat of the nervous storm in epilepsy', as Clark & Prout (1903/4) put it. In their detailed exposition on status, status was viewed physiologically as a sensorimotor reflex involving large cortical areas, the primary cause of which was the cortical pathological changes. They carried out one of the earliest detailed pathological studies of status, comparing pathological findings in 7 cases dying in status and 12 of epilepsy without status. They identified cell loss and gliosis, and recognised a temporal sequence of changes, with acute and secondary histological changes. They dismissed Ammon's horn sclerosis as the essential lesion of epilepsy, along with other current theories which included spasm of the arterioles,

155

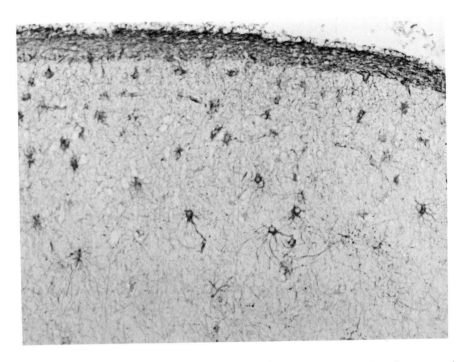

Fig. 4.6. Section through the brain of a male aged 18 years, with chronic temporal lobe epilepsy, and a history of status epilepticus. This specimen shows cortical subpial fibrillary gliosis (Chaslin's gliosis) and numerous hypertrophic astrocytes. These changes are typical of the cortical damage seen in chronic epilepsy, and emphasise the fact that pathological changes are not confined to the hippocampal region. The specimen is stained with glial fibrillary acidic protein immunoperoxidase. (With thanks to Dr B.N. Harding, Institute of Neurology for preparing this specimen.)

disease of a convulsive centre, and disorders of the sympathetic nervous system, the medulla or basal ganglia.

Widespread gliosis and neuronal loss in cortical and basal gangion regions were subsequently recorded in many pathological reports. The epileptogenic nature of cortical scarring was demonstrated by Penfield and colleagues (Penfield 1927; Penfield & Humphries 1940; Foerster & Penfield 1930). Norman (1964), Margerison & Corsellis (1966) and Corsellis & Bruton (1983), although emphasising the Ammon's horn changes, also found in the acute phase of status destructive cerebral changes, degeneration and loss of the Purkinje cells and an acute glial reaction in the cerebellum, patchy massive neuronal destruction and gliosis in the thalamus, and similar damage in the corpus striatum. Acute neuronal necrosis was noted, especially in the middle cortical layers, stretching over wide areas of the cortical mantle in some cases, and only patchily distributed in others

(Corsellis & Bruton 1983). In survivors of the acute lesion, gradual atrophy of the cerebellum was noted, in both the Purkinje cell and the granular layer, and also widespread shrinkage, gliosis and neuronal loss in the neocortex and basal ganglion. In adults dying in status the changes were much less striking than in children. In the worst of the 12 cases examined, acute hypoxic–ischaemic changes were noted, most marked in the hippocampus, but also affecting in a patchy fashion the neocortex, cerebellum and deep grey matter. In 7 of the 12 cases, no acute changes were found, although clear evidence of old scarring, heavy gliosis and neuronal loss, mainly in the hippocampus and cerebellum, was evident. The cellular changes after status were summarised by Meldrum & Corsellis (1984). The nerve cell bodies are hardly visible with a Nissl stain but are eosinophilic with haematoxylin and eosin stains. The cell outline is triangular, the nucleus is small and darkly stained and the nucleolus can no longer be identified. Many nerve cells disappear, leaving only small tags of eosinophilic cytoplasm. In the cerebellum, the Purkinje cells are commonly affected, the cytoplasm loses its Nissl-staining substance and becomes eosinophilic, and the nucleus is dark and shrunken. A later change in affected parts of the brain is a microglial and astrocytic reaction, and eventually dense fibrous necrosis may be laid down. The white matter may show diffuse but slight pallor. In adults similar pathological changes may occur but are usually less severe. These findings largely confirm those of Clark & Prout some 80 years before. Occasionally, more severe pathological damage occurs (see, for instance, the case of Meyer, Beck & Shepherd (1955)).

All the above reports were of convulsive status (where seizure type was stated). A single paper describes three patients without pre-existing epilepsy who died 11–27 days after the onset of non-convulsive status lasting 1–3 days (Wasterlain *et al.* 1993). In all three cases, there were changes similar to those outlined above, with neuronal loss in CA1, CA3 and hilar cells, and also in the amygdala, thalamus, cerebellum and cerebral cortex.

The first golgi study of brain is attributed to DeMoor (1898), who noted diffuse dendritic spine loss and nodulated dendrites, largely in the receptive portion of the neurone, indicating a reduction in afferent nerves. Subsequent investigations have documented loss of dendritic swellings and alteration in dendritic patterns, sometimes in a localised distribution and sometimes more extensive, affecting hippocampal pyramidal and dentate granule cells (Scheibel & Scheibel 1973). The first electron microscopic study was that of Brown & Brierley (1973), who showed loss of synapses in temporal lobe biopsy cases in patients with acute focal epilepsy. Scheibel, Paul & Fried (1983) in a scanning electron microscopic study of the microvasculature in temporal lobe resections observed blood vessel out-pouches, and suggested that blowouts from these could introduce blood elements into tissue, which might induce epileptogenesis. There is no doubt that extraversated iron has potent epileptogenic properties, but this suggestion does not appear to have been followed up.

The mechanisms of the cerebral (especially hippocampal) changes due to status have proved controversial. The earliest were vascular theories. Spielmeyer (1927), noting the similarity of hippocampal damage to that of cerebral ischaemia, suggested that cerebral vascular spasm was responsible. Several workers proposed alternative vascular mechanisms including systemic hypoxia, consumptive hypoxia, hypotension, or cerebral oedema causing mesial temporal tentorial herniation and anterior choriodal and posterior cerebral artery compression. The absence of oedema and of tentorial herniation in pathological specimens, and differences between these pathological findings and those in large series of infants with tentorial herniation, failed to support the latter theory. The next important observations were made by the Maudsley Hospital and Oxford groups (see Falconer *et al.* 1964; Norman 1964; Ounsted *et al.* 1966), who, in a series of surgical and postmortem examinations, concluded that the hippocampal damage was due either to ischaemic or to metabolic damage due to the seizure discharges themselves, especially in childhood, and that primary vascular factors were not relevant. Subsequent research has concentrated upon the features and mechanisms of status-induced damage.

Animal pathological studies

The clearest evidence that status epilepticus per se can result in cerebral damage has come from animal experimentation. The classic studies of convulsive status were carried out in adolescent baboons by Meldrum and co-workers, and have had a profound influence on all subsequent work on status; and for this reason they are here described at length (Meldrum & Brierley 1973; Meldrum & Horton 1973; Meldrum, Vigouroux & Brierley 1973; Meldrum, Horton & Brierley 1974). In ten baboons in whom generalised seizures lasting 82–299 minutes were induced ischaemic neuronal changes of the Spielmeyer type developed. The earliest abnormality was microvacuolation, with normal cell contour and nucleus, increased cytoplasmic staining with cresyl violet, and numerous circular or oval empty spaces, which on examination by electron microscopy were shown to be swollen mitochondria with variable alteration of the cristae. Full-blown changes were most frequent in the smaller pyramidal neurones of layers III, V and VI of the neocortex around the sulci rather than over the crest of the gyri. In the hippocampus, ischaemic changes were seen in the Sommer sector in six of the ten animals and in the end folium in eight, but here the damage was never more than moderate. Thalamic damage was seen in five animals in the anterior and dorsomedial nuclei, and, in two severely damaged animals, the small neurones of the striatum were involved. In seven animals there was mild involvement of the amygdaloid nuclei, and in eight of Purkinje and basket cells of the cerebellum, most marked in the arterial watershed zones. One animal showed foci of status spongiosus disseminated in the outer layer of the neocortex (see table 4.1). It was commented (Meldrum & Brierley 1973) that the distribution of cell loss in specific layers of the neocortex, zones of the hippocampus, and portions of the basal ganglia, and amongst certain cell types in the cerebellum, correspond to the selective pattern of vulnerability in the human brain after status epilepticus, and had the animals survived the dead nerve cells would have been removed by phagocytosis and would have been replaced by glial proliferation resulting in cerebral and cerebellar atrophy and sclerosis of the hippocampus. In the baboons, initially

Table 4.1. *The distribution and severity of cell damage in the brains of 10 baboons after bicuculline-induced status epilepticus*

Baboon	Cerebral cortex				Hippocampus			Thalamus		Striatum	Amygdala		Cerebellum
	Occipital	Parietal	Frontal	Temporal	H1	H3–5	Laterality	Anterior	Dorso-medial		Central-medial	Baso-lateral	
7	++	+	+	+	0	+	L = R	+	+	0	0	0	+(BZ)
9	+	+	+	+	0	+	L = R	++	0	0	0	0	+(BZ)
10	+++	++	++	++	+++	++	R > L	0	0	++R>L	+	++	+(BZ)
15	+	0	0	0	++	0	L = R	+	0	0	++	+	0
16	+	+	+	+	0	+	R	0	0	0	0	+R < L	+
18	++	++	++	++	++	++	L = R	+	+	+	+	+	+(BZ)
19	+	+	+	++	++	++	L = R	0	0	0	0	+	+++(BZ)
23	+	+	+	+	+	0	L = R	0	+	0	0	++	+
25	+	+	+	+	0	0	R > L	0	+	0	0	0	0
27	+++	++	++	++	+++	+	L = R	0	0	0	+	++	+(BZ)

Ischaemic cell change is graded as + signifying involvement of a few scattered cells; ++, involving a large proportion of neurones. BZ indicates ischaemic cell change affecting Purkinje cells at the boundary zone between the superior cerebellar artery and the posterior inferior cerebellar artery. Two baboons showed slight damage in other thalamic nuclei: baboon 9 in the ventrolateral nucleus (+R > L) and baboon 18 in the pulvinar (+). In baboon 16, the entorhinal cortex was symmetrically involved (++). R, right; L, left. +++, involving a moderate number of cells; From Meldrum & Brierley 1973, with kind permission.

there was marked hypertension, acidosis and hyperglycaemia. This phase was followed by increasing hyperpyrexia, and late in the status mild hypotension and in some animals hypoglycaemia, strikingly similar to the changes seen in human status. The neuronal damage caused by status was incurred in the second phase of seizure, from about 25 minutes onward, and, after this time, was worse the longer the duration of the status and the hyperpyrexia, and in the presence of severe arterial hypotension (<75 mmHg), or profound hypoglycaemia.

The experiments were then repeated in eight paralysed and artificially ventilated baboons, in whom hypotension, acidosis, hypoxia and hypoglycaemia were prevented (Meldrum *et al.* 1973). Neuropathological examination revealed a similar pattern of neocortical and hippocampal damage in seven animals, albeit after longer periods of status (seizure durations from 205 to 433 minutes) and the pathological changes were generally less severe. 'Ischaemic cell changes' were found in the small pyramidal neurones of the neocortex, the anterior dorsomedial and ventral nuclei of the thalamus, and the Sommer sector and end folium of the hippocampus. Only the cerebellar damage was totally prevented by paralysis, and was thus thought to be related to the hyperpyrexia and hypertension. In the one animal who had seizures for less than 2 hours, no changes were seen. It was concluded from these experiments that the 'ischaemic' changes were not of vascular origin but due to impaired cellular metabolism.

To explore the metabolic factors further, Meldrum and colleagues studied mechanically ventilated Wistar rats in whom oxygen and glucose levels were maintained. Two hours of bicuculline-induced status produced microvacuolation and ischaemic cell change despite well-maintained oxygenation and glucose levels (Blennow *et al.* 1978); indeed moderate hypotension, hypoxia or hypoglycaemia appeared to impart some protection against neuronal damage, perhaps due to their effect in lessening seizure activity. Blood flow studies in the same experimental model showed marked increases in flow in the hippocampus during seizures, further evidence against a vascular explanation for hippocampal damage (Horton *et al.* 1980). Meldrum and his co-workers then proposed that the neuronal damage was due to oxidative mechanisms in cells with enhanced neuronal activity, a prescient theory, confirmed by later neurochemical investigation (Horton *et al.* 1980).

In a subsequent study of baboons with allylglycine-induced generalised seizures, a pattern of cerebral damage that more closely resembles the changes in human chronic temporal lobe cases resulted after 26–63 seizures in 2–11 hours in eight animals, and in five a period of status epilepticus. The physiological changes were much less severe than those produced by the bicuculline-induced sustained seizures, and in particular the hyperpyrexia was seen only when the seizures were closely spaced. The fall in arterial pO_2 were transient and not severe, and arterial mean pressure fell only in cases where seizure activity was sustained, and respiratory and metabolic acidosis were much less severe than after bicuculline. Sudden cardiovascular collapse occurred late during the status epilepticus cases. Pathological examination revealed ischaemic changes in H1, and H3 and H5 hippocampal neurones, and in pyramidal neurones in the third and fifth layers of the neocortex in those animals with status epilepticus. In the animals who survived long term, usually those without status, there was neuronal loss and gliosis in the vulnerable region of the hippocampus, corresponding to an early stage in the development of Ammon's horn sclerosis (Meldrum *et al.* 1974). It was postulated from this work that, whilst status epilepticus produces widespread neuronal damage, less severe seizures might damage the hippocampus only, and the pattern of damage thus produced was similar to that seen in chronic focal epilepsy.

From this series of experiments, a number of important conclusions were drawn: (a) status can result in cerebral damage; (b) this damage can be due to the seizure activity itself on a metabolic (not vascular) basis, without systemic disturbance; (c) systemic disturbance can worsen the seizure-induced damage, which is thus often due to a combination of excessive neuronal activity and the accumulative effects of secondary changes (e.g. hypoxia, hyperpyrexia, hypoglycaemia, hypotension); (d) the duration of seizure activity is a vital factor; (e) control of the systemic disturbance (in contrast to seizure activity) will only totally prevent damage to the cerebellum; (f) the pattern of damage is similar both to that seen in human status and, in its milder forms, to that encountered in temporal lobe epilepsy. No experiments in status have been as influential, or have advanced knowledge to a greater extent, than these, and this work had dictated the direction of experimental status research, for at least the next two decades. The obvious implications for the management of human status, too, were early recognised.

Succeeding researchers largely confirmed the findings of Meldrum and his colleagues in other animal models of generalised convulsive status epilepticus. Most subsequent research has concentrated on focal status, especially status involving limbic or mesial temporal lobe structures. Again, seizure-induced cell loss has been demonstrated in many other experimental paradigms. A most important discovery was that kainic acid, a rigid analogue of glutamate, with much greater potency as a neurotransmitter or neurotoxin, will induce limbic status epilepticus when administered in rats systemically or by intra-amygdaloid injection (Olney, Rhee & Ho 1974). The seizures are stereotyped, beginning 15 minutes after intra-amaygda injection with staring or facial grimaces, then progressing within a further 10–15 minutes to repetitive episodes of rearing on hindlimbs with copious salivation and sustained clonus of the forepaws and head. These seizure episodes last for more than 1 hour. Pathological examination reveals a disseminated pattern of acute brain damage, including several thalamic and amygdala nuclei, piriform, entorhinal, insular and sensorimotor cortices, the hippocampus and lateral septum. The vulnerability of the hippocampus to the effects of systemically injected kainate was quickly recognised, and has been repeatedly confirmed. The acute changes comprise loss of the spines and branches of dendrites, in the CA3 and CA4 regions particularly, and the neurones most affected are those with the greatest dendritic density of glutamate receptors. The extent of damage correlates with the severity and duration of the seizure activity (Olney, Fuller & de Gubareff 1979; Olney *et al.* 1980; Olney, de Gubareff & Sloviter 1983*a*). Cholinergic agents injected into the rat amygdala produce a similar pattern of brain damage and seizures (Olney, de Gubareff & Labruyère 1983*b*). Ben-Ari

(1985) suggested that the intra-amygdaloid injection of kainic acid produces powerful paroxysmal discharges in the entorhinal cortex, to which the amygdala heavily projects, and that this discharge produces an excitatory action on the CA3 neurones primarily via the granule cells and their mossy fibres. Similar pathological findings have been reported in other experimental status epilepticus models (Ben-Ari *et al.* 1980; Lothman & Collins 1981; Nadler 1981; Collins, Olney & Lothman 1983; Sloviter 1983; Ben-Ari 1985; Soderfeldt *et al.* 1983; Wasterlain *et al.* 1993). In marmosets (*Callithrix* sp.) and baboons, kainate-induced focal seizures produce acute ischaemic cell changes and later neuronal loss and gliosis in the end folium and Sommer sector, and less consistently in restricted regions of the orbitofrontal and occipital cortices (Menini *et al.* 1980; Meldrum 1983). This damage occurs despite the fact that systolic pressure, and blood glucose are unchanged by the seizures, and that seizure activity is restricted to the hippocampus and hypothalamus. This body of experimental work provides strong evidence that restricted focal limbic status can result in neuronal damage, which intriguingly is of the type classically associated with temporal lobe epilepsy. It is known that kainate itself has an excitotoxic action, but this intrinsic cytotoxicity is not responsible directly for cell damage. Ben-Ari *et al.* (1980), for instance, have shown in rats that the remote neuronal damage induced by focal kainate acid injection can be abolished by the anticonvulsant diazepam.

Other experimental models have also shown the potential for seizure-induced neuronal damage, the most convincing of which are those models where 'remote' damage is produced by seizure spread, and thus where the intrinsic damage produced by the experimental lesion can be differentiated from 'epileptic' damage. Sloviter (1983) demonstrated CA3 and hilar neuronal loss following 2–24 hours of electrical stimulation in perforant pathways (a useful model used by others subsequently; see Olney *et al.* 1983*b*). Extratemporal focal seizures also can result in cerebral damage, as shown in the elegant experiments of Collins & Olney (1982), in which thalamic necrosis was observed following penicillin-induced experimental neocortical seizures.

Bertram, Lothman & Lenn (1990) induced status in Sprague-Dawley rats by continuous hippocampal electrical stimulation for 90 minutes and then examined the brains 1 month later. Cell loss was seen in CA1 and also other hippocampal regions, and there was a reduction in overall brain weight, suggesting more widespread damage; interestingly these changes were not seen in rats with induced seizures, without status, even after thousands of seizures. The authors concluded that the cell loss is due to acute damage in status rather than the chronic cumulative effect of epilepsy. Cerebral damage in human status is much more commonly encountered in young children than in adults. Surprisingly, in experimental models of status in the rat and the marmoset monkey, cerebral damage is much less likely in neonatal than in older animals; this may be due to differences in the glutamate receptors in the immature and mature brain. (Fujikawa, Soderfeldt & Wasterlain 1992).

The importance of seizure duration in the production of neuronal damage was reinforced by Nevander *et al.* (1985), who induced status epilepticus by inhalation of flurothyl in well-ventilated and oxygenated rats, of 15–120 minutes' duration. Infarction of the pars reticulata occurred in five of six animals with seizure durations of 30 minutes, and in all animals with longer seizure durations. There was also damage to the central parts of the globus pallidus, but not the substantial nigra. After 45–120 minutes, moderate cell necrosis was observed in the middle layers of the neocortex, and after 60–120 minutes in the amygdaloid and thalamic nuclei and CA4 and CA1 regions of the hippocampus. Rather surprisingly, CA3 neurones and dentate granule cells were not damaged. After 120 minutes of status, damage regularly affected the neocortex and the ventral posterior nucleus of the thalamus. The pattern of hippocampal damage also differs from that induced by kainic acid. Indeed the status epilepticus induced by flurothyl produced much less neuronal damage in the hippocampus than was expected, and this was attributed to adequate blood pressure control and good oxygenation during the status. The authors also speculated as to whether or not the excitatory pathways recruit cell damage in postsynaptic sites. Thus, the damage that occurred in the thalamus was most extensive in the ventral posterior nuclei that project to areas 3 and 4, which also display neuronal loss, and the damage of the hippocampus may represent the affectation of the end station of entorhinal cortex activation via the perforant pathway. These experiments clearly establish that seizure activation is responsible for cell damage. However, some hypermetabolic structures were not damaged, and other factors must also be involved in determining whether or not cell damage will result; Nevander *et al.* speculated that this may relate to the characteristics of postsynaptic receptor function, a proposition yet to be fully explored. However, flurothyl probably acts by opening sodium channels, and the differences in the distribution and type of cellular damage may be due to this specific cellular mechanism, a problem of model and species specificity that complicates all research in this field.

The differences between the cerebral damage induced by seizure activity, hypoglycaemia and hypoxia have also been the subject of intensive study (see Siesjö & Wieloch 1986; Auer & Siesjö 1988). All three insults cause cerebral damage which is distinct in degree, distribution, timing and in mechanism (see table 4.2). Ischaemic damage was the most marked and extensive, and develops most rapidly, the damage due to status was the least severe and slowest to occur. In status, cellular damage is maximal in CA1, CA3 and CA4 regions of the hippocampus, layers III and IV of the cortex, cerebellum, and the substantia nigra; in hypoxia, a different and variable pattern is seen, usually affecting small pyramidal cells in layer III and to a lesser extent other layers of the neocortex, the subiculum, CA1, CA3 and CA4 regions in the hippocampus, substantia nigra, the Purkinje cells in the cerebellum, brain stem and caudate and putamen; in hypoglycaemia, the subiculum, CA1, layers II and III of the neocortex, dentate gyrus, caudate and putamen (table 4.3). At a cellular level, all three share similar excitotoxic processes, which probably form the final common pathway of cell damage; each causes glutamate release, the influx of calcium into cells, lipolysis with accumulation of free fatty acids, and proteolysis. Nevertheless, other neurochemical differences exist; in status, for instance, energy failure does not occur, although cerebral blood

Table 4.2. *Comparison of the extent of cerebral damage caused by ischaemia, hypoglycaemia and status epilepticus in the rat: density of neuronal necrosis*

Condition	Individual animals					
	Mean	1	2	3	4	5
Ischaemia						
6 min	45	12	164	22	1	—
10 min	2657	3500[a]	7000[b]	87	43	600
Hypoglycaemia						
10 min	5	19	0	33	0	0
40 min	635	871	40	1007	624	1481
Status epilepticus						
30 min	0	0	0	0	0	0
60 min	34	70	5	26	79	2
90 min	30	90	0	0	12	7

[a]Cells/coronal section, level of subfornical organ.
[b]Infarcted, hence estimated from neuronal counts of cortical material in identical area.
From Siesjö & Wieloch 1986, with kind permission.

Table 4.3. *Distribution of neuronal necrosis in the rat brain in cerebral ischaemia, hypoglycaemia and status epilepticus (a comparison of three published reports)*

Brain area	Ischaemia	Hypoglycaemia	Status epilepticus
Cerebral cortex			
Layer 1	0	0	0
Layer 2	+ +	+ + + +	+
Layer 3	+ + + +	+ + +	+ + + +
Layer 4	+ + +	+ +	+ + + +
Layer 5	+ +	+	+
Layer 6	+	+	+
Caudate nucleus	+ + + +	+ + +	0
Substantia nigra	+ + +	0	+ + + +
Thalamus	+ +	+	+ +
Hippocampus			
CA1	+ + +	+ + +	+ + +
CA3	+ +	0	0[a]
CA4	+ + +	+	+ + + +
Dentate gyrus	+	+ + +	0
Subiculum	+ + + +	+ + + +	+
Cerebellum	+ + +	0	+ +

0, damage not observed; +, vulnerable to maximal insult; + +, vulnerable to moderate insult; + + +, vulnerable to mild insult; and + + + +, vulnerable to minimal insult.
[a] In most models, severe damage also occurs in the CA3 region of the hippocampus in status. The absence of damage in this example may be model-specific.
Adapted from Siesjö & Wielock 1986, with kind permission.

flow is increased and metabolism is greatly enhanced, and acidosis is moderate; in hypoxia, there is ischaemia and almost complete cessation of cellular metabolism, a loss of ionic homeostasis, redox reduction, reduction in blood flow and marked acidosis; in hypoglycaemia, metabolism is reduced but present, redox systems are oxidised, cerebral blood flow is increased and there is no acidosis. To what extent the differences in the distribution of cellular damage are due to regional vulnerability to these various insults is unclear. Acidosis may be particularly important. It has also been postulated that the distribution of cellular damage is dependent on presynaptic inputs, and that the specific pattern seen in status is due to the pattern of neuronal activation. The selective vulnerability of CA1 and CA3 in status, for instance, may be due to the high concentration of N-methyl–D-aspartate (NMDA) and kainate receptors distributed to the mossy fibre inputs in this region. A specific form of human ischaemia which has attracted neuropathological attention has been near-hanging, where hippocampal damage is prominent especially in the region of the subiculum and Ammon's horn (see Markowitsch 1992), and which in at least one case has resulted in status (Dinsmore *et al.* 1985).

Seizure activity also induces long-term (plastic) changes in neuronal function. These include sprouting (reactive synaptogenesis), loss of neurones, synaptic reorganisation, and changes in cellular structure. Whether such changes are important in status are uncertain. Secondary foci in chronic epilepsy have been clearly demonstrated in animal models, and again may predispose to status. These are active areas of current research.

Another question of great importance is whether status-induced cerebral damage leads to chronic epilepsy, and if so under what circumstances. In clinical studies, the confounding factor of underlying cause has complicated almost all attempts to investigate the problem, but experimental studies in animals have been more informative. Recurrent seizures have been repeatedly observed after kainate-induced status in primates, cats and rodents (see Lothman & Bertram 1993). Age may be an important factor, as shown by Holmes & Thompson (1988), who found an enhanced hippocampal kindling response in adult rats who had had status induced during the fourth week of life, even though no cerebral damage was observed on pathological examination. The epileptogenic effect of status has also been reproduced in the model of self-sustaining limbic status proposed by Lothman and co-workers (see Lotham 1990; VanLandingham & Lothman 1991*a,b*; Lothman & Bertram 1993). Here, chronic epilepsy develops in association with neuronal loss (reminiscent of the changes in human temporal lobe epilepsy), and the chances of developing epilepsy are greater the longer the duration of the status episode. Chronic epilepsy can be induced by status in the mature or immature rat, and these experiments at least do not support the view that the immature brain is particularly resistant to the effects of status.

Neurochemistry of status epilepticus

This brings us to the biochemical basis of status epilepticus and of status-induced neuronal damage, both of which have been intensively researched in the past two decades. A recent review identified at least 69 neurotransmitters or neuromodulators (Fisher & Coyle 1991), and this can be considered only an interim list, in this fast moving field. Epileptic seizures can, at the most simple level, be considered the result of inbalance between inhibitory and excitatory influences (either a defect in the former or an excess of the latter), and it is not therefore surprising to find that actions of GABA and glutamate have been most extensively studied. Each has been implicated in epilepsy and in status (for a definitive review of the pathophysiology and neurochemistry of status, see Wasterlain *et al.* 1993).

Caution is necessary in interpreting many of these studies for several reasons. First, there is the danger of a circular heresy; the fact that one substance is intensively studied and found to be implicated in epilepsy does not mean that other substances, not investigated, are not more important. As new chemical compounds are being uncovered in epileptic brain this frequently becomes an important proviso. Indeed, it is perhaps not overly cynical to note that abnormalities have been found with almost all neurotransmitters that have been studied. This is not surprising as the complex clinical expression of epilepsy involves many different systems, and different types of epilepsy have different basic mechanisms. Furthermore, the thrust of research often depends most on the availability of tools and experimental models. Second, study of glutamate will by necessity emphasise excitation, and that of GABA inhibition. Whilst both may be important, the individual studies may not be able to place their findings in the correct context. The principle that epilepsy is 'due' either to increased excitation or decreased inhibition is in a sense a truism, and is too simplistic. A third central problem for researchers in this field is that chemical mechanisms do not result only in epilepsy; epilepsy also alters neurochemistry. The perennial question of chicken or egg, or cause or effect, is nowhere more perplexing. Fourth, is the fact, again unfortunately all too likely, that many of the chemical changes noted in status may simply be epiphenomena, unrelated to the primary epileptic process. Fifth, researchers need to be wary of the regional nature of many pathological events in epilepsy. Chemical changes in the hippocampus may be very different from those in the neocortex, and furthermore observed focal changes may be the result of spread from other distant cerebral events; an example is the thalamic damage due to neocortical seizure discharges, mediated through corticothalamic projection pathways (Collins & Olney 1982) or the distant damage demonstrated in the perforant path model of status (Sloviter 1983). Observed changes may thus be secondary. Finally, the results of animal experimental studies too should be interpreted with caution, as there is no animal model which is an entirely satisfactory mimic of human epilepsy. The generalised seizures of the Senegal baboon *Papio papio* are physiologically closer to humans than other species, but even this epilepsy has no exact human counterpart. Genetically prone rodent models have been a fruitful source of experimental data, but rodents have crucial biochemical and physiological differences from humans. The injection of convulsant drugs to produce status is another animal approach, and, as discussed above, kainic acid, penicillin, allylglycine, flurothyl and bicuculline have been used, producing different pathological and physiological effects. The direct neurotoxic effect of injected convulsants, however, complicates their use in experimental epilepsy. Animal experiments provide data which are specific to the model and the experimental paradigm and the differing findings in the differing animal models of epilepsy are surely an indication of the complexity of epileptic cerebral mechanisms. There are few ways in which the neurochemist, with currently available tools and experimental models, can untangle these complex webs and the interpretation of neurochemical findings and their extrapolation to the human situation should be circumspect.

Inhibitory mechanisms

A recurring theme in neurochemical studies of epilepsy is that seizures develop because of either inadequate neuronal inhibition or excessive excitation. Studies of inhibition have been centred upon the inhibitory neurotransmitter GABA and those of excitation on the potent excitatory neurotransmitter glutamate, and to a lesser extent on aspartate and acetylcholine.

GABA is the major inhibitory cerebral neurotransmitter, and thus almost certainly has an important role in epilepsy. About 30–50% of all central nervous system synapses are GABAergic, and the highest concentrations are found in the substantia nigra, basal ganglia, hypothalamus, periacqueductal grey and dentate nuclei (Fahn & Cote 1968; Fisher & Coyle 1991). There is also a high concentration of GABA in all cortical grey matter and in the cortical interneurones. A large body of experimental evidence supports the involvement of GABA in seizure mechanisms and the production of status, work which can be divided into three categories. First, it has been demonstrated that increasing GABAergic activity in certain brain sites increases the threshold for epilepsy and inhibits the spread of epileptic activity. This has been shown in a variety of animal models. Gale (1989) suggested on the basis of experiments in rodent models that GABAergic transmission in the substantia nigra has a 'gating' action which inhibits seizure spread, and increasing GABAergic activity in the substantia nigra will inhibit limbic seizures and status, neocortical seizures or seizures induced by maximal electroshock (see Gale 1989). Wasterlain *et al.* (1993) have also noted a 50% reduction in the rate of GABA synthesis after 60 minutes of pilocarpine-induced status epilepticus in the substantia nigra of kindled rats, suggesting a rapid utilisation of GABA in sustained seizures. A second strand of evidence comes from immunocytological studies which show loss of GABAergic action in epileptic zones. A loss of GABAergic terminals in epileptic tissue has been demonstrated in primates (Macaque monkey, *Macaca* sp.) (Ribak *et al.* 1986), and also in isolated cat cortical slabs (Ribak & Reiffenstein 1982). Ribak *et al.* showed further by electron microscopy that this GABAergic cell loss is of at least two neuronal types, basket and chandelier cells, and suggest that the subsequent reduction in inhibitory synaptic control over pyramidal neurones may underlie the production of epilepsy. In cobalt foci in cats, Balcar *et al.* (1978) demonstrated lower GABAergic uptake, with no alteration in glutamate uptake compared with normal controls and contralateral control tissue, and concluded that there was a selective loss of GABA-mediated inhibition in the epileptic tissue, although other work has not confirmed this (see Craig & Colasanti 1986). Sloviter (1987), however, failed to demonstrate a similar

167

loss of GABAergic neurones in rats after status epilepticus produced by stimulation of the perforant path. In these studies, although there was damage to CA1 and CA3 pyramidal neurones and dentate hilar cells, immunochemical analysis showed somatostatin rather than GABAergic immunoreactivity. Sloper, Johnson & Powell (1980) demonstrated in monkeys that the induction of hypoxia produces selective loss of the GABAergic cells which form symmetrical synapses in the neocortex, although similar studies from human surgical tissue are less easy to interpret (Morin & Westerlain 1983; Sherwin *et al.* 1984; Babb & Brown 1986; Lloyd *et al.* 1986; de Lanerolle & Spencer 1991). Third, GABA agonists and prodrugs are generally anticonvulsant and GABA antagonists generally convulsant. Indeed, it was on this basis that drugs such as γ-vinyl-GABA and progabide were developed for clinical use. There are, however, exceptions even to this simple rule (Fariello *et al.* 1991). Although effective in preventing some focal seizures, muscimol and THIP (4,5,6,7-tetrahydroxyisoxazolopyridine), both potent GABA agonists, induce epileptic discharges in the baboon model (Meldrum & Horton 1980), and the infusion of muscimol into rat substantia nigra enhances seizure activity (Sperber *et al.* 1987). These and other paradoxical findings may be due to differences in the mechanisms of focal and generalised seizure models (especially in absence seizures) or to variations in regional susceptibility to GABA; nevertheless, they are evidence against the unitary theory that loss of GABAergic inhibition is the basis of seizure generation (Roberts 1986). In the genetically epilepsy-prone rat and gerbil, GABAergic cell numbers and immunoreactivity are increased, and the epilepsy may be due to enhanced GABAergic inhibition of other inhibitory cells (Ribak 1986). To confound the situation further, it is possible in human epilepsy at least that the loss of GABAergic neurones is the result, not the cause of seizures. Many therapies used in status potentially modify GABA receptor activity, and it seems likely that GABA-mediated inhibition is important in either the generation or termination of status or in inhibition of spread of seizures (Gale 1989), and the ubiquitous inhibitory role of GABA in cerebral function would support this contention. It has to be admitted though that in view of the sizeable body of conflicting animal and human evidence, the simple hypothesis that epilepsy is solely due to loss of GABAergic inhibition is clearly untenable (Fariello *et al.* 1991).

Excitatory mechanisms

In the past decade, the attention of experimental neurochemists has turned from inhibitory to excitatory mechanisms (Olney 1985; Fisher 1991*b*) in the quest to uncover the basis of seizure generation and of seizure-related neuronal damage. The amino acid glutamate has a concentration in mammalian brain of about 5 mM. It is present in many parts of the brain, and has many functions, amongst which is its role as the primary excitatory neurotransmitter in the central nervous system; although only a small part of intracerebral glutamate is involved in synaptic transmission. Since the observation by Hayashi (1954) that the topical cerebral application of glutamic acid in animals and humans produced paroxysmal discharges, there has been interest in its role in both the generation and spread of epileptic activity both in seizures and in status, and its role in status-related cell damage. In the past decade or so, this work has been at the centre of basic neurochemical research in status, not least because of the discovery that kainic acid (a glutamate analogue) can produce a useful animal model of limbic status epilepticus (Olney *et al.* 1974).

The neurotransmittor actions of glutamate are complex, and to date at least five subtypes of the glutamate receptor have been demonstated (Wasterlain *et al.* 1993). The most studied is the NMDA receptor, perhaps largely because a family of potent selective antagonists such as 2-amino-5-phosphonopentanoic acid (AP5) are available. Glutamate (and the closely related amino acid aspartate) are endogenous ligands in mammalian brain, but it also likely that other compounds have actions at the same receptor sites, and the neurochemistry of these excitatory receptor regions is not fully understood (Lehmann *et al.* 1991).

Three strands of neurochemical evidence can be adduced for implicating glutamate in the process of epileptogenesis. First, there is the repeatedly demonstrated point that glutamate, aspartate and related compounds are potent convulsants. The intracerebral injection of glutamate (Stone & Javid 1983), quisqualate, NMDA and homocysteic acid (Coyle 1987) result in fulminant seizures or status, and the systemic or local administration of kainic acid produces focal seizures and status (Olney *et al.* 1974; Nadler 1981; Ben-Ari 1985). There can be no doubting the convulsant potential of any of these compounds. The second line of evidence has been more difficult to interpret. A series of studies have attempted to show increased synaptic release of glutamate or an increased concentration of glutamate in epileptic tissue, with variable success. Differing results have been reported in different species and animal models, with some studies reporting increases, decreases or absence of change (van Gelder 1986; Fisher 1991*a*; Lehmann 1987). For instance, after 2 hours of status induced by folate injection into amygdala in a rabbit, a 50–75% increase in extracellular glutamate concentrations was measurable in the hippocampus, by using small-diameter brain dialysis probes (Lehmann 1987). However, Lehmann *et al.* (1985) in both kainic acid and bicuculline-induced seizure models, and Fujikawa & Cheung (1991) in pilocarpine-induced seizures, failed to detect any increase in extracellular glutamate levels. This might have been due to efficient reuptake, and until a more satisfactory method of determining glutamate turnover is developed this question remains unresolved (Lehmann *et al.* 1985). Similarly, in surgically excised human epileptic tissue, reports of glutamate concentrations are conflicting (van Gelder, Sherwin & Rasmussen 1972; Perry & Hansen 1981; Sherwin *et al.* 1984; Sherwin & van Gelder 1986). In the large series of cortical excisions from Montreal (Sherwin *et al.* 1988), however, glutamate (and aspartate and glycine) concentrations were increased in spiking areas, whereas GABA (and taurine) levels were unchanged. There are critical methodological issues in both the animal and human work which also may strongly influence the validity and interpretations of the published findings (see Sherwin 1988; Fisher 1989, 1991*a,b*). The third line of research has concentrated upon the potential anticonvulsant action of glutamate receptor antagonists. Both competitive and noncompetitive NMDA antagonists (including AP5, AP7, ketamine, dextrophan, dextromethorphan, γ-D-glutamylaminomethylsulphonic acid, CPP-ene, CGS 19755, MK-801) have shown anticonvulsant activity *in vitro* and in a variety of animal seizure models (e.g. Ormandy, Jope & Snead 1989; Bertram & Lothman 1990; Sparenborg *et al.* 1992). There is to date only a single trial of an NMDA antagonist in human epilepsy (Troupin *et al.* 1986) where subtoxic doses of MK-801 showed a modest effect. The matter is complicated by the fact that the anticonvulsant value of the NMDA receptor blockers does not strongly correlate with the receptor affinity of the drugs, which also have other neuropharmacological effects.

In status epilepticus, neurochemical research has been focused not only on the mechanism of seizure activity but also on the role of excitatory transmission in the cellular damage induced by status, and the findings have been of great interest. The simple postulation is that glutamate and aspartate, excessively released during status, act as chemical mediators of status-induced cellular damage. There are a number of strands of evidence supporting this view. First, the pattern of cellular damage induced by excitatory neurotoxic seizure models (e.g. kainic acid-induced status) has been repeatedly shown to resemble that found in human status, both microscopically and ultrastructurally (see Olney *et al.* 1979; Meldrum & Corsellis 1984; Ben Ari 1985; Ben-Ari *et al.* 1986; Nadler *et al.* 1986; Olney 1986; Sloviter 1986; Fisher 1989; Holmes 1991). These effects can be demonstrated, with identical ultrastructural findings (Olney 1986), by local injections of glutamate receptor agonists, systemic administration of drugs such as kainic acid, and also by stimulation of distant sites (for instance the perforant path which is the principal putative glutamate excitatory input pathway to the hippocampus; Sloviter 1983). Second, NMDA receptor antagonists can inhibit the neuronal damage in experimentally induced status; again demonstrable in a variety of animal models with focal, systemic and distant epileptogenic excitation (see Ben-Ari *et al.* 1979, 1980, 1986; Nadler *et al.* 1986; Olney, Collins & Sloviter 1986; Sloviter 1986). Ben-Ari *et al.* (1980), for instance, in rats with status induced by intra-amygdaloid kainic acid injection, found that diazepam abolished both the epileptic events and the neuronal loss usually seen in the lateral septum, claustrum and contralateral cortex and hippocampus. The lesions in the mesial thalamic structures and the ipsilateral hippocampus were also reduced. Prior transection of the perforant path, ipsilateral to the kainic acid injection also decreased the severity of the electrographic and motor effects of the toxin and reduced the extent of the distant (remote) pathological brain damage. Neither diazepam nor perforant path transection reduced the damage at the site of the kainic acid injection. On this basis, it was concluded that the anticonvulsant and neuroprotective effects were interrelated. More recently, however, the neuroprotective actions of NMDA antagonists have been shown to be, at least in part, distinct from the anticonvulsant effects. In Wistar rats, Fujikawa (1988), Fujikawa *et al.* (1989*b*) and Wasterlain *et al.* (1993) injected the NMDA antagonist AP7 into one amygdala and buffered saline into the other, induced seizures for 3 hours and found widespread cellular damage which included neurones on the buffered-saline but not the AP7 side. Similarly intraventricular AP5 lessened CA1 neuronal damage resulting from kainate-induced status

(Lason, Simpson & McGinty 1988), and TCP protected rat hippocampus from kainate-induced damage without suppressing seizure activity (Lerner-Natoli *et al.* 1991). Fariello *et al.* (1989) in a well-controlled experiment using Wistar/Furth rats with chronically implanted hippocampal electrodes showed that MK-801 pretreatment worsened the electrographic seizure activity induced by systemic kainic acid, yet protected against neuronal damage. Fujikawa *et al.* (1989*b*) induced status with pilocarpine in entorhinal-kindled rats, half of which received ketamine 15 minutes prior to the pilocarpine injection: 3 hours of status was induced. The rats without ketamine pretreatment showed neuronal damage in the piriform and entorhinal cortex, amygdala and CA1–4 regions of the hippocampus. Despite continuous EEG spike–wave discharges for 3 hours, the pretreated rats showed no neuronal necrosis. Similarly, Clifford *et al.* (Clifford, Zoramsky & Olney 1989; Clifford *et al.* 1990) showed that in bicuculline-induced status in rats, ketamine and MK-801 administered systemically prevented the degeneration of thalamic neurones caused by persistent seizure activity in the corticothalamic tracts, despite the failure of these agents to eliminate persistent EEG seizure activity. To what extent the excitotoxic effects of seizures are related to seizure activity per se or to related excitatory transmission is at present uncertain; however, these experiments conclusively demonstrate the potential for preventing status-induced neuronal damage, which may prove to be of great clinical importance.

The cellular damage induced by glutamate and other excitotoxic compounds is possibly related to high intracellular calcium concentrations, which have been repeatedly shown to cause cell death (Farber 1981; Meldrum 1986). Calcium entry activates calcium and calmodulin-dependent protein kinases, and cell damage is mediated largely though second and third messenger mechanisms. Griffiths, Evans & Meldrum (1983) were the first to suggest this to be the mechanism of status-induced cellular damage. They showed that, during 2 hours of status induced by bicuculline or L-allylglycine in rats, calcium accumulates in the swollen and disrupted mitochondria in basal dendrites and selected neuronal cell bodies in the CA1, CA3 and CA4 regions, and is associated with largely reversible cell swelling and dark cell degeneration of pyramidal neurones. A more recent autoradiographic study has showed calcium accumulating unilaterally in the CA3 region, the lateral septal nucleus and thalamic reticular nucleus, 2 hours after an ipsilateral intra-amygdala kainate injection which produced limbic status (Tanaka *et al.* 1989). On histological examination, neuronal damage was noted at 4 but not 2 hours after kainate injection, demonstrating that calcium accumulation precedes observable cell damage. The neurotoxicity of glutamate and other excitatory amino acids has been correlated with the extracellular calcium concentrations (Choi 1987), supporting the view that the neurotoxicity of these agents is calcium dependent. Calcium entry into cells may depend on a number of factors of which NMDA receptor function is only one (Weiss *et al.* 1990). However, there is conflicting evidence. Michaels & Rothman (1990), for instance, found that the cytotoxic effects of glutamate on cell culture could be blocked by MK-801, yet the intracellular calcium concentrations of neurones at the end of exposure to glutamate corresponded poorly with eventual survival, and indeed MK-801 actually elevated

Table 4.4. *Cerebral neurotransmitters and receptors which might be involved in status epilepticus*

Neurotransmitter	Cerebral distribution	Receptor types	Action
Cholinergic Acetylcholine	Basal nucleus of Meynert with projections to frontal and parietal cortex, the habenulointer-peduncular cholinergic system, septohippocampal cholinergic system, the striatum (caudate and pallidum), motor nuclei of the cranial nerves	Nicotinic, muscarinic	Excitatory
Aminergic Dopamine	Midbrain: nigrostriatal and mesolimbic systems. Hypothalamus: tuberoinfundibular and hypothalamospinal system	$DA_1–DA_4$	Inhibitory
Noradrenaline	Projections from lateral tegmental area, and locus coeruleus	$1,2,\beta_1,\beta_2$ adrenergic receptors	Inhibitory
Adrenaline	A minor transmitter in the CNS	$1,2,\beta_1,\beta_2$ adrenergic receptors	Inhibitory
Serotonin	Cell bodies in midbrain raphe and diffuse projection to brain and spinal cord	$5HT_{1a}$, $5HT_{1b}$, $5HT_{1c}$, $5HT_2$	Inhibitory
Amino acid GABA	Small interneurones, intracortical circuits via stellate neurones, and projection fibres, e.g. striatonigral tract, hippocampal basket cells, Purkinje and basket cells of the cerebellum	$GABA_A$ and $GABA_B$	Inhibitory
Taurine	Highest concentrations in cortex and cerebellum	Undefined	Inhibitory
Glycine	Highest concentrations in lower brain stem and spinal cord, also in the substantia nigra	Strychnine-sensitive, strychnine-insensitive (NMDA coupled)	Inhibitory
Glutamate	Probably the major excitatory transmitter in the CNS. Ubiquitous distribution within the CNS, including corticostriatal pathway, cerebellar granule cells, olfactory bulb, entorhinal	NMDA (modulated in at least 4 sites), quisqualate, AMPA, kainate, L-aminophosphono-butyrate	Excitatory

Table 4.4. *contd.*

Neurotransmitter	Cerebral distribution	Receptor types	Action
Aspartate	cortex hippocampal–septal pathways Ubiquitous in the brain (distribution as with glutamate)	Unidentified	Excitatory
Other Opioid	Distribution not known. A large concentration in the limbic system, especially the hippocampus	Delta, kappa, mu	Inhibitory

CNS, central nervous system; DA, dopamine; 5HT, 5-hydroxytryptamine (serotonin); NMDA, *N*-methyl-D-aspartate; AMPA, α-amino-3-hydroxy-5-methylisoxazole. GABA, γ-aminobutyric acid. VIP, vaso-intestinal peptide; ACTH, adrenocorticotrophic hormone; TRH, thyrotrophin-releasing hormone.

This list is of the principal neurotransmitters thought to be involved in epilepsy. Other neurotransmitters of possible importance in epilepsy include: the purines (adenosine, ATP); the neuropeptides (cholecystokinin, encephalins, endorphins, melatonin, neuropeptide Y, neurophysin, neurotensin, pancreostatin, secretin, somatostatin, substance P, VIP); and hormones (ACTH, gonadotrophin-releasing hormone, growth hormone, luteinising hormone, melanocyte-stimulating hormones, oxytocin, prolactin, thyrotrophin, TRH, vasopressin).

intracellular calcium concentrations. Similarly, Dubinsky & Rothman (1990) found no correlation between calcium concentrations and outcome in hypoxic cell cultures treated with glutamate. In elegant magnetic resonance spectroscopic studies, Bachelard *et al.* (1994) showed, first, that the increase in intracellular calcium caused by low concentrations of NMDA in the absence of magnesium was slower than the decrease in phosphocreatine, with no changes in ATP, and second, that NMDA caused no rise in intracellular calcium in the presence of magnesium despite a decrease in phosphocreatine. It was thus concluded that NMDA perturbs neuronal metabolism by mechanisms which are independent of the magnesium-gated calcium channels. The situation is more complex than a simple unifying theory will allow. Nevertheless, there is undoubtedly a maze of interconnecting metabolic changes in status, in which calcium has an important if not exclusive role.

In summary, the exact roles of glutamate, aspartate and other endogenous excitatory compounds in the production, maintenance and termination of status is currently uncertain. There are tantalising clues to the central importance of these compounds, but our understanding of the exact mechanisms is imprecise. Excitatory mechanisms seem to play a role in epileptogenesis and also have a part in status-induced neuronal damage, and this second action may be distinct from the first. In the next decade, excitatory receptor antagonists will be developed for

173

human use, and their role in the treatment of seizures and status epilepticus, both as anticonvulsants and also as neuroprotective agents, will be defined.

Other neurotransmitters have been implicated in epilepsy, some in status, although their exact role is uncertain; excitatory transmitters include aspartate and acetylcholine, and inhibitory transmitters taurine, dopamine, noradrenaline, adrenaline, serotonin and opioids (see table 4.4). Status is also associated with breakdown of membrane phospholipids, giving rise to massive increases in the concentrations of arachidonic acid and other free fatty acids, which could be involved in the pathogenesis of epileptic brain damage (Bazán *et al.* 1983). Calcium-mediated changes in calmodulin activity affect neuronal excitability, and could be involved in the prolongation of seizure activity in status (De Lorenzo 1983). Calmodulin kinase activity is also linked to the genetic susceptibility to epilepsy and thus a propensity to status, and also varies in parallel to electrographic intensity as status progresses (Perlin *et al.* 1992). Free-radical release in status is another potential cause of status-induced cerebral damage (see Wasterlain *et al.* 1993). Impairment of protein and DNA synthesis in status has been observed in rats, which could play a part in the cellular damage induced by status and also affect brain development in the neonate or young child (see Dwyer & Wasterlain 1983; Giuditta *et al.* 1983).

CHAPTER 5

Emergency treatment of status epilepticus

There is not a substance in the materia medica, there is scarcely a substance in the world capable of passing through the gullet of man, that has not at one time or another enjoyed a reputation of being an anti-epileptic

(Edward Sieveking 1857)

Sieveking's ironic commentary on the lack of scientific study of therapy in epilepsy is nowhere more pertinent than in the treatment of status. In this chapter I attempt to review objectively the evidence on which to base effective therapy, yet in doing so am aware of the subjective nature of much of this testimony. The main body of this chapter is concerned with the emergency treatment of tonic–clonic status. The specific treatment approaches to the other forms of status are discussed on pp. 287–92.

Tonic–clonic (grand mal) status epilepticus is a feared condition, and rightly so for death or serious morbidity are common sequels. Treatment is urgent because outcome is related directly to the duration of status, and because therapy becomes progressively more hazardous the longer seizures continue. There are two basic objectives in the treatment of status: first, to stop seizure activity as quickly as possible; second, to maintain adequate respiratory and cardiovascular functions (avoiding particularly hypoxia and hypotension), and to minimise the other adverse metabolic, systemic and medical complications. These objectives are to an extent competitive. Successful therapy is essentially a balance between these conflicting requirements, and attention to one may compromise others. The morbidity of status is often iatrogenic, and much of the difficulty of treating status is in the maintenance of this balance. Treatment should involve the clinical pharmacologist as well as the neurologist, and, if drug-induced coma is required, also the anaesthetist or intensive care physician; the treatment issues are often complex, and there are great advantages to a team approach to management.

General measures

The treatment of tonic–clonic status is not simply the correct application of antiepileptic drugs. Of equal importance are general measures (listed in table 5.1) necessary to minimise adverse physiological changes (see pp. 54–61 and table 3.6), to maintain adequate cardiorespiratory function and metabolic homeostasis,

175

Table 5.1. *General measures in the emergency management of tonic–clonic status epilepticus*

Stage 1 (0–10 minutes)
Assess cardiorespiratory function (especially hypoxia and hypotension)
Secure airway, administer oxygen, resuscitate

Stage 2 (0–60 minutes)
Initiate emergency antiepileptic drug therapy
Initiate regular monitoring
Set up intravenous lines in large veins
Draw 50–100 ml of blood for emergency investigations (see the text)
Administer glucose (50 ml of 50% (w/v) solution) and/or thiamine (250 mg as i.v. High
   Potency Parenterovite) where appropriate
Treat acidosis, where appropriate

Stage 3 (0–60 to 90 minutes)
Establish aetiology
Initiate pressor therapy, where appropriate
Correct physiological derangements and medical complications

Stage 4 (30–90 minutes)
Transfer to ITU, and establish intensive care monitoring
Initiate seizure and EEG monitoring
Initiate intracranial pressure monitoring where appropriate
Initiate maintenance antiepileptic therapy

These four stages should be followed chronologically. The above measures are a guide
only, and apply to a typical patient presenting as an emergency to an accident and
emergency department. Requirements clearly vary and in other clinical circumstances
transfer to ITU might be needed earlier or, occasionally, later.

i.v., intravenous.

to establish aetiology and to monitor medical and neurological function. Clinical
circumstances will dictate action, but in the typical new patient in severe status,
presenting to a hospital accident and emergency department, it is helpful to consider management in a series of stages.

Cardiorespiratory function and resuscitation

Hypoxia is the first physiological variable to attend to in status. In all new patients,
cardiorespiratory assessment and resuscitation should precede other activity. The
airway should be secured and oxygen administered. Almost always, hypoxia is
more severe than is anticipated on usual clinical grounds and artificial ventilation
is needed earlier than expected (particularly in settings where most respiratory
failure is pulmonary in origin, where assisted ventilation is a late requirement).
The principles and methods of resuscitation are similar to those in any other
conditions. Hypotension, which if present early carries a poor prognosis, may also
need urgent correction at this stage (see below).

Patient monitoring

Regular neurological observations, measurements of pulse, blood pressure, electrocardiograph (ECG), and temperature should be made, and the usual surveillance of patients requiring intensive care. In severe established status, more intensive monitoring is mandatory and includes intra-arterial blood pressure, capnography, oximetry, central venous pressure and Swan–Ganz monitoring. Metabolic abnormalities may cause status, or develop during its course, and biochemical, blood gases, pH, clotting and haematological measurements should also be taken regularly.

Rigorous attention to nursing care of the convulsing, sweating, comatose patient is vital to prevent pressure sores. Tracheobronchial secretions may be profuse, and bronchial obstruction is a significant risk in status. The airway must be carefully protected, nutrition maintained (parenterally if necessary) and medical complications avoided.

Intravenous lines

Secure intravenous lines should be set up for fluid replacement and drug administration. Most drugs used in status are more likely to be precipitated if added to 5% glucose than to 0.9% sodium chloride (normal saline) solutions. Drugs should not be mixed, and if two antiepileptic drugs are needed (e.g. phenytoin and diazepam) two intravenous lines should be sited. The lines should be in large veins, as many antiepileptic drugs cause severe phlebitis and thrombosis at the site of infusion. Arterial lines must never be used for drug administration, as intra-arterial injection of most of the antiepileptic drugs used in status can cause severe arterial spasm and necrosis.

Emergency investigations

Blood should be drawn for the emergency measurement of blood gases, sugar, renal and liver function, calcium and magnesium levels, full haematological screen (including platelets), and anticonvulsant levels. Serum (50 ml) should also be saved for future analysis especially if the cause of the status is uncertain. Blood clotting measurements should be made if there is any suspicion of disseminated intravascular coagulation, or other clotting abnormalities. Other emergency tests may be necessary, depending on the clinical setting.

Intravenous glucose and thiamine

Hypoglycaemia (usually due to insulin overdose) may precipitate status, and glucose (50 ml of a 50% glucose solution) should be given immediately by intravenous injection if this is suspected, preferably after blood is drawn for sugar estimation. Intravenous glucose will very rapidly halt seizures in this situation. If there is a history of alcoholism, or other compromised nutritional states, 250 mg of thiamine (e.g. as the high potency intravenous formulation of Parenterovite, 10 ml of which contains 250 mg) should also be given intravenously. This is particularly important if glucose has been administered, as a glucose infusion increases the risk of

Wernicke's encephalopathy in susceptible patients. Intravenous high dosage thiamine should be given slowly (e.g. 10 ml of High Potency Parenterovite over 10 minutes), with facilities for treating anaphylaxis, as occasionally the infusion causes an acute allergic reaction. Routine glucose administration in non-hypoglycaemic patients should be avoided as there is often a transient hyperglycaemia at the onset of status, and iatrogenic hyperglycaemia can aggravate neuronal damage. Later in prolonged status, hypoglycaemia is common, and glucose supplementation should be given if glucose concentrations fall below normal.

Acidosis

Lactic acidosis is almost invariable in status and can contribute to cardiovascular collapse. Intravenous bicarbonate therapy has been advocated to prevent shock, but its value is unproven in status. Adequate respiratory and metabolic support, and the abolition of convulsive movements will usually suffice to prevent pronounced acidosis.

Aetiology

The underlying cause of the status should be established (see tables 3.7 and 3.8 and pp. 66–76). Investigations depend on clinical circumstances, and particularly on whether or not prior epilepsy was present, and on age. If the cause of status is obscure, computed tomography (CT) scanning is advisable, and where this can be carried out safely, examination of the cerebrospinal fluid (CSF).

If the status has been precipitated by drug withdrawal, the immediate restitution of the withdrawn drug, even at lower dosages, will usually rapidly terminate the status. The drug should be given by the most rapid route of absorption (e.g. intravenously or rectally for benzodiazepines, intravenously for phenytoin, valproate or barbiturates, or by mouth for carbamazepine).

Pressor therapy

After 30 minutes or so of continuing seizures, cerebral autoregulation begins to fail, and as a result cerebral perfusion becomes increasingly dependent on systemic blood pressure. It therefore becomes imperative to maintain blood pressure at levels which provide adequate cerebral blood flow. For the first hour or so of continuing seizures, systemic blood pressure is normal or even elevated, but in prolonged untreated status, hypotension develops and can become severe. This tendency to hypotension can be exacerbated by all the drugs used intravenously in status, especially at rapid infusion rates, and also by coexisting cardiorespiratory failure. In prolonged status, measures to maintain an adequate systemic blood pressure become crucial. If drug infusion is responsible for hypotension, the rate should be slowed, and if respiratory failure is present this should be urgently corrected; persisting hypotension is an ominous sign. Pressor agents are often necessary in protracted status. Dopamine is the most commonly used, given by continuous intravenous infusion. Dose requirements vary considerably, and dose should be titrated to the desired haemodynamic and renal responses. The usual initial dose is between 2 and 5 µg/kg per minute, but this can be increased to over 20 µg/kg per minute in severe hypotension. Dopamine should be given into a large vein as extravasation causes tissue necrosis. If signs of peripheral ischaemia develop, the infusion should be reduced. ECG monitoring is required, as conduction defects may occur, and particular care is needed in dosing in the presence of cardiac failure. Dopamine does not cross the blood–brain barrier, and so does not sedate. It is available in vials (40 and 80 mg/ml in 5ml volumes), and infusion bags ready for intravenous use (in 5% dextrose, at 0.8, 1.6 and 3.2 mg/ml strengths). It should not be added to alkaline diluent.

Other physiological changes and medical complications

In general, hypoxia and hypotension are the physiological variables which first require urgent attention, but status produces other acute metabolic, autonomic and cardiovascular disturbances which may also need active treatment. The commonest are:

Hypercapnia, which may complicate status, *pari passu* with hypoxia, but (in the threatening; in the setting of intensive care, temperature can usually be lowered by simple non-pharmacological measures.

Hypercapnia, which may complicate status, *pari passu* with hypoxia, but (in the absence of coexisting pulmonary disease) will be reversed when hypoxia is treated, and seldom requires specific therapy.

Pulmonary artery hypertension and pulmonary oedema, which are common in status, have a variety of contributing causes, and may be fatal; therapy should be aimed at lowering pulmonary artery presure, reversing autonomic changes and inducing diuresis.

Cardiac arrhythmias, which can result from injudicious drug therapy, seizure-induced autonomic changes, systemic hypoxia or hypotension.

Disseminated intravascular coagulation, which may develop rapidly, and may require urgent correction.

Renal or hepatic failure, which are both common in status; hepatic disease may be precipitated by drug therapy, and renal failure is usually due to hypotension or severe metabolic disturbance.

Electrolyte and fluid balance, which may be deranged; the fluid requirements of the convulsing and hyperpyrexic patient may be greatly increased, and fluid balance should be impeccable. Dehydration can compromise renal function and overhydration may precipitate pulmonary oedema.

Other potentially serious medical complications can occur and those reported in the status literature are listed in table 5.2. There is no statistical information about their frequency or timing, but in general they are more likely the longer the status continues, the more complex the drug treatment, and the deeper the level of coma. Most could be prevented or minimised by skilful treatment. The longer-term sequelae of status are discussed in chapter 6.

Table 5.2. *Medical complications in tonic–clonic status epilepticus*

Cerebral
Hypoxic/metabolic cerebral damage
Seizure-induced cerebral damage
Cerebral oedema and raised intracranial pressure
Cerebral venous thrombosis
Cerebral haemorrhage and infarction

Cardiorespiratory and autonomic
Hypotension
Hypertension
Cardiac failure, tachy- and brady-arrhythmia, cardiac arrest
Cardiogenic shock
Respiratory failure
Disturbances of respiratory rate and rhythm, apnoea
Pulmonary oedema, hypertension, embolism
Pneumonia, aspiration
Hyperpyrexia
Sweating, hypersecretion, tracheobronchial obstruction
Peripheral ischaemia

Metabolic
Dehydration
Electrolyte disturbance (especially hyponatremia, hyperkalaemia, hypoglycaemia)
Acute renal failure (especially acute tubular necrosis)
Acute hepatic failure
Acute pancreatitis

Other
Disseminated intravascular coagulopathy/multi-organ failure
Rhabdomyolysis
Fractures
Infections (especially pulmonary, skin, urinary)
Thrombophlebitis, dermal injury

Included in this list are only those complications reported in the published literature, and there are undoubtedly others. There are no statistical data regarding frequency or severity.

Seizure and electroencephalographic monitoring

Decisions about drug treatment depend on seizure activity, and so the timing and duration of overt epileptic seizures should be carefully recorded. In prolonged status, the motor manifestations of seizures may be subtle or even absent, and in comatose ventilated patients, motor activity can be suppressed by therapy. In these situations, some form of continuous EEG monitoring is mandatory. Some intensive care units (ITUs) have hard-wired EEG, which provides most information, but a full EEG requires substantial hardware and personnel and in the ITU setting EEG artefacts are common, complicating interpretation. The practical problems of full EEG can be mitigated to some extent, for monitoring purposes, by a customised scaled-down EEG recording using only one or two suitably placed EEG channels. The electrode placement of the customised EEG must first be chosen by characterising the EEG seizure pattern in the individual patient on a full EEG. Alternatively, a *cerebral function monitor*, can be used. This instrument collects data via two electrodes from a single EEG channel. The signal is amplified, filtered to select high frequencies, and then passed through an amplitude compression network to allow recording of wide ranges of amplitude without gain or frequency response adjustment, and finally written out on paper at a rate of 30–60 cm/hour. A typical seizure produces an abrupt increase in the amplitude of the ongoing activity, which returns to normal as the seizure terminates (fig. 5.1).

Burst suppression can also be identified by the monitor, showing a dog tooth pattern (fig. 5.1). If cerebral function monitoring is to be used, it is necessary to customise the recording to recognise the seizure patterns, in every individual case. It has been claimed that the cerebral function monitor is as effective as full EEG in detecting generalised and subtle seizures in status, including nonconvulsive status and prolonged ictal activity masquerading as postictal confusion, but is less effective in focal status (Altafullah, Asaikar & Torres 1991). In my experience, however, it remains true that the less clinically obvious the seizures, the less conclusive is the cerebral function monitor trace. Cerebral function monitoring

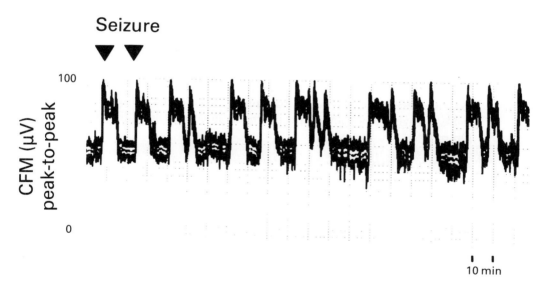

Fig. 5.1. Cerebral function monitor (CFM) trace from a 30 year old female with *de novo* tonic–clonic status epilepticus of uncertain aetiology. On the vertical axis is a logarithmic plot of peak-to-peak amplitude of EEG (μV), and on the horizontal trace time is plotted (the total trace representing 3 hours 40 minutes). The tracing was from early status, showing 15 discrete generalised seizures, manifest by intermittent increases in EEG amplitude. (With thanks to Dr Shelagh Smith, National Hospital for Neurology and Neurosurgery, for preparing this illustration.)

has also been successfully applied in neonatal seizures (Hellström-Westas *et al.* 1985).

BURST SUPPRESSION: This curious and intriguing EEG pattern, first described in 1949 and encountered in various conditions, is a prominent feature of the EEG in patients sedated with barbiturate or nonbarbiturate anaesthetics. It has been suggested that burst suppression may be due to functional (i.e. during barbiturate anaesthesia) or anatomical disconnection of the cortex from underlying white matter, allowing the de-afferented cortical neurones to exhibit spontaneous activity (Fischer-Williams 1963). Whatever the mechanism, the importance of burst suppression in status is that it provides a physiological target for the titration of barbiturate or anaesthetic therapy. It is common practice to advocate a level of drug dosing which will produce burst suppression with interburst intervals of fixed durations of between 2 and 30 seconds (for modern examples, see Young *et al*; 1980, Rashkin, Youngs & Penovich 1987; Lowenstein; Aminoff & Simon 1988 Van Ness 1990). Loading and maintenance dosages of the drugs can be gauged by titration against the EEG, to sustain stable burst suppression activity. It is not clear from what source this arbitrary advice arose, but there seems little reason why the burst suppression pattern should be inherently related to antiepileptic effect; in fact, the two are probably quite distinct. Burst suppression does indicate a certain level of cerebral depression, but epileptic discharges can sometimes be seen against a background of burst suppression. In status, prognosis has not been correlated with achieving or maintaining burst suppression nor indeed have other clinical measures, and there is little theoretical basis for striving to attain this pattern. One suspects its popularity resides in the expedience and practical convenience of a clearly observable measure against which to titrate dosage. Even so, interburst intervals in barbiturate therapy may be quite variable, on stable dosages, especially if the interburst interval is long (Beydoun, Yen & Drury 1991).

Intracranial pressure monitoring and cerebral oedema

Persisting elevation of intracranial pressure (ICP) can occur in prolonged status. Continuous ICP monitoring is advisable especially in children, whenever this is severe or progressive. The need to lower intracranial pressure is usually determined by the underlying cause, rather than by the severity of the status. Intermittent positive pressure ventilation is commonly used, as is high dose corticosteroid therapy (4 mg dexamethasone every 6 hours), although steroids can complicate other therapy and their effectiveness is uncertain. Mannitol infusion in adults is usually reserved for temporary respite for patients in danger of tentorial coning and occasionally neurosurgical decompression is required.

Antiepileptic drug pharmacokinetics in status epilepticus

A working knowledge of simple pharmacological principles is essential for successful prescribing in status (see, for instance, Greenblatt & Koch-Weser 1975*a,b*; Levy *et al.* 1989).

Drug absorption

Route of administration

In tonic–clonic status, the first priority is to deliver adequate quantities of a drug *as fast as possible* to the epileptic cerebral tissue (table 5.3). Although this is to state the obvious, it is surprising how often drugs are prescribed via routes of administration quite unsuitable to the emergency setting.

ORAL ROUTE: No drug is absorbed fast enough by the oral route to satisfy this requirement.

INTRAMUSCULAR ROUTE: A few drugs can be given intramuscularly, notably paraldehyde and midazolam. Most, however, can not. Neither diazepam nor phenytoin should ever be given via the intramuscular route because absorption is slow and unreliable (phenytoin may in fact crystallise in muscle); yet this is a woefully common mistake.

RECTAL ADMINISTRATION: The instillation of a solution, but not the use of wax suppositories, of diazepam, midazolam and paraldehyde produces reliable and rapid absorption of the drug (fig. 5.2; the same is probably true of clonazepam and phenobarbitone also). Rectal administration is a safe and convenient method, without the local or systemic risks of intravenous administration.

INTRAVENOUS ADMINISTRATION: Most drugs are given in status intravenously; sometimes intermittently, by bolus or short-term infusion, and sometimes by continuous infusion. The advantages of intravenous administration are obvious: bioavailablity is 100%, T_{max} is very short, and there are no gastrointestinal factors affecting absorption. Caution, though, is vital. Many drugs require dilution, but if diluted in unsuitable concentrations or inappropriate solvents may precipitate out of solution (a common problem with phenytoin for instance). Co-medication may also cause precipitation (e.g. of phenytoin if the pH of the solution is lowered); for this reason, for instance, the combined administration of diazepam and phenytoin requires two separate intravenous lines. Drugs such as paraldehyde react rapidly with plastic giving sets or solvent bags, and diazepam and thiopentone, amongst others do so on prolonged contact. The intravenous injection of decomposed or chemically altered drugs may be dangerous, a particular problem with paraldehyde. The rate of injection is critical; too fast a bolus injection may result in massive cerebral uptake on first pass, causing respiratory arrest (e.g.

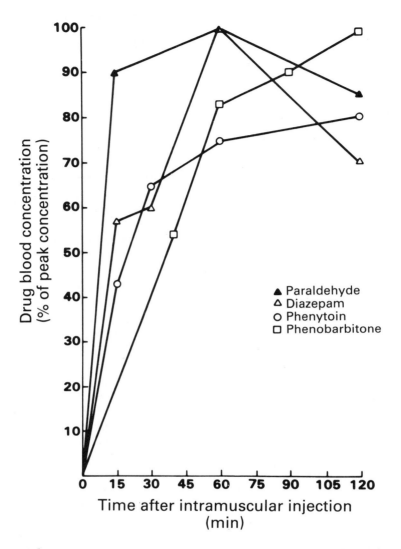

Fig. 5.2. Plasma concentrations of paraldehyde, diazepam, phenytoin and phenobarbitone after intramuscular (i.m.) injection. (From Browne 1983, with kind permission.)

diazepam) or asystole (e.g. phenytoin, by central or peripheral mechanisms). It is essential, when administering any drug intravenously, to monitor clinical and cardiorespiratory function continuously, and be prepared to modify the rate and the dose given.

184

Table 5.3. *Route of administration, lipid solubility and ionisation characteristics of antiepileptic drugs commonly used in status epilepticus*

Drug	Usual route of administration[a]	Lipid solubility[b]	pK_a	Basic/acidic[c]
Chlormethiazole	i.v.	High	3.3	Basic
Clonazepam	i.v.	High	1.5/10.5	Amphoteric
Diazepam	i.v./rectal	High	3.4	Basic
Etomidate	i.v.	High	4.1	—
Isoflurane	Inhale	High	—	—
Lignocaine	i.v.	Mod.	7.9	Acidic
Lorazepam	i.v.	Mod.	1.3/11.5	Amphoteric
Midazolam	i.m./i.v./rectal	Mod.	6.2	Basic
Paraldehyde	Rectal/i.m./i.v.	Low	—	—
Pentobarbitone	i.v.	—	8.1	Acidic
Phenobarbitone	i.v./i.m.	Mod.	7.3	Acidic
Phenytoin	i.v.	High	8.3	Basic
Propofol	i.v.	High	11	Acidic
Thiopentone	i.v.	High	7.6	Acidic

[a] Usual route of administration in status. i.v., intravenous; i.m., intramuscular; rectal, rectal administration.
[b] Lipid solubility figures are based on the octanol/water partition coefficient where this is known. High, >100; Mod., 40–100; low, <40.
[c] pH of the common solution: acidic, anion forming; basic, cation forming.
A dash indicates not known or not applicable.

INTRA-ARTERIAL ADMINISTRATION: No antiepileptic drug in status should ever be given intra-arterially because of the high risk of arterial spasm, necrosis, thrombosis and embolism.

Drug distribution, metabolism and excretion

Drugs are distributed in the body and metabolised in various ways, by processes which can be represented mathematically, and take time to equilibrate. The most important properties determining distribution are lipid solubility, and to a lesser extent the degree of ionisation (table 5.3).

Blood–brain barrier, lipid solubility and ionisation

Cerebral blood vessels are lined with a unique arrangement of endothelial cells (the blood–brain barrier), which allows less molecular transfer than elsewhere in the body, and poses a barrier to egress into brain tissue of blood-borne substances. Only small molecules or ions, molecules for which there are specific transfer systems, or highly lipid-soluble molecules cross the barrier readily. In status, it is the lipid solubility properties of a drug which usually determine the rate of entry into brain and thus the value of a drug. The higher the lipid solubility, the faster will be the time to peak brain levels after intravenous injection. Strongly ionised drugs also will not enter cerebral tissue easily. Ionisation can be predicted from the acidity or basicity of the compound, its pK_a (see table 5.3) and the ambient pH. In status, pH levels can fall progressively, increasing the ionisation of basic drugs (e.g. diazepam) and decreasing the ionisation of acidic drugs (e.g. thiopentone). For amphoteric drugs, such as clonazepam and lorazepam, where neither pK_a value is close to physiological pH, status-induced changes in pH will have little effect.

Distribution of drugs and half-lives

None of the drugs given in status is distributed equally and instantly throughout the body (i.e. the body acting as a single compartment); this is particularly true of lipid-soluble drugs, which are preferentially concentrated in lipid tissue. For this reason, mathematical modelling is necessary to understand pharmacokinetic data, and for most of the drugs given in status, the two-compartment or three-compartment models reasonably accurately describe intravenous distribution data (see fig. 5.3). The central compartment comprises blood and the extracellular fluid of the highly perfused organs (e.g. brain, kidney, liver); the peripheral compartments comprise the less perfused tissues (e.g. muscle, fat). Drugs distribute rapidly throughout the central compartment, and establish an equilibrium between blood and tissue concentrations, but exchange between blood and tissue in the peripheral compartments occurs much more slowly. This movement of drug between compartments can be defined mathematically by identifiable kinetic constants. A two-compartment model will consider all peripheral compartment tissues together, and the three-compartment model will divide the peripheral compartment into a shallow compartment (e.g. muscle) and a deep compartment (e.g. fat). The mathematical models explain the drug concentration curves over time following intravenous administration.

For most lipid-soluble drugs (with linear kinetics) after an intravenous bolus, blood concentrations fall biphasically over time (fig. 5.4). Two-compartment model mathematics provide an explanation for this phenomenon. The first phase largely represents *distribution*, and the second *elimination*. Distribution refers to the rapid transfer of the drug from blood into peripheral compartments, accounting for the initial rapid fall in blood (and brain) level. In the elimination phase, the removal of drug from the blood is dependent on metabolism, which for drugs with moderate or slow clearances (see table 5.4) is a slow process. The rate of fall of blood concentrations over time in this second phase is thus much slower. The three-compartment model is a mathematical refinement, showing differences in drug concentrations in different peripheral tissues. The mathematics of these process have two consequences of the greatest practical importance in status:

1. After a first intravenous injection of lipid-soluble drugs, concentrations are initially very high and then fall rapidly. Initial drug effects are therefore often transient.
2. The concentration v. time curves after initial and subsequent dosages differ

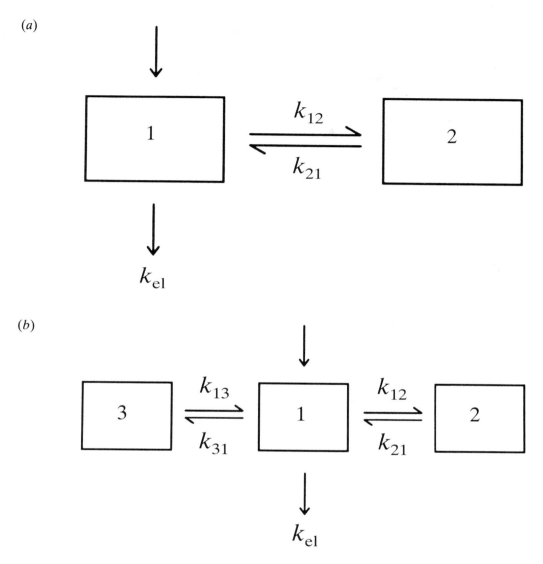

Fig. 5.3. The two- and three-compartment models. In (*a*) the two-compartment and (*b*) the three-compartment models, drug passage in and out of the body is via the central compartment. Transfer occurs between compartments, defined by rate constants (k_{12} and k_{21} in the two-compartment model, and k_{12}, k_{21}, k_{13}, k_{31} in the three-compartment model). Elimination from the central compartment is governed by rate constant k_{el}. The peripheral compartments act as drug reservoirs (lipid stores). Drug concentrations in compartments 1, 2 and 3 can be represented by the symbols C_1, C_2 and C_3. (a) In the two-compartment model, there is considered to be a single peripheral compartment (b) In the three-compartment model there are considered to be two peripheral compartments (one deep and one shallow).

187

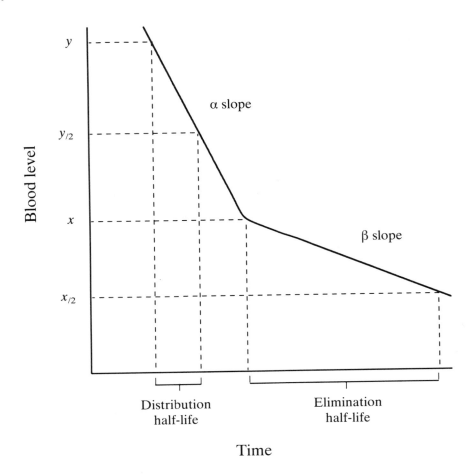

Fig. 5.4. The fall in blood (and brain) levels of a drug after a single intravenous injection (modelled by compartment kinetic theory; and assuming first-order kinetics). The blood levels fall in two phases. The first is rapid (distribution or α phase) and the second more slow (elimination or β phase). The half-life of the first phase (distribution half-life, $α_{1/2}$) and of the second phase (elimination half-life $β_{1/2}$) is the time taken for blood concentrations to fall from y to $y/2$ and x to $x/2$, respectively. Thus, in this double exponential decay, the concentration in the central compartment C_t at time t can be represented by the following equation: $C_t = Ae^{-αt} + Be^{-βt}$ (where $A + B$ is extrapolation of the α slope to time zero, and B is the extrapolation of the β slope to time zero; α is the α slope; β is the β slope).

From this, the approximate α and β half-lives can be calculated by: $t_{1/2α} = 0.693/α$ and $t_{1/2β} = 0.693/β$.

Clearance ($C1$) can also be derived from the area under the curve (AUC), by the following equation: C1 = dose/AUC $_{(0 \rightarrow \infty)}$.

The volume of distribution (V_d) of a drug can be derived from the clearance: $V_d = t_{1/2β} \times$ C1/0.693; thus, the relationship between half-life, clearance and volume of profoundly – even if elimination processes are unchanged. This is because, after repeated dosages, the peripheral tissues contain a larger proportion of the cumulative dose and constitute a 'reservoir' of drug. C_2 can even exceed C_1 so that central compartment (and thus brain) levels are sustained by drug returning from peripheral reservoirs. With administration of further drug, the rapid distribution from blood to peripheral compartments will thus not readily occur, and at this stage, further intravenous injections will cause blood levels to peak as before, but there will be no rapid fall in blood levels. These persisting high levels can produce profound sedation, coma or respiratory depression (fig. 5.5).

The three-compartment model is a closer mathematical model of events for some drugs, and becomes more relevant after prolonged infusion. The skeletal muscle acts as a moderate capacity and rapidly accessible lipid store (a shallow compartment), but other lipid compartments have much greater storage potential (deep compartments, particularly fat tissue). Thus, although a drug may be initially rapidly dispersed to muscle after a bolus dose, there is a strong tendency for the drug then to be distributed slowly to these other lipid areas. When these alternative lipid stores become saturated after repeated dosing, they represent a very substantial reservoir of drug which slowly returns to the circulation, giving very high and persisting concentrations in blood and brain.

The above is a description of conventional compartment theory, which is based on the disposition of drug in volunteers at rest. If an intravenous bolus is given to a subject who is exercising, and there may be a parallel here with a convulsing subject, the pattern of distribution is altered, as the high rate of muscle blood flow brings it effectively into the central compartment; drug concentrations therefore are unexpectedly low and do not decay biphasically (G. Mawer, unpublished observations). In this situation, drug disposition in the convulsive stage of status may be very different from that expected on theoretical grounds, a possibility which has not been explored.

The half-life of a drug is the time taken for its level in the blood to fall by 50%. Where blood concentration decay is biphasic, the half life in the first phase is known as the distribution (or α) half-life ($T_{1/2\alpha}$) and in the second as the elimination (or β) half-life ($T_{1/2\beta}$) (table 5.4).

These considerations are of critical importance in the treatment of status, where large doses of lipid-soluble drugs are being given intravenously over long periods of time. The shorter the distribution half-life, the more transient the initial effectiveness of the drug is likely to be; the longer the elimination half-life, the more likely is accumulation. The dangers of high cerebral concentrations and slow elimination are greater the longer the duration of therapy, and as time passes very careful monitoring is essential.

Caption for fig. 5.4 (*cont.*).
distribution can be represented as follows: $t_{1/2} = 0.693 \times V_d/C1$.

These relationships do not apply to drugs, such as phenytoin or thiopentone, with nonlinear kinetics.

189

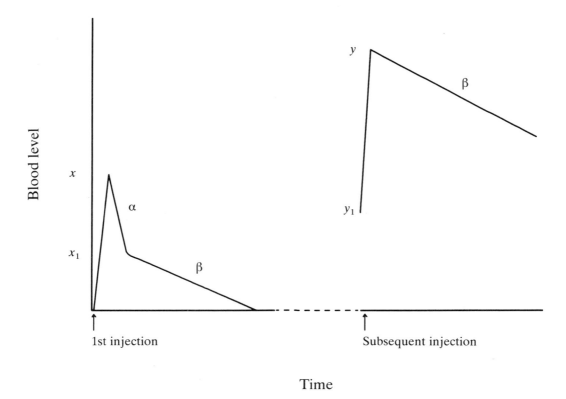

Fig. 5.5. Lipid-soluble drugs: pharmacokinetic differences between an initial and subsequent intravenous injections. After an initial dose, blood levels peak (to *x*), fall biphasically (by distribution) from x_1 to *x*, and then slowly (by elimination). After repeated doses, as the drug accumulates in peripheral compartments, distribution will not occur. Thus, when a subsequent intravenous injection is given, not only is the baseline level higher (y_1), but levels rise to a peak (to *y*) and then fall only slowly (by elimination). Thus persistingly high drug levels result. Such levels will often carry a serious risk of toxicity (e.g. of sedation, hypotension, coma or apnoea). See also figs. 5.9 and 5.10.

Apparent volume of distribution

The volume of distribution is defined as the fluid volume in which the drug would be distributed if a one-compartment model is assumed (i.e. if the body was simply a fluid bag), and can be derived mathematically (fig. 5.4). It is a proportionality constant which relates the total amount of the drug in the body to the plasma concentration. It provides an estimate of the extent of distribution of a drug in tissues (table 5.4). The larger the volume, the greater the distribution (i.e. the larger the capacity of drug reservoirs and the greater the tendency for the drug

Table 5.4. *Pharmacokinetic properties of antiepileptic drugs used by intravenous injection in status epilepticus: approximate adult values*

Drug	Volume of distribution[a]	Distribution half-life[b]	Elimination half-life[c]	Plasma clearance[d]	Class of drug[e]
Chlormethiazole	V. large	V. short	V. short	V. fast	1
Clonazepam	Large	Short	Mod.	Mod.	2
Diazepam	Mod.	Short	Mod.	Mod.	2
Etomidate	Large	V. short	V. short	Fast	1
Lignocaine	Mod.	V. short	V. short	Fast	4
Lorezepam	Mod.	Long	Short	Mod.	4
Midazolam	Mod.	Short	V. short	Fast	4
Paraldehyde	Small	Short	Short	Fast	4
Pentobarbitone	Mod.	V. short	Mod.	Mod.	3
Phenobarbitone	Small	Short	Long	Slow	3
Phenytoin	Small	Short	Mod./Long[f]	Mod./Slow[f]	3
Propofol	V. large	V. short	V. short	V. fast	1
Thiopentone	Large	V. short	Short[f]	Mod.[f]	2

[a] Very large, >4 l/kg; Large, 2–4 l/kg; Mod., 1–2 l/kg; Small, <1 l/kg.
[b] V. short, <5 minutes; Short, 5–30 minutes; Mod., 30–60 minutes; Long, >60 minutes.
[c] Very short, <5 hours; Short, 5–24 hours; Mod., 24–48 hours; Long, >48 hours.
[d] Very fast, >1.0 l/kg per hour; Fast, 0.1–1.0 l/kg per hour; Mod. 0.01–0.1 l/kg per hour; Slow, <0.01 l/kg per hour.
[e] See text, pp. 196–7.
[f] Non-linear kinetics, so figures vary with blood level.

These values are approximations only as published figures tend to vary widely. The values chosen are, where possible, those based on studies of adult patients with epilepsy.

to accumulate); conversely, small volumes imply that little tissue uptake is occurring. It is a useful concept for predicting the dangers of accumulation and determining loading dosages.

Clearance

The clearance of a drug is the rate of elimination divided by the level of drug in the blood (blood level). It is usually given as systemic clearance which is the rate of elimination by all routes divided by the blood level, or renal or hepatic clearance, which are, respectively, the rates of renal or hepatic elimination divided by blood level (table 5.4). Clearance is dependent upon the elimination rate contant (K_e), and is independent of other rate constants (e.g. K_{12}, K_{21}, K_{13}, K_{31}). Clearance depends on such factors as the rate of blood flow and hepatic enzyme capacity (for drugs metabolised in the liver). For some drugs, e.g. chlormethiazole, with rapid renal or hepatic elimination, renal or hepatic blood flow are the major factors determining clearance. For such drugs, the fall in blood flow, common in prolonged status, can result in a rapid and unpredictable rise in blood levels.

Loading dose

The loading dose of a drug (L_d in mg/kg) after intravenous administration may be defined as the amount of drug required to produce a target level. It can be calculated from the following formula:

$$L_d = C_t \times V_d \times W$$

where C_t is target blood level (mg/l), V_d is volume of distribution (l/kg), W is patient's weight (kg).

Thus, for example, the following approximate loading dosages for phenytoin can be calculated (assuming a target blood level of 20 mg/l and a volume of distribution of 0.7, 0.8 and 1.2 in an 70 kg adult, 30 kg child, and 3 kg neonate): adult 1000 mg (14 mg/kg); children 500 mg (16 mg/kg); and neonate 70 mg (24 mg/kg).

Hepatic metabolism

Almost all the antiepileptic drugs used in status are metabolised in the liver, via cytochrome P450-dependent microsomal and to a lesser extent nonmicrosomal enzymes (table 5.5). Metabolism is often biphasic, first a degradation process (e.g. oxidation, hydrolysis, reduction – mainly, but not exclusively by microsomal enzymes) followed by a synthetic process (e.g. glucuronidation or sulphonation). The enzyme activity in both phases is often age dependent, can vary widely in a population (for genetic or constitutional reasons), can be affected by co-medication (either by induction or inhibition of enzyme activity), and may be saturable at dosages used in status. In status, impairment of hepatic function is not uncommon (and may be precipitated by therapy), and can profoundly alter drug metabolism. For some drugs (notably phenytoin and thiopentone), hepatic metabolism is saturable, and above certain dosage rates drug levels will rise rapidly. The microsomal enzymes are often very highly induced by the massive drug exposure common in

192

Table 5.5. *Pharmacokinetic properties of antiepileptic drugs used in status epilepticus*

	Active metabolite	Route of elimination	Protein binding[a](%)
Chlormethiazole	−	Hep[b]/ren/pul(?)	70
Clonazepam	−	Hep/ren	80
Diazepam	+	Hep/ren	98
Etomidate	−	Hep/ren	75
Isoflurane	−	Pul	
Lignocaine	+	Hep[b]/ren	65
Lorazepam	−	Hep/ren	90
Midazolam	+	Hep[b]/ren	96
Paraldehyde	−	Hep/ren/pul	0
Pentobarbitone	−	Hep/ren	60
Phenobarbitone	−	Hep/ren	50
Phenytoin	−	Hep[c]/ren	89
Propofol	−	Hep[b]/ren/pul(?)	97
Thiopentone	+	Hep[c]/ren	80

+, Clinically relevant active metabolites; −, No clinically relevant active metabolites; Hep, hepatic metabolism; Ren, renal excretion (of parent drug or metabolites).
[a] Approximate values for serum protein binding in young adults.
[b] Metabolism dependent on hepatic blood flow.
[c] Hepatic metabolism saturable at normal doses.

status. This induction may develop after only days of therapy and drug dosages may need to be greatly increased.

Active metabolites

Most drugs are metabolised to less active forms, but there are exceptions to this general rule (table 5.5). Active metabolites may complicate the assessment of the efficacy of an antiepileptic drug regimen, particularly if the pharmacokinetic parameters of the metabolite differ from those of the parent drug. Diazepam, for instance, is converted into the body to *N*-desmethyldiazepam, which has an antiepileptic activity about 30% of that of diazepam, but which accumulates with much slower clearance, and so on long-term therapy assumes considerable importance.

Excretion

Most drugs used in status are excreted through the kidney only after metabolic transformation, a process which is directly dependent on glomerular filtration rate (table 5.5). This process is altered in status only if severe renal disease is present, or if cardiovascular disturbance greatly reduces renal blood flow. Paraldehdye and isoflurane are also excreted by the pulmonary route (by exhalation), and are totally unaffected by renal mechanisms.

Blood levels and interactions

Relation of blood level to activity

The blood level achieved by a drug depends on the combined processes of absorption, distribution and elimination; it provides a measure of the amount of drug available for a pharmacological effect. For many drugs the relationship between effect on the brain and blood level is presumably direct, although data are lacking and acute tolerance complicates the issue. For such drugs, target blood levels can be derived, which are often different from those of chronic therapy. The blood level routinely measured comprises both bound and unbound drug. Only the unbound (free) drug is available for uptake and thus for pharmacological effect, which means that, if the bound:unbound ratio changes, the target range of blood levels may not be valid. This effect is relevant in status only in the presence of severe hepatic or renal disease, in which situations the measurement of free levels is sometimes advised.

Steady-state blood levels are those that are reached when drug absorption equals elimination. These have been used to derive most pharmacokinetic measures. In status, as treatment timescales are often short, and as drug dosages are often altered before equilibrium has been reached, steady-state blood levels are not usually relevant. Non steady-state pharmacokinetics make it difficult, however, to predict therapeutic or toxic effects.

Blood levels may be an unreliable indication of activity in status for various other reasons. A bolus dose may expose the brain to very high drug concentrations on the first pass, and venous blood levels may be very misleading. Furthermore, the cerebral effects of some drugs outlast drug exposure. Active uptake or selective binding in brain tissue can also occur, with cerebral levels higher than blood levels, and drugs can also be differentially concentrated within different brain regions. Phenytoin for instance is less concentrated in epileptogenic than in other cerebral tissue, because of gliosis or abnormal receptor binding, which may partly explain its ineffectiveness in some situations despite high blood levels.

Drug interactions

Pharmacokinetic interactions in epilepsy have been the subject of intensive study. Provided that blood level measurements are monitored carefully, interactions are of less importance in the treatment of status than in chronic therapy, because of the large dosages used and the short duration of therapy. Pharmacodynamic interactions (e.g. potentiation, inhibition) may also be important, although little is known or understood about them. Potentiation can result in enhanced efficacy or (more likely) enhanced toxicity; an example of the latter is respiratory depression caused by concomitant diazepam and phenobarbitone therapy. Although most of these effects are recorded anecdotally, there have been few formal clinical studies.

Ideal antiepileptic drug in tonic–clonic status epilepticus

The perfect antiepileptic drug for the treatment of status epilepticus does not exist. The choice of drug therapy in status depends as much upon pharmacokinetics and toxicity as on efficacy, and all the available compounds have drawbacks. The principles of treatment are very different from those of chronic epilepsy; indeed, in status, most of the maxims governing chronic therapy can be ignored. Comparative studies of treatment in status are few, and there is little consensus about optimal drug regimens. It is important to recognise that most published regimens are based on very limited clinical or experimental experience, and much of common practice is arbitrary and unsubstantiated.

Physical characteristics

The ideal antiepileptic drug in status should be suitable for parenteral administration by a route able to provide reliable, fast and complete absorption. This usually means intravenous injection, and of all currently available drugs only midazolam can be given by intramuscular injection, nevertheless, even with midazolam, rates of absorption vary. The drug should be stable in solution, should not react with plastic giving sets, and should not be precipitated by, or otherwise react with, co-medication. No available drugs fulfil all these criteria.

Side-effects and selectivity of pharmacological action

The perfect drug would have a wide therapeutic index: low toxicity at therapeutic doses. In practice, this applies to none of the commonly used drugs in status, which have more or less unselective properties. Three related cerebral side-effects are particularly problematic: *central nervous system (CNS) depression* (sedation), *cardiorespiratory depression* and *hypotension*. Some medications are particularly likely to sedate at initial dosages (e.g. midazolam, chlormethiazole, all anaesthetics); others sedate on prolonged therapy (e.g. diazepam, clonazepam, phenobarbitone). Phenytoin and lignocaine are relatively mild sedatives only. Respiratory depression is a particularly feared complication, not surprisingly, as it may develop quickly and without warning on repeated injections when lipid-soluble drugs saturate lipid stores, or if the intravenous bolus of a drug with rapid distribution is injected too fast. The risk of respiratory depression on initial dosing is highest with drugs with short distribution half-lives (e.g. chlormethiazole, general anaesthetics). On longer term therapy, only paraldehyde, lignocaine and phenytoin seem reasonably free of this effect. Hypotension does not seem to be a significant problem with initial doses of lorazepam, paraldehyde, lignocaine or chlormethiazole, but is a risk carried by all the other commonly used drugs.

Other toxic side-effects of antiepileptic drugs are generally of little importance in the setting of status, where the need to control seizures urgently is of overriding priority, and where intensive drug treatment is short term. Occasionally, however, acute allergic reactions to drugs may complicate management in status (thiopentone and Parenterovite carry a particular risk in this regard).

195

Pharmacokinetics

It is not possible to list 'ideal' kinetics for a drug used in status, although this has been attempted, as different kinetic combinations confer different advantages and disadvantages to individual drugs.

A first essential feature is that the drug enters cerebral tissue rapidly. Usually this implies high lipid solubility and relative lack of ionisation at physiological pH, but not always. The lipid-soluble drugs which enter cerebral tissue most rapidly are those with short distribution half-lives (see table 5.4) and this explains the very short duration of action of, for instance, the intravenous anaesthetics and chlormethiazole. High lipid solubility has other drawbacks, outlined below, and sometimes a drug with modest lipid solubility but with strong cerebral binding characteristics will still have an acceptably fast onset of action, with the added advantage of a more prolonged duration of action (lorazepam and phenobarbitone are examples). Unfortunately, drugs with strong cerebral binding often show a marked tendency to tachyphylaxis, for example lorazepam or thiopentone.

A second desirable feature in status is that the antiepileptic action should be long lasting. Highly lipid-soluble compounds have a tendency to distribute from cerebral tissue almost as rapidly as they have entered it, and, if given by bolus injections, the duration of action may be short (e.g. diazepam, midazolam, intravenous anaesthetics). Obviously, this tendency can be overcome by continuous infusion, but drugs with high lipid solubility given in continuous infusion have a tendency to accumulate dangerously, when infusion exceeds elimination rates. Four classes of drugs useful in status can be identified, based on pharmacokinetic properties and the selectivity of action (see table 5.4):

Class 1: Drugs with a very large volume of distribution, very short elimination and distribution half-lives and rapid clearance (e.g. chlormethiazole, etomidate, propofol). A single bolus will have a rapid onset and short duration of action. The drugs are therefore best given by continuous infusion (or repeated boluses), and the dose can be continuously titrated against response. There is a variable tendency to long-term accumulation that depends largely on clearance.

Class 2: Drugs with moderate/large volumes of distribution, moderate elimination half-lives and clearances, and short distribution half-lives. These drugs will act quickly, have a short initial action, but have a pronounced tendency to accumulate on prolonged therapy and are potentially dangerous where there is low selectivity of action (e.g. diazepam, clonazepam, pentobarbitone, thiopentone).

Class 3: Drugs with a small volume of distribution, and short distribution half-lives. In spite of the short distribution half-lives, the speed of action of such drugs is relatively slow as very high cerebral concentrations are not rapidly achieved. The danger of accumulation is, however, greatly reduced, unless elimination is very slow. The drugs thus act relatively slowly, but are safe on prolonged administration both because of this lack of accumulation and because of their relatively selective action (e.g. phenytoin, phenobarbitone, paraldehyde). The duration of action is long if elimination is slow (e.g. phenytoin, phenobarbitone).

Class 4: Drugs with a moderate volume of distribution, but fast elimination and fast (or moderate) clearance. These drugs carry less danger of accumulation than class 2 drugs, the onset of action is satisfactory, and the duration of action after a single injection is longer than that of class 1 drugs unless elimination is very fast (e.g. midazolam, lignocaine and lorazepam).

Drugs with a combination of large volumes of distribution and slow elimination are not used in status as the tendency to accumulation on prolonged therapy would be too great (e.g. nitrazepam, flurazepam). Ideally also, standard drug doses, should reliably produce therapeutic levels, without great individual variation, although in practice this is seldom the case.

Ideal metabolic properties for drugs used in status are easier to define. First, metabolism should not be saturable, and kinetics should be linear at normal dose ranges (phenytoin and thiopentone are drugs with saturable kinetics). There should be plenty of metabolic reserve, and metabolic parameters should be as little affected by hepatic or renal dysfunction as possible (chlormethiazole is an example of a drug whose metabolic profile is severely affected by hepatic disease). There should be no tendency to rapid autoinduction (barbiturates and phenytoin, for instance, are subject to intense autoinduction), nor should a drug interact with other medication (paraldehyde is a drug with few interactions). In drugs with fast clearance, elimination would ideally not be overly influenced by changes in hepatic or renal blood flow, for instance, as occurs with chlormethiazole or lignocaine (this is an ideal largely unattainable in practice, as the clearance of all high extraction drugs is by definition blood-flow limited). Ideally, metabolites should be inactive, or if active should contribute little to overall antiepileptic effect (diazepam, midazolam, clonazepam, lignocaine and thiopentone all have significant active metabolites). There should be no drug pharmacokinetic interactions.

Antiepileptic action

The ideal drug would be one with proven antiepileptic properties, a very rapid onset of action, and a long duration of action, without acute pharmacodynamic tolerance. In practice, no such drug exists. There have been few if any satisfactory comparative studies in status, and thus comparative efficacy data are scarce. To complicate the issue, some nonbarbiturate anaesthetics used in refractory status have no intrinsic antiepileptic action at all! Nor is it known whether different antiepileptics have specific actions in different seizure types, syndromes or aetiologies.

In the published reports of individual drugs, there is a natural tendency to recommend the drug under scrutiny, a loyalty which renders critical comparison difficult. Thus, diazepam, chlormethiazole, diazepam + phenytoin, phenobarbitone, clonazepam, midazolam, lorazepam, lignocaine, and pentobarbitone all have effusive advocates, as indeed even in recent times have chloral and magnesium. The popularity of certain drugs has undergone changes over time that have more to do with fashion than scientific advance. The most publicised regimens often become the most popular, whether or not backed by solid scientific evidence.

197

Whatever else is needed in status, a rigorous comparison of the current therapy is a pressing exigency.

Stages of drug treatment in tonic–clonic status epilepticus, and drug treatment regimens

It is sensible to divide the drug treatment of tonic–clonic status into stages. There is little divergence of opinion about optimum treatment in the premonitory and early stages, which is simple and usually successful. As status becomes more prolonged, treatment becomes more difficult, outcome worsens, and therapy is based on largely unsubstantiated opinion and prejudice. The need to suppress seizures must be balanced against the risks of heavy sedation and drug-induced coma. In some clinical situations it might be better to vary this balance, sometimes proceeding straight to anaesthesia, perhaps where intensive care measures are already in place; and sometimes delaying sedation in situations where this would be hazardous.

The choice of drugs for each stage is shown in table 5.6 and a scheme of therapy for newly presenting cases in the typical emergency setting, based on my current practice, is outlined in table 5.7 (Shorvon 1993). This scheme is essentially arbitrary, inevitably so in the absence of comparative studies. It is as subjective as others, but based as far as possible on the best published evaluations.

Premonitory stage

In patients with established epilepsy, tonic–clonic status seldom develops without warning. Usually, a prodromal phase (the premonitory stage) during which seizures become increasingly frequent or severe (see p. 53), presages status. Emergency drug treatment in this premonitory stage will usually prevent the evolution into true status. One of three drugs are used, and each is highly effective:

Diazepam is the usual drug of first choice, given intravenously or rectally.
Midazolam is a popular alternative, which can be given intramuscularly, intravenously or rectally.
Paraldehyde is a third alternative, usually given rectally.

The earlier treatment is given the better. It is easier to contain seizures at the onset of status than it is to treat the established condition. If the patient is at home, some antiepileptic drugs can be administered before the patient is transferred to hospital, or in the casualty department before transfer to the ward. The acute administration of either diazepam or midazolam causes drowsiness or sleep, and occasionally cardiorespiratory collapse. Facilities for resuscitation should therefore be available, and the patient continually supervised.

Stage of early status epilepticus (0–30 minutes)

Once status epilepticus has developed, treatment should be carried out in hospital, under close supervision. For the first 30 minutes or so of continuous seizures,

Table 5.6. *Antiepileptic drugs used in status epilepticus*

Antiepileptic drug	Usual method of administration
1. *Premonitory stage*	
Diazepam	i.v. bolus or rectal solution
Midazolam	i.m., i.v. bolus, rectal solution
Paraldehyde	Rectal solution, i.m.
2. *Early status*	
First line	
Lorazepam	i.v. bolus
Diazepam	i.v. bolus
Second line	
Lignocaine	i.v. bolus and short infusion
Clonazepam	i.v. bolus
Midazolam	i.v. bolus
Paraldehyde	Rectal solution, i.m.
Phenytoin	i.v. bolus
3. *Established status*	
First line	
Phenobarbitone	i.v. loading and then repeated i.v./oral bolus
Phenytoin (± diazepam)	i.v. loading and then repeated i.v./oral loading
Chlormethiazole	i.v. bolus and continuous infusion
Second line	
Clonazepam	i.v. short infusion
Paraldehyde	i.v. infusion
Diazepam	i.v. infusion
Midazolam	i.v. infusion
4. *Refractory status*	
First line	
Thiopentone	i.v. bolus and infusion
Propofol	i.v. bolus and infusion
Second line	
Pentobarbitone	i.v. bolus and infusion
Isoflurane	Inhalation
Etomidate	i.v. bolus and infusion

i.v., intravenous; i.m., intramuscular; rectal, rectal administration.
  The list is based on conventional practice, and is by no means exhaustive. In some patients, drugs used in established status may be given earlier.

physiological mechanisms compensate for the greatly enhanced metabolic activity, and cerebral damage is unlikely (see p. 54). This is the stage of *early status*, and one of the following drugs should be used:

Diazepam given by intravenous bolus.
Lorazepam given as an intravenous bolus (the drug of choice at this stage).
Lignocaine given by intravenous bolus and short-term infusion.

Table 5.7. *A recommended drug regimen for status epilepticus in newly presenting adult patients*

Premonitory stage
Diazepam 10–20 mg given i.v. or rectally, repeated once 15 min later if status continues
  to threaten. The injection rate should not exceed 2–5 mg/min
If seizures continue, treat as below

Early status
Lorazepam (i.v.) 4 mg bolus, repeated after 10 min if necessary. The rate of injection is
  not critical
If seizures continue 30 min after first injection, treat as below

Established status
Phenobarbitone bolus of 10 mg/kg at a rate of 100 mg/min (e.g. about 700 mg over 7 min
  in an average adult)
or
Phenytoin infusion at a dose of 15–18 mg/kg, at a rate of 50 mg/min (e.g. about 1000 mg
  in 20 min; with 10 mg diazepam if not already given, infused over 2–5 min). The
  phenytoin can also be given after a phenobarbitone infusion, if this has not controlled
  status.
If seizures continue for 30–60 minutes or longer, treat as below

Refractory status
Anaesthesia, with either propofol or thiopentone. Anaesthetic continued for 12–24 h after
  the last clinical or electrographic seizure, then taper the dose

In the above scheme, the refractory stage (anaesthesia) is reached 60 or 90 min after the
initial therapy. This scheme applies to the typical patient in severe status, presenting as an
emergency. It should be used only as a general guide, suitable for usual clinical hospital
settings. In other clinical settings: the timings may be varied; the early or established
stages can be omitted; and general anaesthesia can be initiated earlier, or occasionally
delayed or avoided altogether.

This scheme is the personal choice of the author for first-line antiepileptic drug
treatment.

Paraldehyde by rectal administration.
Clonazepam: by intravenous bolus.

Each drug has advantages and these are discussed in the relevant sections
below. In most clinical settings, lorazepam and then diazepam (but not both
together) are the drugs of choice. Paraldehyde is a useful alternative to the benzodiazepine drugs in early status, where facilities for intravenous injection or for
resuscitation are not freely available, for instance in nursing homes, where it can
be administered by nursing staff. In patients in respiratory failure, lignocaine may
be preferable. The properties of clonazepam are very similar to those of diazepam.
Phenytoin is sometimes given with diazepam (see below), although in the stage
of early status this is usually unnecessary.

In most patients, therapy will be highly effective. In-patient observation for
24 hours should follow. In previously nonepileptic patients, chronic antiepileptic

therapy should be introduced, and in those already on maintenance antiepileptic therapy this should be reviewed.

Stage of established status epilepticus (30–60 or 90 minutes)

The *stage of established status* can be operationally defined as status which has continued for 30 minutes in spite of early-stage treatment. This time period is chosen, for in most cases, physiological decompensation will have begun after about 30 minutes of seizure activity, and at this stage ITU facilities are mandatory. There are three possible first-line treatment options, all with significant drawbacks, and status by this stage carries an appreciable morbidity.

Phenobarbitone given by intravenous loading at subanaesthetic doses, and then continued by intravenous or oral supplementation.

Phenytoin given by slow intravenous loading, and continued by intravenous or oral supplementation. It is often given at the same time as diazepam (either at this stage or in the early stage of status).

Chlormethiazole given by intravenous bolus and then continuous infusion.

Numerous second-line treatment options exist, including continuous intravenous infusions of *clonazepam*, *diazepam*, *paraldehyde*, or *midazolam*, at various dosages and regimens. Although once popular, continuous benzodiazepine infusions are now not generally recommended. Lorazepam and lignocaine, which are essentially short-term therapies, should not be employed at this stage.

Good comparative studies of these first-line or second-line options do not exist. My personal preference is for phenobarbitone, for reasons given below, although both phenytoin and chlormethiazole are useful alternatives.

If one of these medications does not rapidly control seizures, or if seizures remit and then relapse, a second can be tried, or general anaesthesia (see below) can be employed. It is difficult to be categorical about timing, as this will depend greatly upon local circumstances. Generally speaking, though, general anaesthesia should be initiated if seizures have continued for 60–90 minutes without remission despite appropriate therapy.

Stage of refractory status epilepticus (after 60 or 90 minutes)

If seizures have not responded or have remitted only temporarily, in spite of therapy with one or two of the treatment regimens listed above, the stage of *refractory status* is reached. This is defined operationally as occurring when seizures continue 60–90 minutes after the initiation of therapy in the established status stage, and full anaesthesia is usually required (although as mentioned above, in some situations anaesthesia can and should be introduced earlier, or occasionally delayed). Prognosis will now be much poorer, and there is a high mortality and morbidity. Anaesthesia can be induced by barbiturate or nonbarbiturate drugs.

A number of anaesthetics have been utilised although few have been subjected to formal evaluation and all have drawbacks; five are described in this chapter:

201

Intravenous barbiturate anaesthetics: *thiopentone, pentobarbitone.*
Inhalational anaesthetic: *isoflurane.*
Intravenous nonbarbiturate anaesthetics: *propofol, etomidate.*

The anaesthetics of choice are probably intravenous, of which my preference is for the barbiturate thiopentone which has been widely used, or the nonbarbiturate propofol, which has very promising but essentially untried properties. The patients should be treated with the full range of ITU facilities, including EEG monitoring, and care shared between an anaesthetist and a neurologist. Experience with long-term administration (hours or days) of the newer anaesthetic drugs is very limited. One possible role for these drugs would be to provide initial control while definitive antiepileptic therapy is established. In patients already receiving assisted ventilation and intensive care (e.g. postneurosurgical cases), status is best treated immediately with anaesthetic drugs (without recourse to earlier stage treatment), sometimes given for relatively short periods of time. The nonbarbiturate anaesthetics have little if any intrinsic antiepileptic action (indeed some are proconvulsant), and whether or not this is relevant for anaesthesia in status is quite unknown; this is a conundrum of great importance, yet has not been formally investigated.

Long-term maintenance antiepileptic therapy

Long-term maintenance anticonvulsant therapy must be employed in tandem with emergency treatment in all cases of status. The choice of drug depends on previous therapy, the type of epilepsy and the clinical setting. If phenytoin or phenobarbitone have been used in emergency treatment, maintenance doses can be continued orally (through a nasogastric tube) guided where necessary by blood level monitoring. In the early stages of treatment, however, seizure control has priority, and it may therefore be appropriate to accept blood concentrations which are well above the upper limits of the usual 'therapeutic' ranges. Other maintainance antiepileptics can be started also, given by oral loading doses. It is imperative to establish effective long-term therapy, for seizures frequently recur after initial control in status, and be more difficult subsequently to contain.

Failure of antiepileptic drug treatment

If seizures continue despite emergency therapy, it is important to reassess the clinical circumstances, as there are often complicating remediable factors:

Inadequate emergency antiepileptic drug therapy: The administration of antiepileptic drugs at too low a dose is a common cause of failure of treatment.

Failure to initiate maintenance antiepileptic drug therapy: A failure to provide long-term maintenance therapy, usually by loading dosages given via a nasogastric tube, is a common cause of seizure recurrence after successful initial emergency therapy.

202

Hypoxia, hypotension, cardiorespiratory failure or metabolic disturbance: A failure to reverse hypoxia, hypotension, cardiorespiratory failure or metabolic disturbances will worsen the seizure disorder. It is important to monitor these frequently, as they can develop during the course of the status.

Failure to identify or treat the underlying cause: If a progressive aetiology has been overlooked or undertreated, seizures will continue or worsen. This is particularly true of acute structural or infective disorders.

Other medical complications: A failure to identify and treat complications such as hyperthermia, disseminated intravascular coagulation, or hepatic failure will result in failed seizure control.

Misdiagnosis: The misdiagnosis of pseudoseizures is perhaps the most common cause of treatment failure, at least in specialist hospital practice.

Antiepileptic drugs used in status epilepticus

In the following sections, aspects of the pharmacology and therapeutics of the antiepileptic drugs commonly used in status are outlined. Only those aspects of relevance to the emergency treatment of status are considered and, for a more comprehensive description of antiepileptic drug pharmacology, the reader is referred to the standard texts (e.g. Levy *et al.* 1989; Eadie & Tyrer 1989; Dollery 1991) to which the following is heavily indebted.

Premonitory status epilepticus

Three drugs are commonly used in the premonitory stage of status; all are highly effective: diazepam, midazolam and paraldehyde.

Diazepam

When diazepam (7-chloro-1,3-dihydro-1-methyl-5-phenyl-2H-1,4-benzo-diazepin-2-one; ($C_{16}H_{13}ClN_2O$); molecular weight 284.8) was introduced into clinical practice in 1963 (see Sternbach 1980), a new pharmacological era was entered. Diazepam is a very lipophilic substance, and relatively insoluble in water. The parenteral solution is therefore prepared in propylene glycol and alcohol (Korttila, Sothman & Andersson 1976; intravenous formulation, Valium) or in cremophor EL (for injection or rectal tube formulation, Stesolid), or as an emulsion (Diazemuls). The pK_a is 3.4 (3.2–3.7). Diazepam of course has other clinical uses, for which oral administration is sufficient, but for status it must be given either intravenously or rectally. A knowledge of its pharmacokinetics, which have been subjected to intensive study, is essential for safe and effective use in status. Commonly used commercial preparations of diazepam include Valium, Vival, Diazemuls and Stesolid.

Absorption

Following an intravenous injection of 10–20mg, blood concentrations peak at 700–1600 µg/l within 3–15 minutes in volunteers (Baird & Hailey 1972; Hillestad *et al.* 1974), and sufficient cerebral levels are reached within about 1 minute. In children, peak blood concentrations of about 500 µg/l are obtained at doses of 0.2 mg/kg (Kanto, Pihlajamaki & Tisalo 1974; Agurell *et al.* 1975). In neonates, peak levels of about 10 800 µg/l were recorded after intravenous administration of 1 mg/kg, and 6450 µg/l after 0.5 mg/kg (Langslet *et al.* 1978).

In contrast, intramuscular injection produces variable levels (Gamble, Dundee & Assaf 1975; Meberg *et al.* 1978), which at a dose of 10–20 mg often peak below 500 ng/ml, and peak levels may be lower and more delayed than after oral dosages (levels of 293 ng/ml after intramuscular dosing compared with 492 ng/ml after oral dosing in nine subjects; Hillestad *et al.* 1974). Intramuscular injection into adipose tissue (e.g. the buttocks) should be especially avoided. Intramuscular injection should therefore not be used in status, at least not in adults, although in young children absorption may be better (Meberg *et al.* 1978).

Peak levels are higher and produced more rapidly following administration of a rectal solution of diazepam than after either oral or intramuscular administration. The instillation of 1 mg/kg of the rectal tube solution produces peak plasma levels of 600–1400 µg/l within 10–60 minutes, 10–20 mg levels of 40–340 µg/l, and 30 mg mean peak levels of 342 µg/l (Meberg *et al.* 1978; Knudsen 1979; Magnussen *et al.* 1979; Milligan *et al.* 1982; Rémy *et al.* 1992). In adults, levels peak at about 20 minutes following rectal instillation (Rémy *et al.* 1992); absorption is faster in children, and effective blood levels are usually reached within 5 minutes or so. Suppositories should not be used because of delayed peaks and low peak levels (Agurell *et al.* 1975; Knudsen 1977, 1979; Milligan *et al.* 1982). Bioavailability after rectal administration is variable, in one study being as low as 50% (Magnussen *et al.* 1979). That rectal administration is not totally reliable was also shown by Rémy *et al.* (1992), who measured peak blood levels below 120 ng/ml in 3 of 39 rectal instillations. Bowel movements may also impede absorption and complicate therapy. Nevertheless, in premonitory or early status, rectal instillation is a convenient alternative to intravenous injection; it is safe and can be administered by unskilled personnel, a valuable asset where speed is crucial.

The minimum blood level required to suppress seizures probably depends on seizure type, duration of therapy and other clinical factors, but ranges between approximately 200 and 600 ng/ml in most emergency settings (Ferngren 1974; Rémy *et al.* 1992). It has been suggested more recently, on the basis of preliminary data, that blood levels of 500 ng/ml are required for initial seizure control and 150–300 ng/ml to maintain control (Booker & Celesia 1973; Agurell *et al.* 1975; Schmidt 1985), but in a comparative study in 39 adults with serial seizures, lower levels (mean 257 µg/l) were successful (Rémy *et al.* 1992). Celesia, Booker & Sato (1974) found, in cats, that focal seizures were abolished by brain levels of 4 µg/g (2 µg/ml in serum), generalised seizures were suppressed at lower levels, but interictal cortical spikes at the primary or mirror focus were unaffected by much higher levels.

Distribution

A two-compartment model approximately describes the distribution of diazepam in the acute phase after intravenous administration. After a single intravenous injection (5–10 mg), blood levels initially fall rapidly, and then more slowly, from a high peak to subtherapeutic values (below 200 ng/ml) within 20 minutes (depending on peak concentrations). The initial rapid fall is due to distribution into peripheral compartments (particularly muscle); only 3–5% of the total dose remains in brain tissue (Friedman *et al.* 1985). After repeated dosing, baseline levels are high because of the previous infusions and, as the lipid stores are substantial, decay of concentration by redistribution does not occur. The much slower process of metabolism then becomes largely responsible for the decline in blood levels. Thus, repeated bolus injections produce high peak levels which persist, carring an attendant risk of sudden and unexpected CNS and cardio-respiratory depression. After a single intravenous dose, the distribution half-life is about 60 minutes (reported values between 20–240 minutes; Magnussen *et al.* 1979), although blood levels may rise paradoxically to a smaller peak 6–12 hours after a single intravenous injection, due to remobilisation of the drug and a build-up of *N*-desmethyldiazepam (Baird & Hailey 1972; Meberg *et al.* 1978). CSF and blood levels are equivalent.

The apparent volume of distribution (V_d) of diazepam is 0.8–2.6 l/kg (mean 1.1 l/kg), it is higher in children and in obese individuals (Abernethy *et al.* 1981).

Both diazepam and *N*-desmethyldiazepam are strongly protein bound (quoted values usually between 96% and 98%, with a range of 90–99%). Binding is reduced in hepatic disease and in neonates, but is otherwise little affected by age.

Brain levels of diazepam are about twice those of blood concentrations (Van der Kleijn *et al.* 1983), the drug concentrating in white matter and brain stem structures rather than in grey matter or hippocampus. Both brain level and brain level:blood level ratio fall rapidly (in contrast to lorazepam) in the first 60 minutes after infusion, demonstrating the relatively weak binding of diazepam to

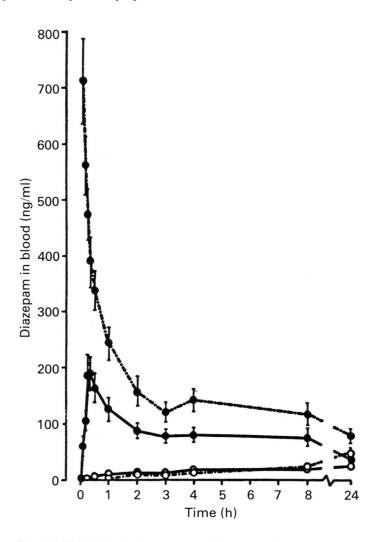

Fig. 5.6. The biphasic decay curve of diazepam after intravenous injection (and a comparison with rectal administration). Blood levels of diazepam (closed circles) and *N*-desmethyldiazepam (open circles) in six adult patients following the administration of 10 mg of diazepam by rectal tubes (continuous line) and intravenous injection (broken line). Note the rapid fall of diazepam following intravenous injection which is due to the redistribution of this lipid-soluble drug. Blood levels fall below 400 ng/ml within 20 minutes. The rectal dose produces levels which are also inadequate (bioavailability was only 50%, which is lower than often found, and might have been due to local factors). Magnussen *et al.* (1979) also instilled 20 mg rectally, and obtained satisfactory peak levels at 15 minutes of 439 (±157) ng/ml. (From Magnussen *et al.* 1979, with kind permission.)

benzodiazepine receptors. The rapid fall in levels is responsible for the relatively short duration of action after a single intravenous injection (fig. 5.6).

Biotransformation and excretion

Diazepam is metabolised by hepatic microsomal enzymes. The major metabolite is *N*-desmethyldiazepam (nordiazepam), which has itself antiepileptic activity of about one third the potency of the parent drug. *N*-desmethyldiazepam has a longer half-life, and if administration is prolonged this metabolite is responsible for a greater proportion of the antiepileptic action (steady-state levels of diazepam occur at about 7–8 days and of nordazepam at about 15 days; at steady state, diazepam levels are about 20–70% lower than those of nordazepam). *N*-desmethyldiazepam levels are generally of little significance in the emergency treatment of status, unless the drug is given by continuous infusion for prolonged periods. Other active metabolites do not contribute much to the effect of the drug.

The elimination half-life is between 18 and 100 hours (mean 20–40 hours). It is about 30% shorter in patients already receiving enzyme-inducing antiepileptic drugs, is not dependent on blood level, shorter in infants (approximately 10 hours) and children (approximately 20 hours), and increased in the elderly (mean about 80 hours) and in the obese. In hepatic disease, the half-life has been found to be greatly increased to a mean of 99–164 hours compared with control values of 23–32 hours. (Andreasen *et al.* 1976; Klotz *et al.* 1977). Both diazepam and desmethyldiazepam can be detected in the blood 6 days after a single 10 mg injection.

Less than 0.5% of diazepam is excreted unchanged (Kaplan *et al.* 1973), between 2.5% and 9% is excreted as *N*-desmethyldiazepam and the rest as 3-hydroxy metabolites and their glucuronide conjugates.

The reported values for diazepam clearance vary from about 0.02 to 0.03 l/kg per minute, but these values fall sharply with repeated dosing, and also are much lower in neonates and infants (see Eadie & Tyrer 1989; Schmidt 1989), and in renal and hepatic disease.

Clinical effect in status epilepticus

Soon after its introduction into clinical use, diazepam was recognised to be a drug of first choice in status (Naquet *et al.* 1965). Gastaut *et al.* (1965, 1967), treating 23 cases, reported 'spectacular and extraordinary' results. Sawyer, Webster & Schut (1968) treated 26 patients, intractable to other medications, and terminated seizures rapidly in 16 and less satisfactorily in 10, noting that acute rapidly progressing cerebral disorders fared worst. Prensky *et al.* (1967) found the drug to be highly effective in 19 of 30 intractable patients, and was uniformly successful in cases without acute cerebral pathology. In five patients, three of whom had received intravenous barbiturate previously, severe respiratory depression occurred. This experience is the basis for the often quoted anecdote that phenobarbitone potentiates the sedative effects of the benzodiazepines. Other reports confirmed these excellent findings in adults and children (Lombroso 1966; Jaffe & Christoff 1967; Lalji, Hosking & Sutherland 1967; Bailey & Fenichel 1968;

Howard, Seybold & Reiher 1968; Wilson 1968; Bell 1969; McMorris & McWilliam 1969; Nicol, Tutton & Smith 1969; Carter & Gold 1970). In 1973, Browne & Penry reviewed all published reports (35 articles detailing 76 case reports), finding lasting control (defined as an uninterrupted control of seizures for 24 hours or more from three or fewer bolus injections of diazepam) in 68% of 188 cases of grand mal status, and temporary control in 20%. Lasting control was also obtained in 73% of focal motor status, 83% of absence status and 62% of complex partial status. The control of primary generalised seizures (at blood concentrations of 0.3–0.8 mg/l) is better than that of secondarily generalised status, and of patients without acute or rapidly progressive cerebral conditions. Schmidt (1985) reviewed all previously published data (table 5.8), and subsequently reported (Schmidt 1989) that a dose of 5–10 mg i.v. at a rate of 1–5 mg/minute will stop seizure activity in 88% of patients. In the only double-blind prospective study, 10 mg of diazepam given intravenously over 2 minutes controlled 76% of seizure episodes and caused side-effects in 12.5% of patients (Leppik *et al.* 1983*a*). A diazepam bolus of 2 mg/minute stopped convulsions in 32% of patients after 3 minutes, 68% after 5 minutes and 80% after 10 minutes, in another study (Delgado-Escueta & Enrile-Bacsal 1983). The large variation in blood levels achieved after a bolus dose of diazepam was emphasised by Treiman *et al.* (1992), who found levels to range from 48.4 to 297 (mean 190.7) ng/ml, at a mean of 38 minutes in 11 drug-naive patients after an infusion of 0.15 mg diazepam/kg. After the rectal administration of diazepam solution, the onset of action is about 10 minutes; seizures were halted in 72% of those receiving 30 mg, and 29% of those receiving 20 mg instillations (Remy *et al.* 1992). Diazepam in common with all the benzodiazepine drugs has a rapid and spectacular effect on EEG, and electrographic activity is usually suppressed within seconds of infusion.

Although clinical seizures are usually rapidly controlled, a substantial number of patients relapse unless additional therapy is also given (55% of initial responders to a single injection by 2 hours; Prensky *et al.* 1967). Mattson (1972) demonstrated this transient effect on EEG graphically. The tendency to relapse is due to a fast initial fall in blood levels. To counter this, it soon became common practice to institute a continuous infusion of the drug after an initial bolus injections. Parsonage & Norris (1967) reported doses of up to about 900 mg over 7 days with a maximum of 200 mg in a single 24 hour period. Although no serious respiratory depression was noted, artificial ventilation was instituted in some patients receiving the higher doses, and acute tolerance to the sedative effects occurred within 24 hours of therapy. More recently, a regimen of 4–8 mg/hour for 3 hours has been recommended in patients who have been electively ventilated (Delgado-Escueta & Enrile-Bascal 1983), and in whom blood levels do not exceed 3 mg/l. Published reports suggest such regimens are safe, but there has been no rigorous evaluation and my own experience suggests that the risks are appreciable. It is quite unclear from the literature how long diazepam infusions can be given safely, although one exceptional patient with eclampsia has received 1.3 g of diazepam by continuous infusion over a 3 day period (Tassinari *et al.* 1983). Delgado-Escueta & Enrile-Bascal (1983) recommended video-EEG monitoring

Table 5.8. *Summary of published reports of the effectiveness of intravenous diazepam in tonic–clonic, absence and partial status epilepticus*

	Total no. of patients	Patients rendered seizure free	
		(*n*)	(%)
Tonic–clonic status epilepticus	224	177	79
Absence status epilepticus	72	44	61
Partial status epilepticus	67	59	88

Some patients had multiple diazepam injections or continuous infusion, and most had additional therapy.
Derived from Schmidt 1989.

and the regular assay of blood levels of diazepam and *N*-desmethyldiazepam in this situation – highly impractical suggestions, the benefits of which are anyway unclear. There are safer alternatives to prolonged continuous benzodiazepine infusions, and this practice has quite rightly largely fallen from favour, at least in situations where intensive monitoring is not possible or facilities for immediate resuscitation are not available. More recently, the combined use of diazepam and phenytoin has been proposed, with the slow-onset long-lasting action of phenytoin complementing the rapid-onset but short-lasting action of diazepam, and this is discussed on p. 251).

Toxic effects in status epilepticus

From its inception as first-line therapy in status, caution has been advised in the prescription of large doses of diazepam. Respiratory depression, hypotension and sedation are the principal risks. Browne & Penry (1973) recorded 16 cases of severe respiratory depression on prolonged usage, including three patients who had also received barbiturates and other predisposed patients. In a consecutive series of 33 patients, respiratory arrest was seen in only one patient, after 15 mg, and mild to moderate respiratory depression in three others at doses of 10 mg (Leppik *et al.* 1983*a*); in another series of 98 patients, apnoea was produced after intravenous injections of 5 mg and 10 mg in two patients with aminophylline-induced and lignocaine-induced seizures (Aminoff & Simon 1980). Although the literature is reassuring about this risk, in normal clinical practice this is still an important problem. The rate of bolus injection is a critical factor, and it is claimed that an injection rate below 2–5 mg/minute will seldom result in serious respiratory depression. The rectal administration of 10–20 mg of diazepam in adults has not been reported to alter respiratory function. Hypotension was noted in 10 patients in the review of Browne & Penry (1973), and is usually severe only when associated with respiratory depression. Nevertheless, occasionally unexpected and profound hypotension can occur, an example is the patient reported by Sawyer *et al.* (1968), whose blood pressure dropped from 160/80 to 85/40 after a second

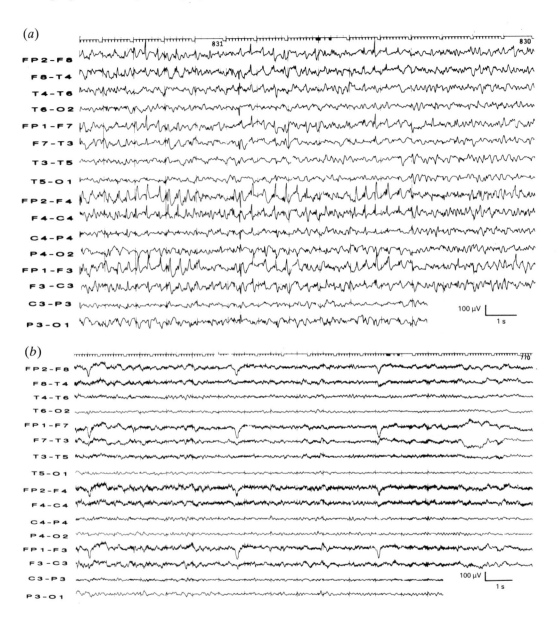

Fig. 5.7 (*a*) and (*b*). Scalp EEG from a 37 year old male with a history of cryptogenic complex partial and secondarily generalised seizures, of frontal lobe origin, since the age of 2 years. He experiences frequent serial seizures and episodes of complex partial and tonic–clonic status epilepticus. The EEG shows the effect of diazepam in a period of complex partial status. The patient was obtunded and confused and the EEG showed generalised epileptic activity (trace a). Diazepam (10 mg) was given

10 mg intravenous injection of diazepam given 10 minutes after a first (the patient had received 200 mg of amylobarbitone 4 hours earlier). Mild to severe hypotension or temporary respiratory depression was reported in 5.2% of 246 patients receiving multiple therapy, including one fatal case (Schmidt 1985). Sedation is common following intravenous or rectal administration of diazepam. Mild sedation is seen in over half of patients given 10 mg intravenously, although rapid tolerance is observable within 24 hours. In a well-controlled study of 15 nonepileptic patients undergoing cardiac catheterisation, light sleep followed 5–10 mg injections (given over 3 minutes) within 2 minutes, lasting 10–30 minutes in all cases. In 8 of the 15 patients, arterial blood pressure dropped by 10 mmHg or more. Pulmonary artery pressure, heart rate, stroke volume and pulmonary or systemic resistances did not change. Hypoventilation was noted in all cases, with a mean 28% decrease in ventilation, and 23% in tidal volume. Although the respiratory consequences are potentially serious, the cardiac effects of diazepam infusion were considered mild (Dalen *et al.* 1969). Facilities for resuscitation are clearly advisable when giving intravenous diazepam.

Thrombophlebitis occurred in 3.5% of over 1500 intravenous injections given during gastroscopy by Langdon, Harlan & Bailey (1973), and may have been due to precipitation caused by rapid injection (Jusko, Gretsch & Gassett 1973). The incidence of phlebitis is minimised by using Diazemuls. Other side-effects are insignificant.

Administration and dosage in status epilepticus

In status, bolus intravenous doses of the Diazemuls preparation of diazepam should be given in an undiluted form at a rate of 2–5 mg/minute.

If an intravenous infusion is administered, the solution should be freshly prepared, as diazepam is absorbed by polyvinylchloride plastics. In a study of this problem, 95% of diazepam activity was lost after standing in dilution in an intravenous fluid bag for 24 hours (MacKichen, Duffner & Cohen 1979). Furthermore, the infusion should be carefully mixed, and 20 mg of diazepam (Valium) should not be dissolved in less than 250 ml of solvent (4% dextrose, 0.18% sodium chloride), as there is a danger of precipitation at higher concentrations. Diazemuls can be diluted in 5% or 10% dextrose solution to a maximum concentration of 200 mg in 500 mg, and Stesolid to a maximum 10 mg in 200 ml of dextrose-saline. Whichever preparation is used, a fresh solution should be made up within 6 hours.

Diazepam may be given rectally, either in its intravenous preparation infused

Caption for fig. 5.7 (*cont.*).
intravenously, and within 10 minutes the EEG became almost normal and the patient's clinical condition resolved (trace b). This is a classical response of status to diazepam. In other cases the effect is less clear cut, and the benzodiazepine drug will normalise neither the EEG nor the clinical state (see for instance figs. 3.9 and 3.16). Furthermore, the correlation between EEG and clinical resolution may not be as clear cut as in this example. (With thanks to Dr David Fish, National Hospital for Neurology and Neurosurgery, for preparing this illustration.)

Table 5.9. *Diazepam*

Indications (stage of status)
Premonitory, early (and established) status

Usual preparations
i.v. formulation: Diazepam emulsion (Diazemuls), 1 ml ampoule containing 5 mg/ml *or*
    i.v. solution 2 ml ampoules containing 5 mg/ml
Rectal formulation: 2.5 ml rectal tube (Stesolid) containing 2 mg/ml *or* instillation of the
    i.v. solution, 2 ml ampoule containing 5 mg/ml

Usual dosage
i.v. bolus (undiluted) 10–20 mg (adults); 0.2–0.3 mg/kg (children). Rate not to exceed 2–
    5 mg/min. Can be repeated
Rectal administration 10–30 mg (adults); 0.5–0.75 mg/kg (children). Can be repeated
i.v. infusion 8 mg/h (now not generally recommended)

Advantages
Pharmacology and pharmacokinetics extensively studied
Long clinical experience in adults, children and the newborn
Proven efficacy in many types of status
Rapid onset of action
Can be given by i.v. or rectal administration

Disadvantages
Accumulation on repeated administration, with risk of sudden respiratory depression,
    sedation, hypotension
Short duration of action, tendency to relapse following single injection
Active metabolite
Pharmacokinetics affected by hepatic disease
Physical properties: precipitation from concentrated solutions, interaction with other
    drugs, reaction with plastic on prolonged contact

---

i.v., intravenous.

from a syringe via a plastic catheter, or as the ready-made proprietary rectal tube preparation (Stesolid 2 mg/ml) which is a convenient and easy method. Diazepam suppositories should not be used, as absorption is too slow.

The initial adult dose in status is 10–20 mg bolus intravenous injection or 10–30 mg rectal instillation. Boluses (10 mg intravenously) can be repeated after 15 minute intervals, to a maximum of 40 mg. In children, the equivalent bolus dose is 0.2–0.3 mg/kg. A continuous infusion of 8 mg/hour has also been used, but is now not recommended except in ITU settings.

Summary of use in status epilepticus (table 5.9)

Diazepam has a time honoured place as a drug of first choice in premonitory or early stages of status. Its pharmacology and clinical effects have been extensively studied in adults, children and the newborn, and it is highly effective in a wide range of status types. It has the advantage of ease of administration via intravenous bolus injections or by the rectal route in the premonitory stage, and has a rapid onset of action. Its pharmacokinetic properties, however, are not ideal. It is highly lipid soluble, is avidly taken up by cerebral tissue and then rapidly redistributed to lipid stores. Its duration of action after initial doses is therefore short. On repeated administration, as concentrations in lipid stores increase, this redistribution does not occur, and further drug doses will result in high brain concentrations which persist, carrying a serious risk of sudden cardiorespiratory collapse, hypotension and CNS depression. These are the only common toxic effects in status. As duration of action of diazepam is relatively short, relapse after initial therapy is common, and longer-term antiepileptic therapy is often required once the transient effects of diazepam have worn off. A combination of diazepam with phenytoin (with its longer-lasting action) is a popular approach which largely prevents late relapse. Diazepam has an active metabolite which accumulates on prolonged therapy, and its pharmacokinetic properties can be affected by hepatic or renal failure. Care should be exercised in preparing diazepam solutions, as it has a marked tendency to precipitate, can interact with other drugs, and is sorbed on to plastic tubing if left standing for long periods.

Midazolam

Midazolam (8-chloro-6-(2-fluorophenyl)-1-methyl-4H-imidazo [1,5-a][1,4] benzodiazepine; $C_{18}H_{13}ClFN_3$; molecular weight 325.8) is an imidazobenzodiazepine drug, basic and water soluble at physiological pH, with a pK_a of 6.2. At physiological pH the ring structure closes, the drug becomes lipid soluble and crosses the blood–brain barrier readily. It was introduced into clinical practice in 1982, as a short-term sedative for minor operative procedures. Antiepileptic action was recorded soon after this, and in the past 5 years the value of midazolam in the early treatment of status has been recognised. Its pharmacology and pharmacokinetics are well understood because of its extensive use in anaesthetics (Dundee *et al.* 1984). The drug is presented usually in ampoules of 10 mg of midazolam base in 5 ml of aqueous solution. Commonly used commercial preparations of midazolam include Hypnovel, Dormicum and Versed.

Absorption

In status, midazolam can be given intravenously, rectally or intramuscularly. It is indeed the only drug in early status which can be given by intramuscular injection, and this property confers a singular advantage over other drugs. After intramuscular injection, 80–100% is absorbed and peak effects are reached after about 25 minutes, although there is marked variation, with much slower absorption in some patients (Patsalos *et al.* 1991). Maximum sedative effects in 166 patients after 0.3 mg/kg given intravenously over 20 seconds were recorded within 2 minutes, and within 40 seconds in the elderly. Rectal administration is also widely used, although pharmacokinetics have not been extensively studied.

Distribution

After intravenous injection, midazolam is very widely and rapidly distributed. The distribution half-life of only 15 minutes reflects its relatively high lipid solubility at physiological pH. As the pH falls, however, the drug becomes less lipid soluble, a potential problem in established status. The volume of distribution is 0.6–1.7 l/kg, and is higher in women, the obese and the elderly. The drug is 96% (range 94–98%) bound to plasma proteins.

Biotransformation and excretion

Midazolam is almost completely metabolised in the liver via α-hydroxylation and then glucuronidation. Although the principal first metabolite, α-hydroxymidazolam, is active, it has a shorter half-life than midazolam, and probably contributes little to the overall antiepileptic action. At steady state, the blood concentration of the metabolite is about one third that of the parent drug. Plasma clearance is 268–630 ml/minute and body clearance 5.8–11.1 ml/minute per kg. Clearance is largely dependent on hepatic blood flow and is greater in supine than in ambulant subjects. The elimination half-life is 1.5–3.5 hours, and is markedly prolonged in the elderly (up to 10 hours). Chronic renal failure does not strongly affect pharmacokinetics, and although severe hepatic disease might be expected to slow elimination, this has not been demonstrated in practice.

Clinical effect in status epilepticus

The antiepileptic action of midazolam was recognised from the early experimental studies (de Jong & Bonin 1981). Brown *et al.* (1979) noted an effect on EEG similar to that of diazepam. Raines *et al.* (1990) showed intramuscular midazolam to be superior to intramuscular diazepam in experimental status in the mouse. Kubová & Mareš (1992) demonstrated its effect in rats of all ages, and Janovich *et al.* (1990) the abolition of seizure activity without significant cardiorespiratory depression in pentylenetetrazol-induced seizures in domestic swine.

The clinical application of midazolam has to date been largely confined to the

214

premonitory or early stage of status. Kaneko *et al.* (1983) reported the successful treatment of status with intravenous midazolam in a 14 year old female. Galvin & Jelinek (1987) then recorded 12 adults in status (in some due to alcohol withdrawal, head injury or hypoglycaemia), treated with intravenous midazolam. The initial dose was 2.5 mg, followed by further increments to a maximum of 15 mg (mean dose 7.4 mg) until seizures were controlled. Immediate seizure control was obtained within 1 minute in all cases. The effectiveness of intramuscular administration was first demonstrated by Egli & Albani (1981) at a dose of 0.15– 0.3 mg/kg in 10 chronic epileptic patients with status or serial convulsive seizures. In 8 patients, seizure control was achieved within 2–3 minutes of a single dose, and in some improvement in EEG was noted within 30 seconds. Jawad, Richens & Oxley (1984) then showed that midazolam doses of 10 and 15 mg abolished EEG spikes within 5 minutes to an extent equivalent to that of 20 mg of intravenous diazepam, and greater than that of 10 mg of intravenous diazepam (Jawad *et al.* 1986; fig. 5.8). Ghilain *et al.* (1988) gave intramuscular midazolam at a dose of 0.2 mg/kg on 18 occasions to 14 patients. Seizures were abolished in all cases within 5–10 minutes, the response was complete on 15 occasions (82%) and partial in three. EEG epileptic activity was abolished within 10 minutes in five of nine patients (but reappeared at the end of the recording in one), was diminished in three and was unchanged in one. Seizures recurred after 3–4 hours in three patients and 18 hours in one, and were controlled in two by repeat midazolam adminstration. Midazolam has also been successfully used to abolish seizure activity in the emergency room and in patients with traumatic brain injury (Mayhue 1988; Wroblewski & Joseph 1992). There are no reported studies confined to children, although the drug is frequently given to children in institutional care in the UK for serial seizures.

Midazolam has also been occasionally used in established status, by continuous infusion. Crisp, Gannon & Knauft (1988) used a 5 mg bolus followed by a 3 hour infusion in an elderly woman. Kumar & Bleck (1992) record the successful treatment of seven patients, refractory to other antiepileptic drugs, in advanced and severe status (including two with status due to drug overdose). Mild hypotension was noted with rhabdomyolysis in one case, but no other side effects. On the basis of this experience, midazolam was considered a useful alternative to anaesthetic barbiturates, as the drug is shorter acting and causes less haemodynamic disturbance than the barbiturates. The recommended regimen is for one or two intravenous bolus injections of 0.1–0.3 mg/kg to be followed by an infusion of 0.05–0.4 mg/kg per hour. Its pharmacokinetic properties also confer some advantages on prolonged infusion over other benzodiazepine drugs, but further experience is necessary before this method of administration can be unequivocally recommended.

Toxic effects in status epilepticus

Minor side-effects are infrequent. There is a lower incidence of thrombophlebitis reported than with diazepam. Mild bradycardia and a slight fall in arterial blood pressure may occur at conventional doses (in one and three respectively of the 14

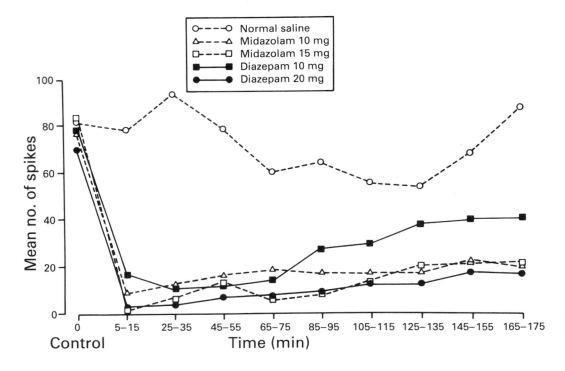

Fig. 5.8. The effect of intramuscular (i.m.) midazolam on electrographic ictal activity; and a comparison with the effects of intravenous (i.v.) diazepam. Comparison of the effect of i.m. midazolam (10 mg, 15 mg) and i.v. diazepam (10 mg, 20 mg) on interictal spikes. The effect of midazolam at both doses was equal to that of 20 mg of diazepam, and superior to that of 10 mg of diazepam. Note the rapidity of onset of the midazolam, administered by the i.m. route. (From Jawad *et al.* 1986, with kind permission.)

patients reported by Ghilain *et al.* (1988). There are no published cases of respiratory arrest after intramuscular injection in status, although in one of my patients apnoea occurred 10 minutes after an intramuscular injection of 10 mg of midazolam after a prolonged grand mal seizure complicated by a mild head injury, an experience which has tempered enthusiasm for the drug. In anaesthetic practice, apnoea occurred in between 10% and 77% of over 300 patients in double-blind studies comparing the induction of anaesthesia by intravenous midazolam (0.2–0.36 mg/kg) and intravenous thiopentone (3.8–6.4 mg/kg, which caused apnoea in 55–83%) (Dundee *et al.* 1984). In status, the intravenous dose is lower and apnoea has not been reported, but clearly this is a potential risk. Toxicity may be more likely in the elderly.

Table 5.10. *Midazolam*

Indication (stage of status)
Premonitory status (and early and established status)

Usual preparation
5 ml ampoule containing 2 mg midazolam hydrochloride/ml

Usual dosage
i.m. or rectally 5–10 mg (adults); 0.15–0.3 mg/kg (children). Can be repeated once after 15 min
In adults, an i.v. bolus dose of 5–10 mg can be given (repeated to a maximum of 0.3 mg/kg). Rate not to exceed 4 mg/min. Can be repeated once after 15 min
i.v. infusion 0.05–0.4 mg/kg per h (after bolus); there is very limited experience of this mode of administration

Advantages
Can be given by i.m. injection, as well as by i.v. injection or by rectal administration
Rapid onset of action
Less tendency to accumulate than diazepam

Disadvantages
Limited experience in status
Cardiovascular depression, hypotension, apnoea, sedation, thrombophlebitis; worse in elderly
No reported studies in children
Danger of accumulation on prolonged or repeated therapy
Short acting, with tendency to relapse following single injection
Elimination dependent upon hepatic blood flow
Lipid solubility falls as cerebral pH falls

---

i.v., intravenous; i.m., intramuscular.

Administration and dosage in status epilepticus

Midazolam is presented in 5 mg ampoules containing 2 mg/ml. It is usually given intramuscularly or rectally in premonitory status, at a dose of 5–10 mg (in children 0.15–0.3 mg/kg), which can be repeated once after 15 minutes or so. A 5–10 mg intravenous bolus injection can also be given (repeated to a maximum of 0.3 mg/kg in adults). Published reports suggest that it can also be given by prolonged intravenous infusion (dose 0.05–0.4 mg/kg per hour), although experience is limited and continuous infusion will undoubtedly carry a risk of accumulation.

Summary of use in status epilepticus (table 5.10)

Midazolam has only recently been tried in status, and clinical experience is limited. It is the only drug in status which can be given by rectal administration or by intramuscular or intravenous injection. Its intramuscular use in premonitory status is a great advantage, and midazolam has an important role at this stage of status. It is effective within 5–10 minutes after intramuscular injection, but there is a strong tendency to relapse after a single injection. It is cleared from the body

217

faster than is diazepam, but on prolonged or continuous administration there will be a substantial risk of accumulation. Bioavailability is about 80% after intramuscular administration, and peak blood levels are reached at about 25 minutes, although there is considerable variation. Its elimination kinetics are dependent on hepatic blood flow. The lipid solubility of the drug, and hence its cerebral action, are reduced as blood and cerebral pH fall. Midazolam exhibits the toxic effects of other benzodiazepines, especially sedation and cardiorespiratory depression, and respiratory arrest may occur occasionally even after intramuscular injection. In current practice, its clinical role is in premonitory status, as an alternative to intravenous or rectal diazepam, but further experience may widen its indications.

Paraldehyde

Paraldehyde, a cyclic polymer of acetaldehyde (2,4,5-trimethyl-1,3,5-trioxane; $C_6H_{12}O_3$; molecular weight 132.2), was introduced into clinical practice in 1882. It has hypnotic, anaesthetic and anticonvulsant properties, and is nowadays used largely for the emergency treatment of epilepsy. It is a colourless liquid with a pungent characteristic odour. Certain physical properties are important clinically; its solubility at body temperature is significantly less than at room temperature, it decomposes in light to acetaldehyde, and then to acetic acid, and it reacts slowly with rubber and plastic. It is not very lipid soluble (octanol:water partition coefficient of 32.6). Its dosage is commonly cited in volume units (e.g. millilitres) as well as mass units (e.g. grams) which for practical purposes can be considered equivalent (strictly speaking 1 ml weighs 1.006 g). An alternative name for paraldehyde is para-acetaldehyde.

Absorption

Although paraldehyde is well and rapidly absorbed following administration by mouth, it has an unpleasant taste, and is usually given in status by the rectal or intramuscular route. Intravenous injection, either as a short-term or continuous infusion, is also possible, but has largely fallen from fashion. Blood concentration after intramuscular injection peaks after 20–60 minutes, and in about 2–4 hours in alcoholics (Anthony *et al.* 1977), although experience suggests that the antiepileptic action is very much faster than this. Rectal administration of the solution is rapid

218

and complete. An oil-based rectal formulation was available, which had a much slower absorption, and is unsuitable for use in status.

Distribution

Paraldehyde is quickly distributed to brain, and anaesthesia is induced within 2–5 minutes of intravenous injection (Gardner, Levine & Bodansky 1940; Thurston *et al.* 1968; Anthony *et al.* 1977; Ramsey 1989). In animal experimentation, the entry of paraldehyde to brain has been shown to be largely determined by cerebral blood flow. In human epileptic foci, there is a high local blood flow, and it is thus possible that the drug is preferentially concentrated in epileptic foci; this would be a very valuable pharmacological property. Clinical effects are noticeable before maximum blood levels are reached. Thurston *et al.* (1968) report sedation within 3 minutes, sleep within 5–15 minutes and maximal blood levels within 20–60 minutes of a single intramuscular injection. Peak CSF concentrations are reached within 20–60 minutes of an intramuscular injection, and at 60 minutes after injection levels are 58–90% (mean 75%) of that of the blood concentration. Brain concentrations are about 25–30% lower than blood concentrations.

A dose of about 100–200 mg/kg is effective in halting status in experimental animals (de Elió, de Jalón & Obrador 1949), which would yield blood levels of about 150–200 mg/l in humans (Bostrom 1982). In neonates, blood levels over 100 mg/l are sufficient to control seizures (Koren *et al.* 1986). Anaesthesia usually can be achieved at levels of 120–320 mg/l (Gardner *et al.* 1940).

Biotransformation and excretion

In 14 neonates, the elimination half-life was 18.1 (± 5.5) hours (Koren *et al.* 1986). In 21 children, elimination half-life ranged from 3.4 to 9.8 hours (Thurston *et al.* 1968), and a mean half-life of 6.2 hours was reported in alcoholic adults (Anthony *et al.* 1977). Blood levels initially fall very slowly; in five children given a single intramuscular injection of 0.25 ml/kg levels were virtually constant between 20 and 120 minutes, and even at 6 hours levels were still 40–60% of the peak level. The mean quoted steady-state volume of distribution is 0.89 l/kg in adults and 3.18 l/kg (range 2.0–7.7) in infants (Lockman 1989).

The drug is 70–80% metabolised by hepatic microsomal enzymes, and the remaining 20–30% is exhaled through the lungs. Liver disease will result in greater excretion by exhalation (Harvey 1985), but the half-life is greatly lengthened. It is assumed that paraldehyde is depolymerised to acetaldehyde, then oxidised to acetic acid and then to carbon dioxide and water. There are therefore no active metabolites. The clearance of paraldehyde in adults is approximately 0.1 l/kg per hour.

Clinical effect in status epilepticus

Although paraldehyde has been available for epilepsy for over 100 years, there are few formal studies of its effectiveness. The intramuscular or rectal injection of 5–10 ml of paraldehyde has been widely used for the initial treatment of status, and this is still its most common indication. Paraldehyde is highly regarded in residential institutions for epilepsy, where many severe cases are treated, and is particularly useful where facilities for intravenous injection and resuscitation are not available. In neurosurgical practice, serious or prolonged status has been terminated by 2–4 ml of intravenous paraldehyde (sometimes repeated once or twice over the course of several hours) without ill effect (de Elió *et al.* 1949).

Koren *et al.* (1986) reported the use of paraldehyde in neonates. Initially an intravenous dose of 200 mg/kg was given over 1 hour (5% in 5% dextrose), followed by 16 mg/kg per hour. On this regimen, the volume of distribution was found to be higher and clearance lower in neonates than in the adults, and so an initial infusion of 400 mg/kg, given over 2 hours, was recommended to obtain blood levels of 100 mg/l or above. All the infants had received prior phenobarbitone and/or phenytoin unsuccessfully. Modest seizure control was achieved with levels between 63 and 101 mg/l, and complete seizure control with levels between 60 and 175 mg/l (mean 118 mg/l). Blood levels of about 100 mg/l were achieved in most neonates with a 2 hour infusion of 200 mg/kg per hour. Where the drug was ineffective, levels were usually found to be lower and an additional 200 mg/kg could be given over the next hour.

An intravenous regimen was described by Whitty & Taylor (1949) in 26 adults, from the Second World War military hospital in Oxford for acute brain injury, and was still being used in peacetime Oxford, in the 1970s. For an average adult, paraldehyde is initially given intramuscularly in a dose of 10 ml followed by 5 ml intramuscularly every 30 minutes if seizures continue. An intravenous glucose–saline infusion is then set up, with glass tubing and a glass side arm, and the paraldehyde is injected intermittently into the side arm at a rate of 6 ml/hour (alternatively a continuous infusion of 18 ml is given in 540 ml of glucose–saline every 3 hours). This regimen was considered to be superior to thiopentone (or chloroform) anaesthesia and safe, although few details were given. Seizures do not often recur on discontinuing paraldehyde, a significant advantage over the benzodiazepines and chlormethiazole. Other encouraging clinical reports of intravenous paraldehyde in status were those of McGreal (1958), Wechsler (1940) and de Elió *et al.* (1949), although the dilution and rate of injection of paraldehyde were not specified. In view of the propensity of the drug to precipitate from solution, however, on no account should the undiluted drug nowadays be given intravenously, and it is usual procedure to dilute the paraldehyde in 0.9% sodium chloride (normal saline) to a 5% strength, before intravenous administration.

Paraldehyde has been especially recommended for use in status due to alcohol withdrawal (Browne 1983), but there have been no comparative studies; both chlormethiazole and phenobarbitone are also effective. It can be safely used in acute intermittent porphyria.

Toxic effects in status epilepticus

In animals, the therapeutic index is narrow. The minimal anaesthetic dose in rabbits and cats is 0.3 ml/kg and the mean lethal dose 0.45 ml/kg (Burstein 1943). Paraldehyde was widely used in the early part of the century, but its popularity waned following a spate of reports of serious adverse reactions. In retrospect, many were probably due to the use of decomposed drug or inappropriate dilutions, and now in human adult practice the drug is widely considered to be safe. At least 95 deaths have been associated with paraldehyde usage, and have been caused by suicidal overdose, alcoholism, the use of decomposed drug, or incorrect dosage or dilutions (Burstein 1943; Browne 1983). Paraldehyde causes drowsiness or sleep when administered, in conventional dosages, but the level of sedation is quite acceptable. Thurston *et al.* (1968) administered the drug at an intramuscular dose of 0.25–0.33 ml/kg in 21 children; in all of whom sedation was observable within 3 minutes and sleep was induced within 5–15 minutes, but vital signs were unaffected. After 6 hours the children were still asleep, but had been roused for feeding in the intervening period, without difficulty. Following intravenous infusion, de Elió *et al.* (1949) were able to record an antiepileptic effect from exposed motor cortex in five patients undergoing neurosurgery for 30 minutes, with excitability recovering slowly after this. Hypotension is rarely if ever a problem, and other rare toxic reactions include pulmonary oedema causing cyanosis and cough, and right heart failure. Metabolic acidosis may occur, particularly in chronic administration, and severe lactic acidosis, far in excess of that due simply to the oxidation of any paraldehyde-derived acetaldehyde, has been recorded following just 40 ml given by intramuscular injection in a 30 year old man (Linter & Linter 1986). One neonate has survived a blood level of 1744 mg/l (Bostrom 1982), although death has also been recorded at only 543 mg/l (Figot, Hine & Way 1952). Pulmonary oedema and haemorrhages and right heart dilatation are postmortem findings in patients and experimental animals dying from paraldehyde poisoning (Burstein 1943).

The solubility of paraldehyde is highly temperature dependent; maximum solubility is 12.8% at 12 °C, and at normal body temperatures paraldehyde is only 7.8% soluble (Robinson 1938). Solutions of greater than 10% may thus precipitate after injection, resulting in the circulation of pure paraldehyde droplets and microvascular thrombosis. A more dilute solution should therefore always be administered by the intravenous route. Rectally, paraldehyde is traditionally given mixed with an equal volume of water (or arachis oil). This clearly will not dissolve the drug, but might be worth while to provide a greater surface area for absorption. The conversion of paraldehyde to glacial acetic acid in light may be very toxic, and may cause death if administered by injection (Anonymous 1954). Outdated paraldehyde may also cause severe proctitis and an excoriating anal rash, if given rectally, or even large bowel perforation (Hutchison 1930; Agranat & Trubshaw 1955; Stanley 1980). Intramuscular injection may cause severe causalgia, if the injection is too close to the sciatic nerve, and sterile abscess; these complications are seen particularly in children (Hutchinson 1930; Woodson 1943).

Administration and dosage in status epilepticus

Paraldehyde is usually given rectally in the premonitory or early stage of status. It can also be given by deep intramuscular injection, and occasionally by intravenous infusion in established status. Whichever route of administration is chosen, however, certain important precautions should be taken. As paraldehyde readily

Table 5.11. *Paraldehyde*

Indications (stage of status)
Premonitory, early (and established) status

Usual preparation
Ampoule containing 5 ml paraldehyde (equivalent to approximately 5 g); in darkened glass

Usual dosage
Rectally (or i.m.) 5–10 ml diluted by same volume of water for injection (adults); 0.07–
    0.35 ml/kg (children). Can be repeated after 15–30 min (premonitory or early status)
In established status in adults, i.v. infusion of 5–10 ml/h (as a 5% solution in 5%
    dextrose). This can be given after i.m. dosing if necessary
In neonates, an infusion of 200 mg/kg per h can be given for at least 3 hours, or an initial
    infusion of 200 mg/kg per h followed by 16 mg/kg per h for 12 h

Advantages
Rapid and complete absorption by i.m. injection or rectally
Rectal or i.m. administration where facilities for resuscitation not available
Seizures do not often recur after control has been obtained
Longer duration of action than other benzodiazepines
Risk of accumulation is low
Small risk of hypotension, cardiorespiratory depression

Disadvantages
The decomposed or inadequately diluted i.v. solutions are highly toxic: rectally causing
    severe proctitis; intramuscularly causing sterile abscess; intravenously causing
    microembolism, thrombosis, cardiorespiratory arrest
Solubility less at body than at room temperature
Cardiorespiratory depression, sedation, metabolic or lactic acidosis, sciatic nerve damage
    if i.m. injection wrongly placed, pulmonary oedema, cardiac failure
Practical precautions: correct dilution, glass tubing and syringes, avoid exposure to light,
    short shelf life
Hepatic disease markedly increases half-life
Lack of recent pharmacological or clinical study

i.v., intravenous; i.m., intramuscular.

decomposes to acetaldehyde and then to acetic acid on exposure to light, it should
always be stored in the dark and is supplied in darkened glass ampoules. A freshly
made solution should therefore always be used. The drug also reacts with rubber
and plastic, and so, if infused, must be given via glass giving sets and syringes.
An injection using a plastic syringe, however, is acceptable if given rapidly after
the solution is drawn up, for instance for intramuscular injection in status. If given
by intramuscular injection, this should be into deep buttock muscles, well away
from the sciatic nerve.

Paraldehyde is supplied in 10 ml ampoules (approximately 10 g), and is diluted
in equal measure with 0.9% sodium chloride (normal saline) for rectal or intramuscular administration (although it must be recognised that this will not render
the compound soluble!). For intravenous administration, it should be given as a 5%

infusion in 5% dextrose, freshly made up every 3 hours. There is now no place for the bolus injection of undiluted paraldehyde even into a fast running drip.

In early status, paraldehyde can be given at a dose of 10 ml of 50% solution rectally or intramuscularly (children 0.07–0.35 ml/kg), which can be repeated once after 15–30 minutes. It is still occasionally used in established status in adults, by continuous infusion of a solution of 3×5 ml ampoules in 500 ml of dextrose saline freshly made up every 3 hours, at a dose of 15–30 ml every 3 hours (i.e. approximately 100–200 mg/kg per hour). An adult bolus dose of 0.3 ml/kg in 10% solution injected 'slowly' has been recommended, repeated after 15 minutes, but in view of its low solubility this carries significant risk, and the doses also seem rather high (Lockman 1989). In neonatal status, an infusion of 200 mg/kg per hour can be given for at least 3 hours, or an initial infusion of 200 mg/kg per hour followed by 16 mg/kg per hour for 12 hours.

Summary of use in status epilepticus (table 5.11)

Although an old-fashioned medication, paraldehyde still has a place in the treatment of status; indeed it is widely given in units experienced in the treatment of epilepsy. It is now used mainly as an alternative or sequel to the administration of diazepam in the stage of premonitory or early status. It is especially helpful in situations where intravenous administration is difficult, or where conventional antiepileptic drugs are contraindicated or have proved ineffective. The drug is usually given rectally or intramuscularly, and absorption is fast and complete. The onset of action is rapid and its antiepileptic properties last for many hours. Seizures tend to recur less after control is achieved than with the shorter-acting benzodiazepines, the anaesthetic drugs or with chlormethiazole. Paraldehyde does not have a strong tendency to accumulate, and the risks of hypotension or cardiorespiratory depression are low. The main drawbacks of paraldehyde are its potential toxicity and the logistical problems associated with its administration. Side-effects are however, unusual, provided the correct dose is not exceeded, the solution is freshly made, the paraldehyde is not decomposed, is diluted satisfactorily, and is not permitted to stay in contact with rubber or plastic tubing for any length of time. The intramuscular injection must be into deep muscle, well away from the sciatic nerve, to avoid iatrogenic damage. In established status, paraldehyde can be given by intravenous infusion, but this is a complicated and fraught procedure, and one which is now very rarely recommended. Intravenous administration carries the risk of potentially serious toxic effects, and careful monitoring is essential. Inappropriately diluted or decomposed paraldehyde is highly toxic by any route of administration, and considerable care should be exercised in its preparation and administration. The drug reacts with plastic or rubber, so glass giving sets and syringes are needed for intravenous infusion.

Early and established status epilepticus

Treatment in these stages of status is controversial, and widely differing drug regimens have been recommended. The following drugs, listed alphabetically, are

223

those that are commonly used in addition to diazepam, midazolam and paraldehyde (described above): chlormethiazole, clonazepam, lignocaine, lorazepam, phenytoin and phenobarbitone.

Chlormethiazole (clomethiazole)

Chlormethiazole (5-(-2-chloroethyl)-4-methylthiazole; C_6H_8ClNS; molecular weight 161.7) is given as its edisylate (ethanedisulphonate) salt (molecular weight 513.5), which is freely soluble in water, virtually unionised at physiological pH, lipid soluble (octanol/water partition coefficient 132), basic in solution, and has a pK_a of 3.3. It is an effective antiepileptic drug which is commonly used in status epilepticus in the UK, Europe and Australia, but almost never in the USA. Jostell and colleagues have carried out detailed pharmacokinetic studies (Jostell 1987; Jostell *et al.* 1978; Pentikäinen, Neuvonen & Jostell 1980; Scott *et al.* 1980). Commonly used commercial preparations of chlormethiazole include Heminevrin, Distrameurin, Hemineurin and Distraneurine.

Absorption

Chlormethiazole is given initially as an intravenous infusion in status epilepticus. Adequate cerebral levels are reached quickly, and the antiepileptic effect of the infusion is very rapid. The blood level required to control seizures is uncertain, but anaesthetic studies have shown a good correlation between blood levels and the depth of sedation; unconsciousness usually occurs with levels above 6–10 mg/l. However, the rate of injection is important, and blood concentrations as low as 2.5 mg/100 ml on fast injections have been shown to be fatal (Horder 1978).

Distribution

Chlormethiazole is rapidly distributed after a single intravenous injection (fig. 5.9). Blood levels follow a biphasic pattern with an (initial) distribution half-life of 2 minutes. The volume of distribution is large, between 4 and 19 l/kg (mean 9 l/kg in young adults, 13 l/kg in elderly). Chlormethiazole is about 70% bound to plasma proteins in young adults and 60% in the elderly (Nation *et al.* 1976; Jostell 1987).

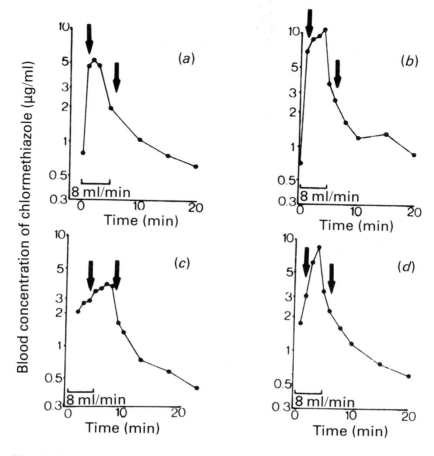

Fig. 5.9. The plasma concentrations of chlormethiazole, after a single intravenous injection in four adult subjects. The plasma concentrations after a single infusion of 320 mg of chlormethiazole ethanedisulphonate given over 5 minutes in four subjects. Arrows represent the times at which the patients lost and regained consciousness. Note the very rapid distribution phase, with an approximately 10-fold fall in serum levels from their peak within approximately 10 minutes in all cases. (From Scott *et al.* 1980, with kind permission.)

Biotransformation and excretion

Less than 5% of chlormethiazole is excreted unchanged in the urine, and there are four major routes of hepatic metabolism. It is very rapidly removed from the circulation. The clearance value of about 1–3 kg/l per hour is close to (and some-times exceeds) hepatic blood flow. This is probably its major determining factor, and variations in hepatic blood flow, common in intensive care situations, can

225

result in unexpected blood level changes. Extrahepatic clearance must occur, perhaps by the pulmonary route, but details are uncertain. There is a danger of accumulation as the lipid compartments become substantial, and the decay of blood (and brain) concentration by re-distribution does not occur. The elimination half-life following a single intravenous dose in healthy young adults has been variously estimated to lie usually between about 3 and 7 hours (Moore *et al.* 1975; Jostell *et al.* 1978; Pentikäinen *et al.* 1980; Scott *et al.* 1980; Seow, Mather & Roberts 1981) and increases with age (Nation *et al.* 1976; Jostell 1987) and is greatly lengthened by severe hepatic disease (Pentikäinen *et al.* 1980). After prolonged therapy, the elimination half-life is greatly increased because of accumulation (values of 3.5–12.1 hours recorded by Scott *et al.* (1980), see fig. 5.10). There are no published data on the elimination half-life in epileptic patients, but clinical experience suggests that it is short, at least in the early stages of treatment. There are no known active metabolites. Renal failure does not have a major effect on the pharmacokinetics of chlormethiazole.

The pharmacokinetics of chlormethiazole (very short distribution half-life, large distribution space, high clearance) convey a significant advantage over the other nonanaesthetic drugs used in status, as blood levels can initially be rapidly manipulated by varying the infusion rate. The dose can be titrated, in a highly responsive fashion, on a minute-by-minute basis against seizure activity. On prolonged administration, however, as chlormethiazole accumulates in the lipid compartments, these pharmacokinetic advantages are lost (fig. 5.10). As accumulation occurs, blood levels no longer fall rapidly in a biphasic fashion, and further administration may cause abrupt hypotension or respiratory depression. One young patient is reported who received 78 g of chlormethiazole over 101 hours with blood levels of 21 mg/l at the end of the infusion, levels which did not fall below 10 mg/l until a further 21 hours had passed, and mechanical ventilation was required for 64 hours (Robson *et al.* 1984).

Clinical effect in status epilepticus

The first report of chlormethiazole in status was in 1963 by Poiré *et al.*, and there have been a number of small uncontrolled series since then. Houdart & Laborit (1965, 1966) reported 23 patients aged 2–75 years with status; in 20 seizures were abolished (ten immediately), in two seizures continued and one died. Three cases histories were given with no other details of dosage regimens or complications. Bentley & Mellick (1975) recorded three patients in whom seizures were rapidly controlled after 100–250 ml of a 9.8% solution of chlormethiazole, given at a rate of 250 ml/hour. Chlormethiazole was continued at reducing doses for a further 4 hours. In the third case, seizures recurred 48 hours later, again to be fully controlled with chlormethiazole. In an influental report, Harvey, Higgenbottam & Loh (1975) gave a continuous infusion in nine episodes (eight patients) which had not responded to a Valium infusion (and in two cases also to thiopentone), in all of which seizures stopped within 6 hours. The drug was used in a continuous infusion with rates up to 0.7 g/hour, which in two patients had to be continued for 3 weeks. Assisted ventilation was not required in either patient when chlor-

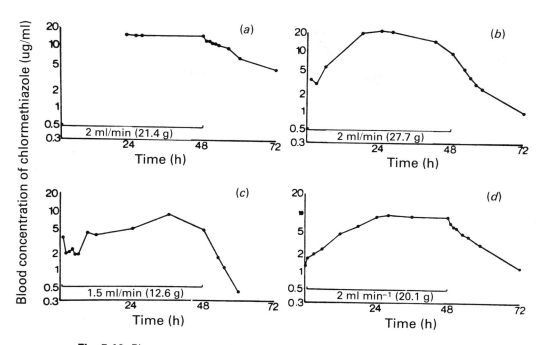

Fig. 5.10. Plasma concentrations of chlormethiazole following a prolonged (48 hours) infusion in four adult subjects. Plasma concentrations of chlormethiazole in four patients during and following continuous infusion for 48 hours (total doses given as chlormethiazole base). Note the much longer recovery phase, compared with that after a single injection (fig. 5.9). After the prolonged infusion, levels fall to subanaesthetic concentrations only after 4–12 hours. The difference is due to the accumulation of drug in peripheral compartments on prolonged infusion, with the result that the plasma level decay curve is dependent on elimination (a much slower process) and not redistribution. This emphasises the potential danger of prolonged infusions of a lipid-soluble drug such as chlormethiazole. (From Scott *et al.* 1980, with kind permission.)

methiazole was substituted for thiopentone, and in two cases the intravenous formulation could be changed to oral chlormethiazole after some days. Doses of 500–700 mg/hour were given without serious impairment of consciousness or depression of respiration. The drug has been successfully used at all ages. Miller & Kovar (1983) successfully treated a neonate, resistant to phenobarbitone, diazepam, paraldehyde and magnesium, with a chlormethiazole infusion for 19 days. Laxenaire, Tridon & Poiré (1966) reported their results with 120 patients treated with status epilepticus, many of whom were retarded children. Chlormethiazole was first infused at a rate of 60–80 drops/minute to control seizures (this dosage also inevitably induced sleep), then slowed down and discontinued after 1.2–1.6 mg had been administered. In every patient, seizures were controlled, partial seizures less easily than generalised seizures. Details of the length of treatment or the total dosages were not given. Stanley (1982) reported two children in whom seizures recurred after initial intravenous control, and in whom oral chlormethiazole was then required.

Toxic effects in status epilepticus

In rabbits, the LD_{50} dose by oral and parenteral administration is very different (800 mg/kg orally and 220 mg/kg intravenously), a variability due to the first-pass effect as the drug is delivered to the liver by the portal venous system. Systemic bioavailability is greatly reduced by this phenomenon. No potentiation of the toxic effects of barbiturate and chlormethiazole has been reported (Svedin 1966), but the drug may potentiate the respiratory depressant effects of benzodiazepines.

Chlormethiazole may cause respiratory depression, although this risk is typically thought to be slight. Laxenaire *et al.* (1966), reporting 120 cases, considered respiratory depression to be a risk only in patients with cardiac, respiratory or hepatic disease, or in those pretreated with other sedative drugs. Apnoea occurred only once, when inadvertently 250 ml had been infused in less than 15 minutes. This optimistic assessment was not shared by Pentikäinen, Valtonen & Miettinen (1976), who reported six deaths due to respiratory depression following intravenous infusion in nonepileptic patients, all of whom had other systemic diseases or alcoholism. Considering the limited use of the drug (about 120 infusions over the period of observation), the risk of death appears particularly high. Cardiac arrhythmia and heart block may occur, and tachycardia is common. I have also observed sudden cardiorespiratory collapse in patients treated for days with chlormethiazole and other drugs. In the complex clinical circumstances surrounding status, it is often not possible to attribute toxicity definitively to prolonged chlormethiazole treatment, but an impression is gained that large doses and prolonged infusion are potentially hazardous.

Chlormethiazole has rather unpredictable effects on consciousness level, but although drowsiness is common it is seldom severe at normal rates of infusion. Light sleep is produced by an infusion rate (0.8% solution) of 7.5 ml/minute in an adult, and unconsciousness by 25 ml/minute. Deep unconsciousness may be produced at high dosages, or with faster rates of infusion. The effect on blood pressure is usually slight, although severe hypotension has been recorded during inadvertently fast rates of infusion.

If the infusion is given over long periods of time (24–48 hours), a significant fluid load without electrolytes is administered. Electrolyte balance should be monitored and electrolytes added to the infusion solution where necessary. Lingam *et al.* (1980) reported the side-effects in five children treated with chlormethiazole; headache occurred in all, as did fever (cause not ascertained) and thrombophlebitis. In the series of Harvey *et al.* (1975) none of the then recognised side-effects of chlormethiazole, namely hypotension, sneezing or gastroenteritis were reported. Thrombophlebitis developed in two patients, and was severe in one. Low, Stephenson & Goel (1980) reported a 27 month old child who was treated at a dose of 10–18 mg/kg per hour successfully for 43 days, without serious compli-

228

Table 5.12. *Chlormethiazole (clomethiazole)*

Indication (stage of status)
Established status

Usual preparation
0.8% solution of chlormethiazole edisylate in 500 ml in 4% dextrose (8 mg/ml) and
   sodium hydroxide

Usual dosage
i.v. infusion of 40–100 ml (320–800 mg), at rate of 5–15 ml/min. Then continuous
   infusion, with dosage titrated according to response (usually 1–4 ml/min, range 0.5–
   20 ml/min) (adults). Initially 0.1 ml/kg per min (0.08 mg/kg per min) increasing
   progressively every 2–4 h as required (children)

Advantages
Very rapid and short-lived initial action
Dose can be initially titrated against response, on a moment-to-moment basis, without
   inducing respiratory arrest or anaesthesia

Disadvantages
Accumulation on prolonged use, with risk of sudden cardiorespiratory collapse,
   hypotension, sedation
Risk of respiratory arrest and hypotension if maximum rate of injection exceeded
Cardiac rhythm disturbances, vomiting, thrombophlebitis
Tendency for seizure recurrence on discontinuing therapy
Risk of fluid overload and electrolyte disturbance on prolonged therapy
Limited published experience in status particularly in children. Insufficient published data
   for neonatal use
Metabolism affected by changes in hepatic blood flow
Hepatic disease markedly reduces clearance and elimination
Slowly sorbed by plastic

cations, and without loss of consciousness or respiratory depression. Other side-effects include nausea, vomiting, urticaria, conjunctival irritation and hiccups. A withdrawal syndrome has also been reported.

Administration and dosage in status epilepticus

Chlormethiazole is usually supplied in 500 ml bottles of a 0.8% solution of chlormethiazole edisylate (8 mg/ml) in dextrose and sodium hydroxide. It may be sorbed by the plastic of the giving set tubing (Lingam *et al.* 1980; Pentikäinen *et al.* 1980). In status, an initial intravenous infusion of 40–100 ml of the 0.8% solution is given (i.e. 320–800 mg) at a rate of 5–15 ml/minute. It is essential not to infuse chlormethiazole too quickly, to avoid the risk of respiratory depression, cardiac arrhythmia or hypotension. The infusion is continued at a minimum dose which will control seizures (commonly 0.5–4 ml/minute, maximum 20 ml/minute in adults). When seizures are controlled (for 12 hours in a case of adult status), the rate of infusion should be slowly reduced. An infusion rate of 0.01 ml/kg (0.08 mg/kg per minute) in children has been recommended, increasing every 2–4 hours until seizures are abolished or drowsiness intervenes.

In view of the risk of accumulation, the prolonged use of the drug should be avoided where possible. If long-term infusion is judged necessary, it would be wise periodically to reduce the dose every few hours to minimise accumulation. It is not uncommon for seizures to recur on chlormethiazole withdrawal, in which case the minimum effective dose should again be determined and continued. Sometimes, switching from the intravenous to oral form (1–3 capsules of 192 mg chlormethiazole base a day; a 192 mg capsule of chlormethiazole is equivalent to a 500 mg tablet of chlormethiazole edisylate or 5 ml of chlormethiazole edisylate syrup) is necessary as status resolves. It must be emphasised that the above dosage regimens are essentially arbitrary, in the absence of formal comparative studies or any published experimental work providing data on dosage. Although published data on prolonged use are limited, the remarkable effectiveness of the drug cannot be doubted. The ability to titrate the dose against seizure activity, by simply turning the drip rate up or down, is unique amongst and in certain situations is a great advantage over, all other nonanaesthetic drugs used in status.

Summary of use in status epilepticus (table 5.12)

Chlormethiazole is widely used in established status, where it is given by continuous intravenous infusion. It is rapidly redistributed, and has a large volume of distribution. Thus, initially, the drug has a rapid and very short-lived effect. At first, therefore, the infusion dose can be titrated continuously, controlling the clinical effects on a moment-by-moment basis without inducing anaesthesia. This is a very useful property not shared by other drugs used in status. On longer-term therapy, though, as drug concentrations in lipid stores increase, this effect is lost. Prolonged infusions carry a substantial risk of accumulation, and sudden cardiorespiratory collapse, cardiac arrhythmia, hypotension or sedation may occur unexpectedly when blood levels are persistently high. Considerable care should be exercised when infusions are continued for more than 12 hours. There is also a strong tendency for seizures to recur as the patient is weaned from the drug, and a switch from intravenous to longer-term oral supplementation is sometimes required. On prolonged therapy there is also a danger of fluid overload, and electrolyte supplementation (with sodium, potassium, calcium and chloride) may be required as the infusion fluid is electrolyte deficient. Chlormethiazole elimination is greatly affected by changes in hepatic blood flow and by hepatic disease, and the drug is adsorbed by plastic on prolonged contact. Although chlormethiazole is undoubtedly a highly effective antiepileptic drug in status, there have been few formal trials of chlormethiazole at any age, and published experience of its long-term use and its role in children or in the newborn is very limited.

Clonazepam

Clonazepam (5-(*o*-chlorophenyl)-1,3-dihydro-7-nitro-2H-1,4-benzodiazepin-2-one; $C_{15}H_{10}ClN_3O_3$; molecular weight 315.7) bears a close structural relationship to nitrazepam and was introduced into clinical practice in 1966. It has broad antiepileptic properties, and a particular place in the treatment of status epilepticus. It is a crystalline powder, highly soluble in lipid but not in water, and virtually unionised at physiological pH. The pK_a is 1.5 and 10.5 as there are two different molecular dissociation sites. The drug is presented in ampoules of 1 mg in 1 ml for dilution with 1 ml of water for injection. The pharmacokinetics have been well reviewed (Pinder *et al.* 1976; Greenblatt, Miller & Shader 1987; Sato 1989). In spite of extensive experience of use of the drug elsewhere, the intravenous preparation in status is not licensed for use in the US. Commonly used commercial preparations of clonazepam include Rivotril, Klonopin, Iktorivil and Lansden.

Absorption

In status, clonazepam is given by intravenous bolus dose at a rate not exceeding 1 mg in 30 seconds. Mean blood levels after intravenous injection of 1.5 mg of 5.0–7.8 µg/l in adults, and of 28–117 µg/l in neonates after doses of 0.1 mg/kg have been reported. Rectal administration in children results in rapid absorption, and although this route of administration is promising, no clinical studies in status have been reported.

Distribution

Clonazepam is very rapidly and extensively distributed following intravenous injection, reflecting high lipid solubility and lack of ionisation. The distribution half-life is less than 30 minutes, and CSF and blood concentrations of the drug rapidly equilibrate. The volume of distribution is 2.4 (range 1.5–4.4) l/kg, a moderately high value reflecting extensive tissue binding. There is clearly a danger of accumulation in lipid reservoirs, although this has not been formally reported. Published values of plasma protein (albumin) binding lie between 47% and 82%. No clear relationship has been established between blood level and therapeutic effect, and the minimum cerebral level required to control acute seizures is not known. Widely varying blood levels have been associated with seizure control (e.g. 5–70 µg/l).

Biotransformation and excretion

Clonazepam is extensively metabolised by the hepatic cytochrome enzyme system, to virtually inactive (amino compounds) and to active (nitro compounds) metabolites, but the circulating blood concentrations of the latter are too small to contribute to the antiepileptic action. Less than 0.5% of clonazepam is excreted unchanged. Reported elimination half-life values of clonazepam have varied between 18 and 49 hours (mean 29 hours) in subjects who have not previously received enzyme-inducing drugs. The clearance of clonazepam in adults is approximately 0.057 l/kg per hour. The half-life is shorter in children, and in epileptic patients (22–33 hours; Dreifuss *et al.* 1975).

Clinical effect in status epilepticus

Gastaut *et al.* (1971) reported, with some excitement, the efficacy in status of clonazepam, which they considered was greater than diazepam. The clinical effects of clonazepam were described in detail in 39 episodes of status in 37 patients (some of whom could not be controlled with phenobarbitone or diazepam); only one patient did not respond. Dosages varied from 1 to 8 mg by bolus injection at lower doses and infusion at higher dosages. The effect was manifest within 1 minute in most cases, without side-effects. The authority of Gastaut and his colleagues resulted in the rapid adoption of clonazepam for status. In the next 2 years, 8 further trials were reported in 385 patients with an overall 82% response rate at doses between 0.5 and 8 mg (usually 1–4 mg) (quoted by Gimenez-Roldán, López Agreda & Martin 1972; Beck & Tousch 1973; Bladin 1973; Ketz, Bernoulli & Siegfried 1973; Kruse & Blankenhorn 1973; Martin & Hirt 1973; Tridon & Weber 1973). The drug was noted to be effective where phenobarbitone and other antiepileptic drugs had failed, and to be particularly useful in tonic–clonic or absence status. The response to intravenous clonazepam is rapid, and lasts for up to 24 hours in most types of seizure; this is significantly longer than is achieved by diazepam, and an important advantage of clonazepam. Myoclonic, tonic, atypical absence and simple partial seizures respond less well (Van Huffelen & Magnus 1976; Mori *et al.* 1977; Tassinari *et al.* 1983; Garcia *et al.* 1987). Congdon & Forsythe (1980) reported the effects of clonazepam in 17 cases of infantile and childhood status. A bolus dose of 0.25 mg was given, and if unsuccessful was repeated at 30 second intervals to a maximum of three injections. In all 17 episodes, seizures ceased, but in six the status recurred at a mean of 24.5 hours later. Blood levels at 10 minutes ranged from 1 to 750 µg/l and at 30 minutes between 0 and 324 µg/l. Because of this variation, the routine measurement of blood levels does not seem worth while. In the six children in whom the status recurred, diazepam was given at a dose of 250–750 µg/kg, and in five of the six seizures were halted, but in each patient the duration of action of clonazepam was longer (mean duration of action of clonazepam was 24.5 hours and of diazepam 8.8 hours). Tassinari *et al.* (1983) found clonazepam and diazepam to be of roughly equal efficacy in 17 patients who had received both; this would certainly accord with my own experience in the treatment of adult status. Occasional patients are encountered who do not respond to diazepam but in whom clonazepam is effective, and vice versa. There are as yet no controlled studies comparing clonazepam and diazepam.

Continuous infusions of clonazepam diluted with physiological saline or dextrose have been recommended in the past for the treatment of status. Clonazepam (3 mg) can be mixed with 250 ml of 0.9% sodium chloride (normal saline) solution, 5% dextrose or dextrose saline (0.45% sodium chloride and 2.5% dextrose), and the infusion should be freshly made up every 12 hours. The total recommended dose used is 10 mg every 24 hours. Much higher doses are sometimes used and I have encountered a patient who received 24 mg over 12 hours, with additional Valium, without ill effect. There are few if any satisfactory published clinical data to support either the effectiveness or safety of a continuous infusion, and in view of the long half-life and the known tendency of benzodiazepines to accumulate, this mode of administration of clonazepam should probably be avoided unless careful monitoring is carried out, and full ITU facilities are available.

Toxic effects in status epilepticus

The early reports emphasised the lack of toxicity of clonazepam when given intravenously (Gastaut *et al.* 1971), although further experience suggests that the side-effect profile in acute therapy is similar to that of diazepam. Its safety has been established both in adults and children (Congdon & Forsythe 1980). Local thrombophlebitis may occur at the injection site, but is usually mild. Respiratory depression is the most important adverse effect, but has been reported in fewer than 5% of treated patients. As with diazepam, the risk of respiratory depression is greatest following acute brain injury (focal or metabolic), in those who have already received barbiturates (Tassinari *et al.* 1983), and in the elderly. Hypotension and cardiovascular collapse are rarely observed, and probably occur only when clonazepam is injected too quickly. The negative inotropic and hypotensive effect of clonazepam and other benzodiazepines is probably less than that of thiopentone and other anaesthetic barbiturates. There is a small but important risk of respiratory arrest and facilities for resuscitation should ideally be available whenever clonazepam (or any other benzodiazepine) is given by the intravenous route. Occasionally diazepam and clonazepam are said paradoxically to exacerbate tonic seizures (and tonic status), but evidence is anecdotal and unconvincing. One published report (Bittencourt & Richens 1981) of a patient with apparent tonic status worsened by diazepam, subsequently turned out to be a case of pseudostatus. Clonazepam sedates and depresses levels of consciousness, and is more potent than diazepam in this regard. Tolerance to the anticonvulsant effects may develop, although in the context of the acute therapy of status this is not usually evident, a particular advantage over diazepam and especially lorazepam.

Table 5.13. *Clonazepam*

Indication (stage of status)
Established (and early) status

Usual preparation
1 ml ampoule containing 1 mg of clonazepam

Usual dosage
1 mg bolus injection over 30 s (adults); 0.25–0.5 mg (children). Can be repeated up to
   four times. The 1 ml ampoule of clonazepam is mixed with 1 ml of water for injection
   (provided as diluent) *immediately* before administration. Rate not to exceed 1 mg in
   30 s.
The drug can also be given more slowly in a dextrose (5%) or 0.9% sodium chloride
   solution[a] (1–2 mg in 250 ml).
Continuous infusion in 0.9% sodium chloride or dextrose (5%) at a dose of 10 mg/24 h
   has been given (3 mg in 250 ml), but is now not generally recommended

Advantages
Rapid onset of action
Longer duration of action than diazepam, midazolam
Acute tolerance less marked than with lorazepam or diazepam
Wide experience in adults and children (not in neonates)
Proven efficacy in tonic–clonic, partial and absence status

Disadvantages
Potential for accumulation on prolonged infusion
Respiratory arrest, hypotension, sedation, thrombophlebitis
Danger of sudden collapse if recommended rate of injection exceeded
Possibly more sedative than other benzodiazepines

---

[a] Normal saline.

Administration and dosage in status epilepticus

Clonazepam is best given by bolus injections of 1 mg over 30 seconds, which can
be repeated if necessary on about four further occasions (childhood dose 0.5 mg).
It is diluted with 1 ml of water, immediately before injection. The drug can also
be given more slowly, diluted in 250 ml of 5% dextrose or 0.9% sodium chloride
(normal saline). Previously, continuous intravenous infusion was popular, but this
is now probably best avoided in view of its long half-life, the risk of toxicity and
the availability of better alternatives.

Summary of use in status epilepticus (table 5.13)

The main indication of clonazepam is as a bolus injection in early status, where
there is wide experience in adults and children in convulsive, absence and partial
status. Although there is little to choose between the two drugs in routine clinical
practice, clonazepam does have a longer duration of action, and a lower incidence
of late relapse. Published experience of clonazepam is, however, less than that of
diazepam. The side-effect profiles of clonazepam and diazepam are approximately

similar, and there is a risk of cardiorespiratory depression, thrombophlebitis and sedation. The continuous infusion of clonazepam in established status has been used in the past, although now (in common with all benzodiazepine infusions) is not generally recommended unless careful ITU monitoring is carried out and facilities for resuscitation are available. These are necessary because of the tendency for clonazepam to accumulate, with the attendant risks of profound sedation and respiratory depression.

Lignocaine (lidocaine)

NHCOCH$_2$N(C$_2$H$_5$)$_2$

CH$_3$

CH$_3$

Lignocaine (2-(diethylamino)-*N*-(2,6-dimethylphenyl)acetamide; C$_{14}$H$_{12}$N$_2$O; molecular weight 234.3) was synthesised in 1943, and has for many years been used as a local anaesthetic and cardiac anti-arryhthmic. It is available for intravenous administration as lignocaine hydrochloride. Lignocaine is insoluble in water (the hydrochloride is highly soluble) and relatively insoluble in lipid (octanol/water partition coefficient 42). The pK_a of lignocaine is 7.86. It has considerable promise as a short-term antiepileptic drug, for initial therapy of status (or for patients resistant to diazepam) by repeated bolus injection and short-term continuous infusion. Its singular advantages are a short half-life and a relative lack of respiratory or cerebral depressant effects. It is widely used in status in Scandinavia both in adults and in children. Commonly used commercial preparations of lignocaine include Xylocaine and Xylotox.

Pharmacokinetics

The pharmacokinetics of lignocaine have been intensively studied in cardiological but to a lesser in extent neurological settings. After intravenous injection, distribution to vascular organs is very rapid, and the drug crosses the blood–brain barrier freely. The apparent volume of distribution in adults is 1.3 l/kg and is 2- to 3-fold greater in infants (Hellström-Westas *et al.* 1992). The drug is 65% protein bound. It is rapidly and extensively metabolised in the liver by the microsomal mixed-function oxidase enzymes, to a variety of metabolites of which the xylidide derivatives (methylethylglycinexylidide and glycinexylidide) have antiepileptic activity, but less so than the parent drug. No unchanged lignocaine is excreted in the urine. The clearance of lignocaine approaches the rate of hepatic blood flow, to which it is therefore very sensitive.

In adults the distribution half-life is often less than 10 minutes, and the elimination half-life about 1.6 hours. In neonates, there is lower plasma protein binding, and the reported elimination half-life is about 5 hours for lignocaine, 9–28 hours for methylethylglycinexylidide and 22 hours for glycinexylidide (Wallin, Nergardh & Hynning 1989). Thus, with prolonged therapy, there is a tendency for the active metabolites to accumulate.

Clinical effect in status epilepticus

Lignocaine was first given in status in 1955, and since then its use has been reported in over 150 patients (Bernhard, Bohm & Hojeberg 1955; Taverner & Bain 1958; Westreich & Kneller 1972; Hariga & Ectors 1974; Lemmen, Klassen & Duiser 1978; Tsukamoto *et al.* 1980; Hellström-Westas *et al.* 1988; Pascual *et al.* 1988, 1992; Wallin *et al.* 1989; DeGiorgio *et al.* 1991). In the only controlled study (Taverner & Bain 1958), lignocaine was superior to placebo in all three patients studied. Pascual *et al.* (1992) reported a detailed study of 42 episodes of status in 36 patients, 22 with limited pulmonary reserve, and 14 in whom diazepam had proved ineffective (to a maximum dose of 20 mg). Lignocaine was administered in a single intravenous dose of 1.5–2 mg/kg (usually 100 mg) over 2 minutes. If no response was observed, a second identical dose was given. If an initial response was followed by recurrence, a continuous infusion of lignocaine was initiated at a rate of 3–4 mg/kg per hour. Of the 42 episodes, 31 responded to the first injection, but seizures recurred in 19 (within 3–30 minutes in 18). Thirty patients (the 11 nonresponders and 19 temporary responders) received a second bolus injection and 19 responded. Twelve showed a permanent response, but in seven convulsions recurred within 10–180 minutes. The same 11 patients who failed to respond to the initial dose failed also to respond to the second bolus. Continuous infusion in the seven temporary responders resulted in complete suppression of seizures in three. Those with secondarily generalised status or acute systemic or focal cerebral disorders showed a poor response to the initial bolus injection, and the overall outcome was worse. Hellström-Westas *et al.* (1988) first reported the use of lignocaine in 46 neonates at various dosages with good effect, and followed this up with a further report of 24 severely ill infants with neonatal seizures (it is not clear whether the same patients were included in both reports; Hellström-Westas *et al.* 1992). A bolus dose of 1.5–2.2 mg/kg was given, followed by a continuous infusion at a dose of 4.7–6.3 mg/kg per hour. In 15 of the 24 neonates, seizures were immediately abolished, in seven seizures were improved but not completely stopped, and in two there was no effect. Blood levels of lignocaine and its two main active metabolites were measured and showed wide individual variation, with little correlation between anticonvulsant efficacy and blood level. Combining the concentrations of lignocaine and its active metabolites, the maximum recommended anti-arrythmic adult level (30 µmol/l) was exceeded after 4 hours of infusion. The drug was completely eliminated within 24–48 hours after stopping the infusion.

These results suggest that lignocaine has efficacy in status similar to that of diazepam, and may also be useful where diazepam has failed to control seizures.

The response to bolus injection is, however, essentially temporary, due to its rapid clearance. Indeed, where prolonged response is reported, this may have been due to concurrent therapy. A second dose has a more prolonged action, and a short-term continuous infusion can be usefully employed, although experience of this in status is limited. Because of the tendency of the active metabolites to accumulate, a lignocaine infusion should probably not be continued for longer than 12 hours, and the risk of adverse effects increases after 4 hours. The main use of lignocaine is therefore as a short-term antiepileptic drug, or as a first-line treatment given before longer-term agents such as phenytoin or phenobarbitone can be employed. Lignocaine may have a particular role for the treatment of status in patients with pre-existing respiratory disease.

Toxic effects in status epilepticus

Data concerning toxicity are sparse, but severe central nervous system or respiratory depression has not been recorded at standard doses. In the controlled study reported by Pascual *et al.* (1992), slight hypotension was noted in two responders, and an 87 year old patient with severe chronic obstructive respiratory disease died following cardiorespiratory arrest. Cardiorespiratory suppression following intravenous injection in patients with severely depressed left ventricular function or cardiac conduction disorders has been demonstrated in cardiological practice, and cardiac monitoring is essential. The total dose of lignocaine which can be given safely by continuous infusion is not known. However, as the drug has proconvulsant effects at doses greater than 300 mg/hour (blood concentrations greater than 6 mg/l), it would seem prudent not to exceed this dose. The rate of intravenous bolus injections should not exceed 750 μg/minute. In their series of neonates treated with lignocaine, Hellström-Westas *et al.* (1992) reported acidosis and bradycardia in one infant where the drug was given as an infusion.

Administration and dosage in status epilepticus

Lignocaine is available in ready-made 0.1% (1 mg/ml) and 0.2% (2 mg/ml) intravenous infusion containers (500 ml) in 5% glucose, or as 5 ml or 10 ml ready-made injection syringes (containing 100 mg of lignocaine), or as 5 ml vials for dilution containing 100 mg and 1000 mg of lignocaine. It is given in early status, by bolus injection of 1.5–2.0 mg/kg (usually 100 mg in adults) over 2 minutes. This can be repeated once if necessary. If seizures continue, a continuous intravenous infusion can be given for several hours (but not for longer than 12 hours) in a dose of 3–4 mg/kg per hour (3–6 mg/kg per hour in neonates). The suggested infusion concentration is 0.2% in 5% dextrose, Ringer's solution or 0.9% sodium chloride (normal saline).

Summary of use in status epilepticus (table 5.14)

Lignocaine has enthusiastic support as a drug of first choice in early status, as an alternative to diazepam. The drug has been used successfully in adult, childhood and neonatal status, given by intravenous bolus or short-term infusion. Its advantages are its rapid action, the low risk of cardiorespiratory or cerebral depression,

237

Table 5.14. *Lignocaine (lidocaine)*

Indication (stage of status)
Early status

Usual preparations
5 ml ready-prepared syringe containing 20 mg lignocaine/ml (2%) *or* 10 ml ready-prepared syringe containing 10 mg lignocaine/ml (1%) (i.e. both syringes containing 100 mg)
5 ml vial containing 20 mg/ml (i.e. 100 mg) of lignocaine (2%)
5 ml vial containing 200 mg/ml (i.e. 1000 mg) of lignocaine (20%)
Ready-made 0.1% (1 mg/ml) and 0.2% (2 mg/ml) infusions (in 500 ml containers in 5% dextrose)

Usual dosage
i.v. bolus 1.5–2.0 mg/kg (usually 100 mg in adults). Rate not to exceed 50 mg/min. Can be repeated once if necessary.
Continuous infusion 3–4 mg/kg per h (usually of 0.2% solution in 5% dextrose, for no more than 12 hours); 3–6 mg/kg per h (neonates)

Advantages
Small risk of respiratory or cerebral depression, or hypotension
Wide experience in adults, children and neonates
Small risk of accumulation
Proven efficacy in tonic–clonic and partial status
Especially useful in patients with respiratory disease

Disadvantages
Short-term effect, with marked tolerance; temporary seizure control only
Possible proconvulsant effect at high levels
Active metabolite which may accumulate on prolonged therapy
Cardiac monitoring essential
Cardiac rhythm disturbances, depression of cardiac function
Clearance dependent on hepatic blood flow

---

and the lack of accumulation. Its effects are unfortunately only temporary, and recurrence of seizures is common unless more definitive long-term antiepileptic drug treatment has been introduced. It may have a particular place in the treatment of patients with pre-existing respiratory disease. Hypotension and cardiac arrhythmia are the most important side-effects, and cardiac monitoring is essential. Its clearance is sensitive to hepatic blood flow, and it has an active metabolite which can accumulate on prolonged therapy (not usually relevant in status). Lignocaine is proconvulsant at high levels, and so caution should be exercised if particularly high doses are given, or in hepatic failure.

Lorazepam

The first reported use of lorazepam (7-chloro-5-(2-chlorophenyl)-1,3-dihydro-3-hydoxy-2H-1,4-benzodiazepin-2-one; $C_{15}H_{10}Cl_2N_2O_2$; molecular weight 321.2) in clinical practice was in 1973. It is now most widely used as an anxiolytic;

its use in epilepsy is confined largely to the emergency treatment of status epilepticus. It is a crystalline substance, insoluble in water, and unionised at physiological pH. It is only moderately lipid soluble, and much less so than diazepam (octanol/water partition coefficient for lorazepam is 73). It has a high affinity for the benzodiazepine receptor, and an antiepileptic efficacy similar to that of clonazepam. Its long duration of action and relative lack of distribution confer substantial advantages over diazepam. The pK_a is 1.3 (and 11.5 for its alternative form). It can be diluted and does not precipitate in glucose or sodium chloride solutions. The pharmacokinetic properties of lorazepam are well characterised (Comer *et al.* 1973; Dundee *et al.* 1978; Greenblatt *et al.* 1979; Ochs *et al.* 1980; Greenblatt & Divoll 1983; Morrison *et al.* 1984; Homan & Unwin 1989) A commonly used commercial preparation of lorazepam is Ativan.

Absorption

In status lorazepam is invariably given by intravenous bolus injection. Whilst this produces high brain levels rapidly, it is noteworthy that, within 2 hours of administration, similar blood levels are produced by intravenous, intramuscular injection or oral administration (thus any of these routes will suffice for nonurgent therapy, for instance in partial status). Promising, but anectodal, results for rectal administration in children have also been reported (Mitchell & Crawford 1990). Continuous intravenous infusions have been advocated, but tolerance renders this approach ineffective. The relatively low lipid solubility means that cerebral uptake is slightly slower than with other more lipid-soluble drugs (for instance diazepam), but the delay is not clinically significant.

Distribution

Lorazepam is slowly distributed because of its relatively low lipid solubility, with a distribution half-life (where this is meaningful) of about 2–3 hours, yet it is

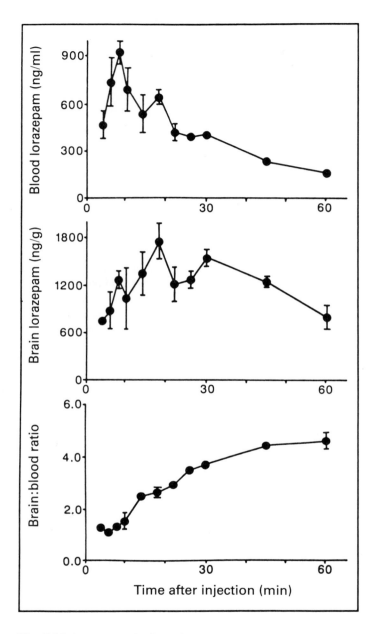

Fig. 5.11. Lorazepam brain and serum concentrations, and brain:serum concentration ratio after intraperitoneal injection of 2.0 mg/kg, in three rats. Note (1) the slow fall in plasma levels (lorazepam is not very lipid soluble, and there is therefore no rapid distribution phase); and (2) the relatively slow rise in cerebral levels, due to the poor lipid solubility of the drug; but (3) the slow rise in the

strongly bound to the benzodiazepine receptor. These properties confer on it a distinct advantage over diazepam and other benzodiazepines; there is little accumulation in lipid stores (muscle, fat), yet it has a relatively prolonged anti-epileptic action, longer than would be anticipated from simple blood level measurements. The volume of distribution is about 1.0–2.0 l/kg, and it is 90% (range 88–92%) bound to plasma proteins. CFS concentration is about 10–15% of that in blood, and this proportion does not vary with blood level. In rats, cerebral concentrations are about 40-fold higher than the free blood concentrations, and cerebral levels decline more slowly over time than blood levels, in marked contrast to the very rapid fall in diazepam cerebral concentrations (Walton & Treiman 1990; fig. 5.11). The minimum effective blood level for seizure control is said to be 30 ng/ml (Walker *et al.* 1979), and after a single intravenous injection of 5 mg, levels generally remain above 30 ng/ml for 18 hours. In 10 cases of status, mean lorazepam levels at 2 hours were 52 ng/ml after 4 mg injections (Walker *et al.* 1979). After a bolus dose of 0.1 mg lorazepam/kg in 32 drug-naive patients, levels ranged from 51.9 to 244.6 (mean 121.1) ng/ml at a mean of 28 minutes after the infusion (Treiman *et al.* 1992).

Biotransformation and excretion

Lorazepam is metabolised by the hepatic microsomal enzymes, largely by glucu-ronidisation, and unlike most benzodiazepines there are no active metabolites. The elimination half-life is about 15 hours (range 8–24 hours). The glucuronide derivative is the main urinary excretory product, and the renal clearance of the metabolite is about 37 ml/minute. The blood concentrations of lorazepam are largely unaffected by even severe hepatic or renal disease, although concentrations of inactive metabolites may vary.

Clinical effect in status epilepticus

Experimental studies have often shown lorazepam to have a greater efficacy than that of other benzodiazepine drugs, and a longer action than its half-life would predict. This can be attributed in large part to the strong receptor affinity of lorazepam, but this does not explain all observed differences between lorazepam and clonazepam; other factors must be involved (Valin *et al.* 1981).

The effectiveness of lorazepam in status has been well demonstrated in studies of over 400 patients (or episodes), with seizure control rates of about 80%. Some reports have been in neonates (Deshmukh *et al.* 1986; Maytal, Novak & King 1991), and others in children and adults (Waltregny & Dargent 1975; Amand & Evrard 1976: Walker *et al.* 1979; Griffith & Karp 1980; Sorel, Mechler & Harmant

Caption for fig. 5.11 (*cont.*).
brain:blood concentration ratio, demonstrating the strong cerebral binding of the drug. The relative persistence of cerebral levels is responsible for the prolonged action of lorazepam. In status epilepticus, target serum levels above 300 ng/ml should be effective in most cases. (From Walton & Treiman 1990, with kind permission.)

1981; Leppik *et al.* 1983*a,b*; Gilmore *et al.* 1984; Levy & Krall 1984; Treiman *et al.* 1985; Lacey *et al.* 1986; Crawford, Mitchell & Snodgrass 1987; Gabor 1990; Andermann *et al.* 1992). Open comparisons have been made with diazepam, phenytoin and clonazepam (Sorel *et al.* 1981; Leppik *et al.* 1983*a*; Treiman *et al.* 1985), and efficacy has been related to blood level in status (Walker *et al.* 1979; Sorel *et al.* 1981). Crawford *et al.* (1987) reported a large retrospective study of 300 episodes of treatment (single and repeated injections) in 77 adults and children, at a mean dose of about 0.1 mg/kg in children under 12 years, and 0.07 mg/kg in older subject. Of the treatment episodes, 79% resulted in cessation of seizures, the results being somewhat better in partial than in generalised convulsive seizures. Prior administration of other antiepileptic drugs did not influence either effectiveness or side-effects. Leppik *et al.* (1983*a*) compared diazepam (10 mg) and lorazepam (4 mg) in a double-blind trial involving 81 episodes (78 adult patients). Seizures of all types were controlled in 89% of lorazepam and 76% of diazepam treatment episodes, and in 91% and 92%, respectively, of generalised seizures. Similar results were repeated by Andermann *et al.* (1992) in a double-blind comparison with diazepam in 62 patients. These differences are not significantly different. In the six neonates with seizures unresponsive to phenobarbitone (40 mg/kg), reported by Maytal *et al.* (1991), lorazepam was given intravenously at a dose of 0.05 mg/kg (repeated to a total dose of 0.15 mg/kg if necessary) and this controlled seizures within 3 minutes, without side-effects.

Aaltonen, Kanto & Salo (1980) noted the peak sedative action of lorazepam to be 30–60 minutes after injection, suggesting a relatively slow penetration into brain, significantly slower than that of diazepam (Elliott 1976). Anxieties that the onset of action might be too slow in status in human subjects have not, however, been realised. The median onset of action of lorazepam is 3 minutes (range 1–15 minutes), similar to that of diazepam (Leppik *et al.* 1983*a*). Seizures usually cease within 15 minutes of injection in successful childhood or adult cases (Amand & Evrard 1976; Walker *et al.* 1979; Crawford *et al.* 1987), and within 3 minutes in the neonatal patients of Maytal *et al.* (1991). Effects on the EEG of normal subjects are noticeable within 30–240 seconds after intravenous injection of 2–5 mg, and CSF concentrations peak within 7 minutes of injection (Comer *et al.* 1973).

A very important potential advantage of lorazepam over diazepam is its longer duration of action, in both adults and children, and in neonates, where effects lasting 12 hours or so are usual (Deshmukh *et al.* 1986; Maytal *et al.* 1991). Although the blood half-life of lorazepam is shorter than that of diazepam, high cerebral concentrations persist for much longer (for hours rather than minutes). Nevertheless, within 24 hours, tolerance becomes a frequent problem, probably more so than with other benzodiazepines, reflecting cerebral binding properties. Repeated doses (and long-term infusions) are thus less effective than single doses (Crawford *et al.* 1987). Seizure control, for instance, was observed for over 3 hours in 83% and over 24 hours in half of the patients reported by Lacey *et al.* (1986). In another series of 22 patients, control was recorded in 19 cases for 12 hours, 17 cases for 24 hours, and 16 for 48 hours (Homan & Walker 1983). Alternative longer-term antiepileptic drug therapy is therefore recommended

242

within 12 hours of the administration of lorazepam in all cases, even by the most enthusiastic advocates (Mitchell & Crawford 1990) an exception may be in acute neonatal status (Maytal *et al.* 1991). The long duration of initial action, however, is a great potential advantage over shorter-acting drugs in early status, and allows time to establish aetiology, and to organise and initiate more definitive longer-term therapy.

Toxic effects in status epilepticus

Lorazepam injection produces relatively few serious side-effects and, surprisingly, prior medication with other antiepileptic drugs does not seem to increase the risk or severity of adverse reactions (Mitchell & Crawford 1990). In a comparative study of lorazepam and diazepam (Leppik *et al.* 1983*a*), significant (but not fatal) adverse effects occurred in 13% (5 of 40 episodes on lorazepam) and 12% (5 of 41 episodes on diazepam) of cases, including respiratory depression in 10% and 9.8%, respectively. Crawford *et al.* (1987) recorded respiratory depression at an unstated frequency, and noted this after the first injection or not at all – a rather different pattern than is common after diazepam therapy. Drug-induced hypotension is rare (one patient reported by Leppik *et al.* (1983*a*)). Cardiac rate or rhythm changes have not been reported in status. Sedation is, of course, common, and postinjection drowsiness or sleep must be anticipated in all cases; severe stupor or coma or prolonged sedation, however, is rare. Agitation, confusion, hallucinations, drowsiness, tremor, ataxia and other transient cerebral side-effects are also reported. Thrombophlebitis or pain at the injection site, common with diazepam therapy, does not occur with lorazepam injection.

Administration and dosage in status epilepticus

Lorazepam is given by intravenous bolus injection. It is usually available as a 1 ml ampoule containing 4 mg of lorazepam. As the drug is only moderately lipid soluble, the rate of injection is not critical. In adults, it is usual to give a bolus dose of 0.07 mg/kg (to a maximum of 4 mg) and to repeat this after 10 minutes if no effect has been observed. In children under 10 years, bolus doses of 0.1 mg/kg are recommended. Long-term infusion is not recommended.

Summary of use in status epilepticus (table 5.15)

Lorazepam is indicated in the early stage of status only. Its pharmacology and clinical effects have been extensively investigated in adults, children and in the newborn, and at all ages lorazepam is highly effective. It binds strongly to cerebral tissue and thus has a longer duration of action than diazepam. It is only moderately lipid soluble, and so the problems caused by redistribution are less than with the other benzodiazepines, the injection can be given rapidly, and there is only a small risk of accumulation. Because of these properties, many now consider lorazepam to have replaced diazepam as the drug of choice in early status. Its main disadvantage is the rapid development of tolerance in most patients. Initial injections of lorazepam are effective for about 12 hours (longer than with diazepam), but later administration is much less useful, and there is no place for longer-term lorazepam

Table 5.15. *Lorezepam*

Indication (stage of status)
Early status

Usual preparation
1 ml ampoule containing 4 mg/ml

Usual dosage
i.v. bolus of 0.07 mg/kg (usually 4 mg), repeated after 10 min if necessary (adults); bolus
  of 0.1 mg/kg (children)
The injection can be given at any rate

Advantages
Extensive clinical experience in adults, children and the newborn
Proven efficacy in tonic–clonic and partial status
Pharmacology and pharmacokinetics well characterised
Single injection produces a long-lasting effect
Little risk of accumulation
Stable compound with little tendency to precipitate in solution
Low risk of hypotension
Pharmacokinetics relatively unaffected by hepatic or renal disease

Disadvantages
Strong tendency to acute tolerance, therefore cannot be used for long-term therapy
  (effective for 12 h only)
Respiratory depression (but lower incidence than with other benzodiazepines), sedation

i.v., intravenous.

therapy in established status. Maintenance antiepileptic drug therapy should, therefore, always be given concurrently with lorazepam therapy. Lorazepam has the sedative effects shared by all the benzodiazepine drugs used in status, but sudden hypotension or respiratory collapse are less likely because of the lack of accumulation after single bolus injections. It is stable in solution, and in the doses used in status its pharmacokinetics are relatively unaffected by hepatic or renal disease.

Phenytoin

Phenytoin (5,5-diphenylhydantoin; $C_{15}H_{12}N_2O_2$; molecular weight 252.3) was first synthesised in 1908, but its antiepileptic action was not recognised until 1938; as Lennox (1960) put it 'for epileptics a year of Jubilee'. A parenteral formulation was prepared in 1956. Its first use in status was in 1958 (Carter 1958), but its value in this clinical situation was not immediately appreciated. It has a pK_a of 8.3, and is highly lipid soluble, but relatively insoluble in water. The phenytoin solutions used for injection are very alkaline, with pH values around 12. A commonly used commercial preparation of phenytoin is Epanutin. Previously the drug was also known as dilantin.

Absorption

In status, the initial doses of phenytoin should be administered only via the intravenous route (although subsequent long-term supplementation can be given orally). It is very poorly absorbed following rectal administration, and very slowly and unpredictably absorbed after intramuscular injection. So much so, indeed, that peak blood levels and rate of absorption are both less after intramuscular than after oral administration. Neither rectal nor intramuscular administration in status should be contemplated. The upper limit of the conventionally quoted phenytoin therapeutic blood level range is 80 μmol/l (20 mg/l), but many patients in status require higher levels (say up to 120 μmol/l (30 mg/l) before seizures can be controlled.

Distribution

In a careful study of the rate of phenytoin entry into brain in adult dogs and cats (Ramsey *et al.* 1979), peak brain levels were reached within 6 minutes after phenytoin infusion, and high levels were well maintained for 60 minutes due to substantial tissue binding. Concentrations in the CSF also peaked at about 6 minutes, suggesting that the drug enters each compartment by an independent mechanism.

After a single intravenous injection in human subjects, phenytoin reaches peak brain levels within 15 minutes. After intravenous injection, the distribution half-life is short (about 6 minutes on initial dosing), and levels fall rapidly before stabilising. Wallis, Kutt & McDowell (1968) found mean blood levels of about 18 mg/l for 24 hours in 26 patients given 300–500 mg 6 hours after 100 mg intravenously and 500 mg intramuscularly. Wilder *et al.* (1977) found mean blood concentrations to be above 10 mg/l (i.e. 'therapeutic levels') in 9 of 14 patients 12 hours after an intravenous infusion of 10–17 mg/kg without oral supplement. Overall, brain levels are maintained better than blood levels owing to preferential binding, and they fall at a slower rate (Ramsey *et al.* 1979; fig. 5.12). Thus, compared to diazepam, for instance, phenytoin is relatively slow to enter cerebral

245

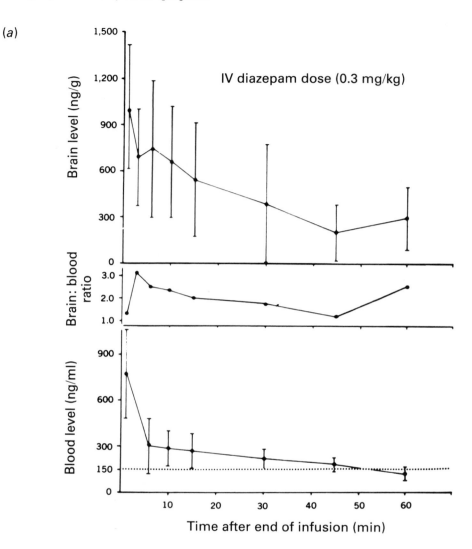

Fig. 5.12. Comparison of (*a*) diazepam, (*b*) phenobarbitone and (*c*) phenytoin blood and brain levels after single intravenous injections. These three illustrations show drug concentrations in brain and blood, and the brain:blood ratio, of phenytoin, phenobarbitone and diazepam, in the adult cat or dog following the intravenous infusion of diazepam (0.3 mg/kg), phenobarbitone (10 mg/kg) or phenytoin (10 mg/kg). Maximum brain levels were achieved at 1 minute for diazepam, 3 minutes for phenobarbitone and 6 minutes for phenytoin. The latter two drugs thus entered brain more slowly, but high brain concentrations were retained for longer periods of time. The rapid entry and exit of diazepam from cerebral tissue explains the

(*b*)

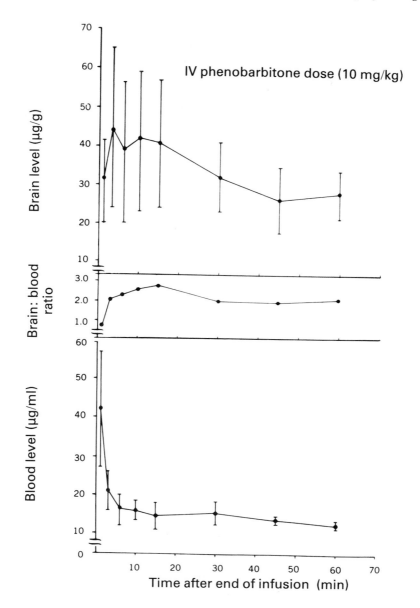

Caption for fig. 5.12 (*cont.*).
relatively rapid onset but short-lived action of diazepam in status. (From Ramsey *et al.* 1979, Brain uptake of phenytoin, phenobarbital, and diazepam, *Archives of Neurology*, **36**, 535–539, copyright 1979, American Medical Association, with kind permission.)

(c)

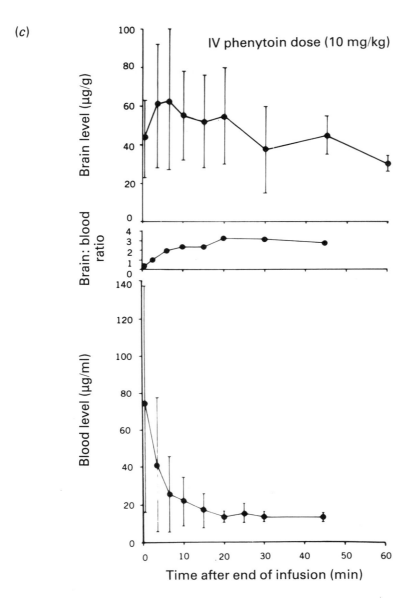

Caption for fig. 5.12 (*cont.*).

tissue but the effects are much longer lasting. The overall concentration of the drug in brain is one to two times that in blood. Concentrations vary in different cerebral regions. High levels are found in white matter, lower levels in grey matter and particularly low concentrations in active epileptogenic areas (Sherwin, Eisen

248

& Sokolowski 1973; Vajda *et al.* 1974; Rapport *et al.* 1975; Sironi *et al.* 1980) and in regions of acute cerebral damage. This distribution may explain the poorer efficacy of phenytoin in acute symptomatic status

The notorious pharmacokinetics of phenytoin have been the subject of intensive investigation (see Woodbury & Swinyard 1972; Eadie & Tyrer 1989; Woodbury 1989). It is a drug which exhibits zero-order kinetics, with saturable metabolism at therapeutic dosages, and marked individual variation in metabolic rates. Dose:blood level ratios therefore vary widely both within populations and also in individuals at different doses. Because of the zero-order kinetics, the elimination half-life varies greatly with blood level, a fact recognised only in 1970; hence, early published blood half-life values are difficult to assess. In any population, elimination half-life values also vary owing to genetic differences in metabolic ability. Published half-life values range between 10 and 160 hours (usually 20–70 hours) after a single intravenous infusion of 15–18 mg/kg (Gugler, Manion & Azaroff 1976; Cranford *et al.* 1978; Leppik *et al.* (1983*b*). In 53 intravenous phenytoin infusions at a mean dose of 16.6 (± 1.8) mg/kg, the mean clearance was 0.0157 (± 0.0132) l/kg per hour, volume of distribution 0.78 (± 0.11) l/kg, and the elimination half-life 51.2 (± 31.6) hours. The value usually cited for volume of distribution is about 0.7 l/kg (Cranford *et al.* 1978; Leppik *et al.* 1983*b*) with less variation than with clearance, although both are dependent on blood level. Because of this population variability and intraindividual variation with blood level, blood level monitoring is required in all patients in status. In a study of intravenous loading in 139 adults on 159 occasions (137 with frequent repetitive seizures), doses of 18 mg/kg produced therapeutic levels for 24 hours after infusion in all cases, 15 mg/kg in most cases, and 12 mg/kg in a few cases (Cranford *et al.* 1978). On continuing oral (or nasogastric) administration after intravenous loading, brain concentrations increase in parallel with blood concentrations and steady-state levels are reached after about 4 days (Woodbury 1989).

Phenytoin is strongly protein bound, about 80%–93% at 37°C, and this varies little with blood concentration. Binding is affected by temperature, is lower in neonates (approximately 70% bound) and also in late adult life, and is slightly decreased by hepatic and renal disease and in late pregnancy (Porter & Layzer, 1975; Painter *et al.* 1987; Woodbury 1989). Brain concentrations are about 10-fold higher than CSF concentrations.

Biotransformation and excretion

Phenytoin is metabolised in the liver, principally by hydroxylation, via the cytochrome oxidase system enzymes arene oxidase and epoxide hydrolase. The major metabolites are p-HPPH (5-(4-hydroxyphenyl)-5-phenylhydantoin) and then a dihydrodiol metabolite (Chang & Glazko 1972; Browne & Chang 1989). Both enzymes are potentially saturable, and both exhibit genetically determined activity which varies widely between individuals. The metabolites do not have significant antiepileptic activity. Less than 5% of phenytoin is excreted unchanged, and after intravenous administration about 50–60% is excreted as p-HPPH (Noach & van Rees 1964; Noach, Woodbury & Goodman 1958).

249

Clinical effect in status epilepticus

When phenytoin was first introduced as intravenous therapy, the recommended dosages were small (100 mg or so). Although initial reports were enthusiastic (Carter 1958; McWilliams 1958), the drug did not gain wide popularity, possibly partly due to inadequate dosing, and also because diazepam had entered clinical practice (to great acclaim) at about the same time. Indeed, many then thought that phenytoin had no effect on acute seizures. When blood level measurements were introduced into clinical research, it became clear that the phenytoin levels obtained either by the intravenous infusion of small doses or by intramuscular injection were too low. Then, in a seminal report, Wallis *et al.* (1968) described the results of intravenous loading of 1000 mg (a seemingly very high dose at that time) in 31 patients with status, of whom 18 immediately responded (including two partial responders). Patients with acute or rapidly progressing cerebral pathology were found to be less likely to respond to phenytoin, or indeed subsequent therapy with other antiepileptic drugs, an observation that has since been made repeatedly. McWilliam (1958) reported control in 10 out of 11 children in status, and Wilder *et al.* (1977) cessation of seizures within 30 minutes of starting a phenytoin infusion in 9 out of 10 cases of major status. Leppik *et al.* (1983*b*) described the use of intravenous phenytoin (0.65–2 g) on 159 occasions in 139 adults. In 87%, seizures were completely controlled by the time the infusion had been completed. Patients with acute cerebral insults or diffuse encephalopathy did significantly worse (complete control in 43% of 37 cases) than those with established epilepsy or alcohol withdrawal (control in 90% of 99 cases). Von Albert (1983) reported a total of 84 patients treated with phenytoin, in 75% of whom seizure ceased during the infusion, in 15% soon after the infusion, but in 10% no seizure control was obtained (included were patients with acute encephalitis or delirium tremens). In an extension of his previous series to over 200 patients, Wilder (1983) reported the cessation of seizures within 10 minutes of initiating the infusion in 30% of the patients, and within 20 minutes in about 80% (phenytoin was infused at a rate of 50 mg/minute to a dose of 15 mg/kg). Thus, by the end of the early 1980s, phenytoin had become firmly established as a drug of first choice in major status, chosen, for instance, by 75% of neurologists from California as first-line therapy (see Lowenstein & Alldredge 1993).

Effective cerebral levels of the drug are maintained for many hours after phenytoin loading, and thus phenytoin loading commonly results in the permanent cessation of seizures; this is a distinct advantage over shorter-acting antiepileptics such as diazepam. It is usual to initiate maintenance therapy with phenytoin (orally or via a nasogastric tube) 6 hours after initial loading at a starting dose of 100 mg every 6–8 hours. This ensures stable blood levels close to 80 μmol/l in the majority of patients, although subsequent dosage should be guided by blood level monitoring. A range of levels of 20.6–53.4 μg/ml was found at a mean of 14.3 minutes after a 17.5 mg/kg infusion in 10 drug-naive patients presenting in status, emphasising the need for blood level monitoring (Treiman *et al.* 1992). The co-administration of diazepam did not make much difference. The need to monitor blood levels in children and infants, from early in treatment, was also stressed by Richard *et al.* (1993).

Delgado-Escueta & Enrile-Bacsal (1983) have popularised a combination drug approach to the treatment of status epilepticus (a concept originally suggested by Sutherland & Tait (1969). The regimen comprises the simultaneous administration of 10–20 mg of diazepam intravenously at a rate of 2 mg/minute together with phenytoin at a rate of 50 mg/minute (to a total dose of up to 18 mg/kg), via separate intravenous infusion sites. The rationale of this approach is that diazepam will control the seizures rapidly (within about 5 minutes) in most patients, but the effects may wear off quickly (after 60 minutes or so). The administration of phenytoin takes about 20 minutes and it may not begin to take effect until after a further 10–20 minutes, but it has a long action. The combination thus provides both immediate and long-lasting cover in a way that the individual drugs do not. Furthermore, 50% of patients who do not respond to the initial diazepam will subsequently respond to the phenytoin. If, after 40 minutes, seizures continue, Delgado-Escueta & Enrile-Bacsal (1983) then recommended the addition of an intravenous infusion of diazepam (100 mg diluted in 500 ml of dextrose 5% and run in at 40 ml/hour (8 mg/hour) for 3 hours, to obtain blood levels of between 0.2 and 0.8 mg/l), although nowadays longer-term diazepam infusion has fallen from fashion. In a series of 50 patients, the initial regimen halted seizures in almost all patients with primary generalised, myoclonic or tonic–clonic status, and 65% of those with secondarily generalised status epilepticus. The subsequent intravenous infusion of diazepam controlled a further 22%, leaving just 12% of all secondarily generalised cases needing further therapy. The phenytoin levels targeted in this protocol are in the region of 15–20 mg/l and diazepam levels in the region of 0.2–0.8 mg/l.

Toxic effects in status epilepticus

The rate of intravenous injection of phenytoin should not exceed 50 mg/minute, to minimise the risk of cardiac arrhythmia. Transient nausea, ataxia, nystagmus and vertigo may occur but are usually unimportant in the emergency setting. Respiratory depression is rare on intravenous loading of phenytoin, although anecdotal evidence suggests a potentiation of the depressant effects of previously administered barbiturate or benzodiazepine. Intravenous loading of phenytoin does not seriously depress consciousness. These are significant advantages of phenytoin over the benzodiazepines, and valuable features in the early treatment of status. More prolonged administration of high dose phenytoin may result in symptoms of intoxication (e.g. drowsiness, mood change, nausea, confusion, ataxia, diplopia) but these can be avoided by monitoring blood concentrations. Wallis *et al.* (1968) infusing phenytoin at a rate of 100 mg/minute reported Cheyne-Stokes respiration in 1 of 31 patients, and a drop of 10–15 mmHg in systolic pressure in three elderly patients, and were the first to recommend an infusion rate of 50 mg/minute. Wilder (1983) recorded hypotension (less than 10% of pretreatment systolic blood pressure) in about 50% of over 200 patients treated with phenytoin at a dose of 15 mg/kg and an infusion rate of 50 mg/minute, and mild slowing of the pulse in 10% . Neither severe sedation nor respiratory depression occurred. von Albert (1983) reported no respiratory depression or hypotension in 84 patients. Cranford *et al.* (1978) reported the results of treatment with phenytoin infused at a rate of 50 mg/minute in 159 intravenous loading episodes. Blood pressure was unaltered in 46%, fell by less than 10 mmHg diastolic or 20 mmHg systolic (infusion rate not altered) in 28%, and fell more severely requiring slowing of infusion rate in 25% and discontinuation in 2%. Hypotension was more common in the elderly, but could be avoided by slowing the infusion rate to 10–30 mg/minute. ECG abnormalities occurred in 2% of infusions, including atrial fibrillation in a patient who developed moderate hypotension. Marked respiratory depression occurred in only one patient, who had a high phenytoin blood level prior to infusion and whose postinfusion level rose to over 240 μmol/l (resulting in Cheyne–Stokes respiration, hiccups and then brief apnoea). The level of consciousness was not significantly altered in any case. Other side-effects were uncommon, and included vomiting, choreoathetosis and nystagmus. With the exception of the patient described above, loading with 18 mg phenytoin/kg caused no complications even in those with substantial preinfusion levels. Thus, unless very high preinfusion levels are suspected, high dose loading can be recommended even in pretreated patients. Higher postinfusion blood levels do of course occur in patients who are already receiving phenytoin, but they are substantially higher only in the early postloading phase. Severe thrombophlebitis can occur at the site of injection, particularly if there is extravasation of phenytoin into tissue; the intravenous infusion should be given into a large vein. The drug should not be used in acute intermittent porphyria.

Administration and dosage in status epilepticus

Phenytoin is usually available as 5 ml ampoules containing phenytoin sodium (250 mg in propylene glycol 40%, ethanol 10% and water), and the pH adjusted with sodium hydroxide. There is a danger of crystallisation (Cloyd, Gumnit & McLain 1980), and an alternative preparation has been produced solubilised in tetraglycol and Tris buffer (von Albert 1983). If injected directly in large quantities, the propylene glycol vehicle can itself cause mild hypotension, and is also occasionally allergenic. The phenytoin solution has a pH of 12, and if added to drip bottles containing large volumes of fluid at lower than physiological pH (e.g. 5% glucose) precipitation may occur in the bottle or tubing. Use in a solution of 0.9% sodium chloride (normal saline) at a concentration of 5–20 mg/ml is safer (Carmichael *et al.* 1980). There is also a serious risk of precipitation if other drugs are added to the infusion solution. Administration via a side arm, or directly using an infusion pump is preferable. Phenytoin should not be given by either rectal or intramuscular injection. The rate of infusion of phenytoin solution should not exceed 50 mg/min, and it is prudent to reduce this to 20–30 mg/minute in the elderly. The usual adult dose is about 1000 mg, therefore taking about 20 minutes to administer. Regrettably, a lower dose is too often given, which results in suboptimal cerebral levels. This is a common and potentially serious mistake. ECG monitoring is advisable whilst phenytoin is being administered. The dose of the intravenous

Table 5.16. *Phenytoin*

Indication (stage of status)
Established (and early) status

Usual preparations
5 ml ampoule containing 250 mg stabilised in propylene glycol, ethanol and water
 (alternatives exist; e.g. phenytoin in Tris buffer or in infusion bottles of 750 mg in
 500 ml of osmotic saline)

Usual dosage
15–18 mg/kg i.v. infusion. Usual dose 1000 mg. Rate not to exceed 50 mg/min (20 mg/
 min in the elderly) (adults); 20 mg/kg i.v. infusion. Rate not to exceed 25 mg/min
 (children)

Advantages
Extensive clinical experience in adults, children and neonates
Proven efficacy in tonic–clonic and partial status
Prolonged action, with stable blood levels
Relatively little respiratory or cerebral depression
Can be continued as chronic therapy
Low risk of accumulation
No tolerance or late relapse
Pharmacology well characterised
Can be continued as chronic therapy

Disadvantages
Delayed onset of action, and administration is time consuming
Zero-order pharmacokinetics, with wide individual variation (so blood level monitoring
 essential on prolonged therapy)
Cardiac monitoring essential
Risk of precipitation if diluted in inappropriate solutions or if mixed with other drugs
Cardiac rhythm disturbances, thrombophlebitis, hypotension
Risk of toxicity if recommended rate of injection exceeded

---

i.v., intravenous.

infusion in children is 20 mg/kg, at a rate not exceeding 25 mg/minute. Recently, a more dilute, less alkaline preparation of phenytoin has been produced (750 mg in 500 ml of 0.9% sodium chloride; Phenhydran) which is given over 2 hours, with fewer side-effects and less tendency to cause thrombophlebitis (Andersen *et al.* 1992). This might be preferable in some cases, although in most the required duration of infusion will be too long. Phenytoin therapy can be continued after intravenous loading by oral or further intravenous dosages of 5–6 mg/kg every 6 hours. Blood level monitoring is essential, from the first day of phenytoin administration (Richard *et al.* 1993).

Summary of use in status epilepticus (table 5.16)

Phenytoin is indicated at the stage of established status, where its pharmacology and clinical effects have been extensively studied in adults, children and the newborn. Phenytoin is a highly effective anticonvulsant in status. It has a long duration of action, and can also be continued as maintenance therapy. It has to be infused relatively slowly, and has a slow onset of action; for this reason it is often given in conjunction with diazepam, which has a rapid onset but short duration, the combination providing a rapid-onset long-lasting effect. Phenytoin has saturable pharmacokinetics at therapeutic doses, and blood level monitoring is essential. Phenytoin causes relatively little CNS or respiratory depression, although hypotension is common. ECG monitoring is essential during phenytoin loading. Phenytoin is an inconvenient drug to administer, as its solution is strongly alkaline, and, if added to large volumes of 5% dextrose, may precipitate. Phenytoin can be used in 0.9% sodium chloride (normal saline), but is better injected via a side arm or an infusion pump. Phenytoin should not be admixed with other drugs and cannot be given by intramuscular injection.

Phenobarbitone (phenobarbital)

The antiepileptic properties of phenobarbitone (5-ethyl-5-phenylbarbituric acid; $C_{12}H_{12}N_2O_3$; molecular weight 232.2) were recognised in 1912, and the drug has been used widely ever since. Remarkably few formal clinical studies have been carried out, however, and the relative merits of phenobarbitone in status are still controversial. It is an acidic crystalline substance with a pK_a of 7.3, only sparing soluble in water (although the sodium salt is much more soluble), and only moderately relatively lipid soluble (octanol/water partition coefficient 60). Lowering the pH of the solution reduces ionisation, a potential advantage in status. For intravenous use, the sodium salt of phenobarbitone is usually prescribed. Phenobarbitone has much greater intrinsic anticonvulsant action than other barbiturate drugs (including pentobarbitone and thiopentone), perhaps because of its cerebral distribution, its high concentration in motor cortex, or its specific physico-chemical membrane-stabilising actions (Raines *et al.* 1979). Commonly used commercial preparations of phenobarbitone include Phenobarb, Luminal and Gardenal.

Absorption

Phenobarbitone can be given in status by the intramuscular, rectal and intravenous routes. The usual mode of administration in status is a short intravenous infusion, which produces high cerebral levels moderately quickly. The peak blood levels after intramuscular administration are reached within 4 hours (often in 1–2 hours) (Graham 1978), with a bioavailability of about 80–100% in adults or children (fig. 5.13) (Viswanathan, Booker & Welling 1978; Wilensky *et al.* 1982). In neonates adequate levels occur within about 1–2 hours after intramuscular loading (Brachet-Liermain, Goutières & Aicardi 1975; Boréus, Jalling & Kållberg 1978). Cerebral levels may be reached sooner, but generally intramuscular administration, in spite of its high bioavailability, is not recommended in convulsive status. Rates of absorption and bioavailability are similar after oral and intramuscular administration, and either route may be quite suitable for less urgent indiciations (e.g. partial status; Wilensky *et al.* 1982). Rust & Dodson (1989) provided a detailed review of the pharmacokinetics of phenobarbitone. Rectal administration is feasible and potentially useful, as an aqueous solution is well absorbed (Boyd & Singh 1967), but this method has not gained popularity, and further clinical studies are warranted. After intraperitoneal injection in rats, blood levels of 21 mg/l or more controlled tonic–clonic status, by extrapolation equivalent to doses of 14.5 mg/kg in humans (Walton & Treiman 1989). Higher levels (in excess of 75 mg/l) were needed to control focal motor activity and all EEG evidence of status.

Distribution

After intravenous administration, phenobarbitone is first concentrated in vascular organs and then is distributed more evenly throughout the body (with a low concentration in fat). The drug has a relatively slow entry into brain when compared to more lipid-soluble compounds such as diazepam or thiopentone. Maximal brain level:blood level ratios are reached after 12–60 minutes (compared to 30 seconds, for example, in the case of thiopentone). Phenobarbitone may gain entry to the more vascular grey matter faster than to white matter, but evidence on this point is conflicting. At steady state, the ratio of brain:plasma concentrations in 16 neonates coming to autopsy was 0.71 ± 0.21 (Painter *et al.* 1981), and in adults or children between 0.35 and 1.13 (Sherwin *et al.* 1973; Vajda *et al.* 1974; Harvey *et al.* 1975; Houghton *et al.* 1975). CSF concentrations are about 50% those of blood.

Early experimental studies suggested that phenobarbitone entered brain relatively slowly after intravenous injection, because of its degree of ionisation at physiological pH and poor lipid solubility (Butler 1950; Mark *et al.* 1958, Domek, Barlow & Roth 1960). This might be thought to render phenobarbitone unsuitable for emergency status treatment, but more recent studies have drawn rather different conclusions. The brain uptake of phenobarbitone was carefully studied during prolonged bicuculline-induced status epilepticus in paralysed and ventilated Suffolk sheep (Simon *et al.* 1987). Much higher cerebral phenobarbitone levels were recorded in animals in early status than in nonconvulsing controls. Similarly, in

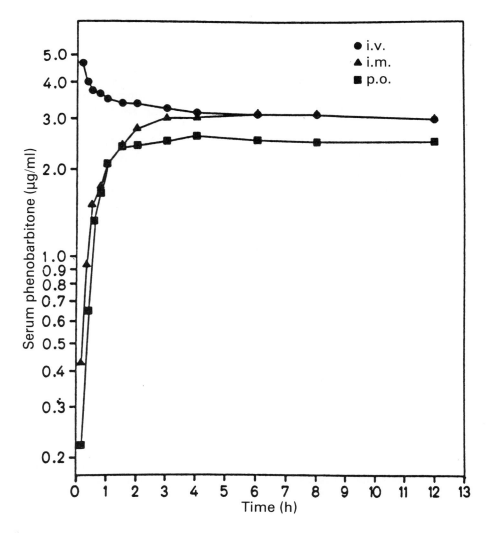

Fig. 5.13. Phenobarbitone concentrations after intramuscular (i.m.), intravenous (i.v.) and oral (p.o.) administration. Absorption of phenobarbitone in six adult subjects, given the drug orally (130 mg), and by i.m. and i.v. injection (130 mg). This demonstrates complete bioavailability by i.m. and p.o. administration, and the i.m. injection produces adequate blood levels within an hour or so (too slow for initial therapy in convulsive status). Results in epileptic patients did not differ from those in controls. Similar complete absorption has been found in infants. (From Wilensky *et al.* 1982, with kind permission.)

generalised status in rats, phenobarbitone cerebral uptake was greater enhanced by seizure activity (Walton & Treiman 1989). The increased rate of uptake during seizures is probably due largely to increased cerebral blood flow and ictal hypertension, and a breakdown in the blood–brain barrier. In established status, the blood pH falls and this too will facilitate phenobarbitone diffusion to the brain. This rapidity of uptake during seizures explains why the onset of action is more rapid in status. The preferential concentration of phenobarbitone in the active epileptic focus confers further advantage over other drugs with less specific patterns of distribution. Another benefit is that high cerebral concentrations are maintained for long periods of time. In a study in adult cats (Ramsey *et al.* 1979), the rate of entry into brain parenchyma was measured following intravenous infusion of phenobarbitone (10 mg/kg), phenytoin (10 mg/kg) and diazepam (0.3 mg/kg). Maximum brain levels of diazepam were achieved within 1 minute, those of phenobarbitone within 3 minutes and those of phenytoin within 6 minutes. High phenobarbitone (and phenytoin) concentrations were maintained for 60 minutes (i.e. no difference between 1 and 60 minute levels), despite falling blood levels, although cerebral diazepam levels fell rapidly (fig. 5.12). Blood and brain levels are found to be similar on long-term therapy (Sherwin *et al.* 1973), but like so many other pharmacological parameters these measurements derived in chronic (steady-state) conditions do not necessarily apply to acute therapy in status.

Following intravenous injections of phenobarbitone, the distribution half-life is 5–15 minutes and the volume of distribution about 0.6 l/kg in adults with epilepsy, and 0.6–0.8 l/kg in children; in neonates reported values have varied widely from 0.39–2.25 l/kg (Lockman 1983; Wilensky *et al.* 1982; Goldberg & McKintyre 1983; Rust & Dodson 1989). About 45–59% (mean 50%) of the drug is protein bound (largely to albumin), and is independent of drug concentration. Protein binding is significantly less in neonates.

Biotransformation and excretion

The main routes of biotransformation in humans are known, although the relative importance of each and the degree of variation are not. Phenobarbitone biotransformation is slow, and is of no clinical relevance in the treatment of status epilepticus.

The elimination half-life of phenobarbitone in adults ranges from about 50–150 hours after a single intravenous dose (mean of about 100 hours; Rust & Dodson 1989), and elimination kinetics are unchanging at normal blood levels (an advantage over phenytoin). In older children the half-life is shorter (mean of about 60 hours, with a reported range of about 20–70 hours). At birth, the capacity to metabolise phenobarbitone is poor, but rapidly develops in the first 4 weeks; half-life values in the first week of life are 77–404 (mean 115) hours compared with 67 hours at 4 weeks. At the age of 6 months, very varied values are cited, e.g. 37–198 hours (Jalling *et al.* 1973; Jalling 1974). The excretion of phenobarbitone is reduced by severe liver or renal disease. Measurements of phenobarbitone clearance in adults have ranged from 0.003 to 0.006 l/kg per hour, and clearance is higher in infants and children (mean value 0.012 l/kg per hour). Clearance is not greatly dependent on hepatic or renal blood flow.

Clinical effect in status epilepticus

Theoretically, phenobarbitone has disadvantages as a drug for status. It is a non-lipid-soluble compound which in normal subjects enters cerebral tissue relatively slowly, it is a powerful sedative, and it has a long elimination half-life and potentially serious side-effects. However, its rate of cerebral uptake is much faster in active epileptic tissue, and it may be preferentially concentrated in epileptic foci. It has a long duration of action, powerful antiepileptic action and possibly also acts as a cerebral-protective agent (Piatt & Schiff 1984). The anticonvulsant effects of phenobarbitone are many times more potent than those of other more lipid-soluble barbiturates such as pentobarbitone or thiopentone at equal CNS depressant levels. It is easy to administer, and has stable pharmacokinetics. These potential advantages of phenobarbitone in the treatment of status have only lately been fully appreciated, and recent clinical trials in status have been very encouraging.

In the only controlled study of phenobarbitone, indeed, one of the very few randomised controlled clinical trials of any drug in status (albeit flawed, see Osorio & Reed 1988), 18 patients were treated with phenobarbitone and 18 with phenytoin + diazepam (Shaner *et al.* 1988). Phenobarbitone was given by intravenous infusion at a dose of 100 mg/minute, until 10 mg/kg had been administered. In 16 of the 18 patients, this simple regimen controlled seizures, although six were given additional phenytoin. In the other two patients, seizures were subsequently controlled by further phenobarbitone therapy, to a total dose of no more than 12 mg/kg, with phenytoin and diazepam. The mean elapsed time from the onset of infusion to cessation of seizures was 5 minutes in the phenobarbitone group, compared with 9 minutes in the phenytoin + diazepam group. No patient on phenobarbitone had convulsions after 25 minutes. Patients responding to phenobarbitone monotherapy had peak blood levels which ranged from 15 to 27 mg/l, and which would be considered only moderate therapeutic levels in chronic therapy. The incidence of hypotension (2 of 18 patients) or cardiac arrhythmia (1 of 18 patients) was low, and similar in both groups, although exact details are not given. The phenobarbitone infusion proved to be technically easier than the combined phenytoin + diazepam regimen, which requires two separate intravenous lines. Furthermore, because of the anectodotal evidence of hypotension induced by the simultaneous administration of phenobarbitone and diazepam, options after failure of the phenytoin + diazepam regimen are less than after a failed phenobarbitone infusion. Evidence from this study indicates that an infusion of phenobarbitone is better initial therapy than that of phenytoin + diazepam. No other satisfactory clinical adult case series have been published, although my own experience and other anectodal evidence confirm these excellent results. The theoretical concern that the onset of action of phenobarbitone is slow – which would be a major drawback in status – does not seem to be confirmed in clinical practice. The need for blood level monitoring of phenobarbitone levels was stressed by Treiman *et al.* (1992), who found a range of blood levels of 15.4–73.7

μg/ml (mean 29.9) at a mean of 22.6 minutes after an infusion of phenobarbitone at a dose of 15 mg/kg in 25 drug-naive patients.

In children, loading doses of 5–20 mg/kg have been traditionally recommended, but in recent years higher dosages of phenobarbitone have been used safely and to good effect. Crawford *et al.* (1988) retrospectively reviewed 48 children (50 episodes of status) in refractory status who had been treated, on the paediatric ITU with high doses of phenobarbitone (defined as phenobarbitone levels in excess of 60 mg/l) given either by repeated bolus injections or continuous infusion. The maximum dose given in a 24 hour period ranged from 30 to 120 mg/kg (by bolus dose, maximum infusion was 40 mg/kg per day). Blood levels varied from 70 to 344 mg/l. Seizures stopped in all but three episodes. Forty patients received respiratory support, but in 39 ventilation was instituted before the start of phenobarbitone therapy. High levels were tolerated by other patients without the need for assisted ventilation. Thirteen patients required pressor agents during the course of the status, in eight prior to the phenobarbitone, and five died. Four of the five patients requiring pressor agents during phenobarbitone loading did so while phenobarbitone levels were rising to very high levels (maximum levels of 162–344 mg/l). Nine patients died, usually as a consequence of the underlying disease, and in 30 there were new severe neurological deficits. Although doses were high in this report, levels were (with few exceptions) only moderate, and maximum levels rose above 200 mg/l in only eight patients. It was concluded that there was no maximum dose above which further doses were ineffective, but evidence based on such a retrospective study design is inconclusive. Prolonged respiratory depression was not observed, and even in the presence of high phenobarbitone levels, respiratory support was not always required. Artificial ventilation was withdrawn in many patients once seizures had been controlled, despite persisting high blood levels. Indeed, there was a striking lack of respiratory depression even at high doses. Hypotension was a hazard especially at high levels or when levels were rising rapidly, but was usually easily controlled. No other serious side-effects were observed. Tolerance to sedation developed quickly, but not to the anticonvulsant effects. The conclusion of this study was that high dose phenobarbitone therapy has many relative advantages over other therapies. Although this may be true, the poor outcome in this retrospective review hardly justifies such optimism. Although high dosages were employed, levels were only moderate, confirming the findings from adult studies that low blood levels (which, it is important to note, do not necessarily imply low cerebral levels) control seizures in most patients. Acute tolerance to the effects of sedation and respiratory depression are commonly encountered, but not to the antiepileptic effect; this is a substantial potential advantage of phenobarbitone over, for example, benzodiazepine drugs.

In the newborn, levels over 15 mg/l (60 μmol/l) are usually needed, although occasionally levels of 45 mg/l or more are required (Gal *et al.* 1982). It is seldom necessary, however, to maintain high levels over an extended period of time. Reported response rates in neonatal seizure series, following intravenous loading, are 32% (Lockman *et al.* 1979), 36% (Painter *et al.* 1981), 85% (Gal *et al.* 1982) and 33% (Van Orman & Darwish 1985).

Toxic effects in status epilepticus

Parenteral administration of high doses of phenobarbitone carries toxic penalties, the most important of which is its inevitable sedative action. Levels above 70 mg/l will compromise the level of consciousness in almost all patients. On prolonged therapy for status, phenobarbitone may contribute to coma, although in the published studies this side-effect is seldom mentioned, and in my own experience sedation is less prominent than might be expected. Hypotension may develop, especially at high or rapidly rising levels, and by repute especially after diazepam co-medication, although formal study of this clinical point is lacking. Respiratory depression is a feared complication of phenobarbitone therapy, but again will usually develop only after severe CNS depression. There are, however, no published data formally reporting the frequency or severity of either CNS or respiratory depression in status; in fact the latter seems rare (Crawford *et al.* 198). Other significant side-effects in the setting of status are rare. Phenobarbitone is dissolved in propylene glycol, as are most other intravenous drugs used in status, and at high doses, especially in the neonate, there is a theoretical danger of propylene glycol-induced hyperosmolality, lactic acidosis, cardiac arrhythmia, hypotension or haemolysis (Crawford & Mitchell 1989). No such effects, however, have been reported in practice. As with other barbiturates, the drug is contraindicated in acute intermittent porphyria.

Administration and dosage in status epilepticus

Phenobarbitone solutions are prepared from the sodium salt, as this is more soluble than crystalline phenobarbitone. The drug is usually presented in 1 ml ampoules containing 200 mg of phenobarbitone in a mixture of propylene glycol (90%) and water (10%). It is a stable preparation which does not easily decompose, nor is the drug absorbed by plastic. Phenobarbitone should not be used in a solution containing other drugs (e.g. phenytoin), as this may result in precipitation. The usual recommended adult doses are an intravenous loading dose of 100 mg/minute until a total dose of 10 mg/kg (i.e. in an adult a total of about 600 mg) is given, followed by daily maintenance doses of 1–4 mg/kg. The initial maximum dose in an adult should probably not exceed 1000 mg (as the drug is not lipid soluble, and in obese patients the mg/kg guide may be unreliable). In neonates, initial phenobarbitone loading doses of between 15 and 20 mg/kg have been recommended to produce therapeutic levels, with subsequent supplementation of 3–4 mg/kg per day, to a maximum dose of 40 mg/kg. As pharmacokinetic values (e.g. volumes of distribution or clearance) alter dramatically in the first days and weeks of life, dose requirements changes, and levels should be carefully monitored. In older children, loading doses of between 5 and 20 mg/kg are often recommended with maintenance doses of 1–4 mg/kg, although much higher doses have been given safely.

Table 5.17. *Phenobarbitone (phenobarbital)*

Indication (stage of status)
Established status

Usual preparation
1 ml ampoule containing phenobarbitone sodium (200 mg/ml) in propylene glycol (90%)
and water for injection (10%)

Usual dosage
i.v. loading dose of 10 mg/kg at rate of 100 mg/min (usual adult dose 600–800 mg),
followed by maintenance dose of 1–4 mg/kg (adults). i.v. loading dose of 15–20 mg/kg,
followed by maintenance dose of 3–4 mg/kg (children and neonates); higher doses can
be given

Advantages
Extensive clinical experience in adults, children and the newborn
Highly effective in tonic–clonic and partial status
Potential cerebral-protective action
Stronger anticonvulsant action than other barbiturates
Rapid and long-lasting action
Safety at high doses established
May be preferentially concentrated in epileptic foci
Can be continued as chronic therapy
No tolerance and no late seizure relapse
Stable in solution

Disadvantages
Long elimination half-life
Sedation, respiratory depression, hypotension
Autoinduction
In neonates and infants, pharmacokinetics change rapidly with age

i.v., intravenous.

Summary of use in status epilepticus (table 5.17)

Phenobarbitone is probably a better drug in established status than is often
believed; indeed it is probably the drug of choice in the established condition. It
is a highly effective broad-spectrum antiepileptic, with rapid onset and prolonged
action. There is extensive experience of its use in adults and in children, and few
drugs have been as well studied in the newborn period. It is only moderately lipid
soluble, does not redistribute widely, and there is a danger of accumulation only
on very prolonged therapy. Phenobarbitone is concentrated preferentially in active
epileptic cortical regions. It has linear pharmacokinetics and stable and nonreactive
physical properties. It may have cerebral-protective action. Once seizures are
controlled, relapse is unusual due to its long action and the absence of acute
tolerance, a marked contrast to the benzodiazepines. Its main disadvantages are
its potential to cause sedation, respiratory depression and hypotension, although
in practice these effects seem slight except at high levels or with rapidly rising

261

levels. In the newborn period, the pharmacokinetics, and hence dosage requirements change rapidly. Phenobarbitone is extensively metabolised in the liver and autoinduction is common.

Stage of refractory status epilepticus: anaesthesia

When conventional antiepileptic drug therapy proves ineffective in status, it is the usual practice to induce anaesthesia in an attempt to control seizures. The principles of therapy are similar for all anaesthetics, and presumably a wide range of barbiturate and nonbarbiturate anaesthetic agents could be used, although only a few have been the subject of published reports. The barbiturate drugs used in anaesthesia in status (thiopentone, pentobarbitone) have the advantages of long experience in status, and strong antiepileptic action. However, their pharmacokinetic properties are problematic and the drugs are potentially highly toxic. The nonbarbiturate drugs (isoflurane, etomidate and propofol) have much more convenient pharmacokinetics, in particular short half-lives, lack of accumulation, nonsaturable kinetics, lack of autoinduction and tolerance. They are also much less toxic, without the cardiorespiratory risks of barbiturate therapy. Experience with these agents in status, however, is meagre. Of the various inhalational anaesthetics, only isoflurane has been used widely in status. Three nonbarbiturate intravenous agents are commonly used in anaesthetic practice: etomidate, propofol and ketamine. The first two have been the subject of published reports in status. A conundrum in the use of non-barbiturate anaesthetics in status is that, although all are powerful anaesthetics, they do not generally have antiepileptic properties; indeeed, at subanaesthetic doses isoflurane, propofol and etomidate, for instance, can exhibit proconvulsant action. Whether nonanticonvulsant anaesthesia is as effective in status as anticonvulsant anaesthesia is quite unclear.

All the drugs are given in doses sufficient to induce deep unconsciousness; therefore assisted respiration, cardiovascular monitoring, and the full panoply of the ITU are essential. The depth of anaesthesia should be that which abolishes all clinical and EEG epileptic activity (often requiring sedation to the point of burst suppression on the EEG), and cerebral electrical activity must by necessity be visualised, either with a formal EEG or a cerebral activity monitor.

The choice of barbiturate or nonbarbiturate anaesthetic depends on local arrangements. The inhalational anaesthetics require delivery systems which are highly inconvenient in the usual ITU settings, therefore intravenous agents are more popular.

Thiopentone sodium (thiopental sodium)

Barbiturates may be used at subanaesthetic dosages in status or as general anaesthetics. Phenobarbitone is commonly used in the former role, but it has fallen from use as an anaesthetic because of more satisfactory alternatives. Barbiturates with a sulphur substitution at C-2 (thiobarbiturates) are more lipid soluble than the parent barbiturates, and have a decreased latency to action, a much shorter duration of action, and are more rapidly metabolised. Thiopentone (5-ethyldihydro-5-(1-methylbutyl)-2-thioxo-4,6 (IH,5H)-pyrimidinedione mono-sodium; $C_{11}H_{17}N_2SNaO_2$; molecular weight 264.3) is the thiobarbiturate commonly used as an intravenous preparation in status, in cases where anaesthesia is desired. It is a hygroscopic powder, alkaline in solution (pH of the 8% solution is 10.2–11.2), highly soluble in lipid and also freely soluble in water (sodium salt), and has a pK_a of 7.6. At pH7.4, the drug is 39% ionised. Commonly used commercial preparations of thiopentone include Pentothal sodium, Intraval and Trapenal.

Absorption

Thiopentone is used in status only by intravenous infusion. Intramuscular injection may cause severe local injury, and sloughing of the skin may follow extravasation of the drug from a poorly positioned intravenous site. Injection near a nerve may cause permanent palsy. Intra-arterial injection should never be used, and causes severe local thrombosis and tissue necrosis (requiring treatment with analgesia, anticoagulation, sympathetic blockade of the limb, and α-adrenoceptor antagonists). Burst suppression occurs with levels of about 30–40 mg/l or above, although there is considerable individual variation. Much higher levels are sometimes required on prolonged treatment, and this 'acute tolerance' to the effects of thiopentone can complicate therapy (Toner *et al.* 1980). Total electrical silence is observed usually with levels over 70 mg/l (Orlowski *et al.* 1984; Turcant *et al.* 1985). Anticonvulsant effects are detectable at levels of 5–15 mg/l. The pharmacological properties of thiopentone are problematic, both because the drug, like phenytoin, has saturable pharmacokinetics and because its pharmacodynamic properties change over time as therapy proceeds.

Distribution

The pharmacokinetics have been extensively studied in anaesthetic practice (i.e. in short-term therapy), but there have been no formal studies in the setting of status. It acts rapidly because of its lipophilic nature and its low degree of ionisation. Following a single intravenous anaesthetic dose of thiopentone, unconsciousness occurs in about 10–20 seconds (first pass of the bolus of the drug

263

through the brain), as the drug is taken up into the most vascular areas of the brain (grey matter first). This uptake is flow determined, and maximal brain levels are achieved within 30 seconds. Sleep is induced with a single circulation time, and the depth of anaesthesia increases for about 40 seconds and then decreases progressively until consciousness is regained about 7–10 minutes later. This sequence reflects the rapid fall in blood levels during the distribution phase. At the time of awakening, blood concentrations are about 10% of peak values. This rapid fall does not occur when lipid stores are sufficiently saturated to prevent rapid distribution; in such cases (i.e. after long infusion), the duration of action is dramatically prolonged. Recovery in this setting may take hours or days even if no further drug is administered (this is a well-recognised occurrence in anaesthetic practice if the total dose exceeds 1g). There is a substantial variability, however, and in some patients consciousness is not lost completely, even after prolonged high dose thiopentone therapy, for instance in the case of Feneck (1981). The tendency to accumulate is of great importance in status, where total dosage may be very large, and where the duration of therapy greatly exceeds that used in other anaesthetic practice. The distribution half-life of thiopentone after initial bolus dosing is very short (about 2.5 minutes). The drug is about 65–85% bound to plasma protein, at all therapeutic levels. The volume of distribution is 1.96 kg/l initially, although it is much greater on prolonged therapy, rising commonly to 5 kg/l or more (9.16 in one patient) (Turcant *et al.* 1985). In status, thiopentone blood levels of about 40 mg/l are usually therapeutic (Becker 1978). Levels of thiopentone in the CSF on acute therapy are usually between 15% and 40% of blood levels.

Biotransformation and elimination

Thiopentone is metabolised in the liver, by the P450 microsomal enzyme system, largely by phase I desulphuration and oxidation. The majority of its metabolites are inactive, but pentobarbitone (produced by desulphuration) has potent antiepileptic action. Thiopentone exhibits saturable pharmacokinetics and, as hepatic metabolism is near saturation at the doses used in status, considerable variation in steady-state blood levels and other pharmacokinetic parameters is to be expected. Thiopentone elimination follows first-order kinetics after initial infusion and at levels below 35 mg/l, and commonly zero-order kinetics at higher levels. The clearance of thiopentone falls and the blood levels increase as hepatic metabolism saturates, and the elimination half-life increases. At levels below about 30 mg/l, the elimination half-life is about 3–11 hours (mean 8 hours), but at high blood levels or after prolonged therapy it may increase to 18–36 hours (Turcant *et al.* 1985); a half-life of 60 hours was recorded in one patient with blood levels between 60 and 70 mg/l (Stanski *et al.* 1980). The usually quoted clearance of thiopentone is about 2.7–4.1 ml/kg per minute following single bolus injections, but at the high dosages and prolonged therapy used in status clearance is lower (e.g. 0.102 l/ minute, in 48 patients reported on prolonged therapy by Turcant *et al.* (1985)). This contributes to the long recovery period sometimes needed on stopping prolonged therapy. In patients on thiopentone infusions, about 10–50% of total barbiturate blood concentrations may be accounted for by pentobarbitone, and this metabolite contributes substantially to the clinical effects (Watson *et al.* 1986). The clearance of pentobarbitone is about one tenth that of thiopentone, and is dependent on hepatic metabolism. Pentobarbitone has a particular tendency to accumulate further on prolonged thiopentone infusion because of saturation of metabolic pathways. Thiopentone and pentobarbitone levels can be measured accurately, and it would be wise to monitor both during prolonged thiopentone therapy (Toner *et al.* 1979; Turcant *et al.* 1985; Watson *et al.* 1986). Indeed, on prolonged therapy (for example 3 days or more), daily or twice-daily levels should be required. Excretion occurs predominantly in the urine as inactive metabolites.

Clinical effect in status epilepticus

Thiopentone is widely recommended for treating status (at least in Europe and Australia, less so in the USA), yet remarkably there have been very few published records of its efficacy in status. Brown & Horton (1967) reported 117 patients, of all ages, with status treated over a 12 year period with small (subanaesthetic) doses of thiopentone, usually after stupyfying doses of phenobarbitone or paraldehyde. Thiopentone was given by intravenous injection of 25–100 mg in Ringer-lactate solution. If seizures continued, a further infusion was given at a rate of 2 mg/minute and continued for an average of about 48 hours. A dose of one gram of thiopentone was usually sufficient in the first 12 hours, although up to 21 g was necessary in some patients. Only two of the 117 patients required therapy for more than 72 hours, and only two died. No side-effects or difficulties in management were encountered, and the authors concluded happily that the regimen never failed, was safe, certain and easy to use, and that depression of consciousness was never observed. An angry response to this report followed, in a letter from a neighbouring unit describing six patients requiring artifical ventilation, including two patients resuscitated following intravenous thiopentone therapy without ventilatory support in whom thiopentone had induced cardiorespiratory collapse. The safety of the treatment, without respiratory support, was doubted and parallels were drawn with the previous vogue for thiopentone in eclamptic fits which resulted in the death of many patients (Dundee & Gray 1967). Partinen, Kovanen & Nilsson (1981) provided details of five patients with severe status treated with thiopentone, refractory to very large doses of other antiepileptic drugs, including diazepam (100–420 mg), phenytoin (1000–1750 mg), paraldehyde (18–24 ml), chlormethiazole (2000–4000 mg) and clonazepam (3–4 mg), and in whom status had continued for at least 4 days. The following regimen was used: first, an intravenous bolus dose of thiopentone (100–250 mg) was given, followed by repeated bolus doses of 50 mg at intervals of 2–5 minutes until the EEG showed no seizure activity. Phenytoin or benzodiazepines were given concurrently by mouth, and intramuscular dexamethasone (5 mg every 6 hours). An intravenous thiopentone infusion was then initiated at a rate of 0.5–1.5 ml/minute, of a solution of 2500 mg in 500 ml of 0.9% sodium chloride (normal saline) regulated by blood pressure monitoring, which was continued until 12 hours after the last EEG paroxysm. The drug was then withdrawn gradually over 12 hours. All patients were artificially ventilated and curarised. In all five patients the seizures abated, in four permanently, but in one seizures recurred and were successfully treated subsequently with lignocaine and chlormethiazole. The duration of thiopentone therapy was not stated. Young *et al.* (1980) briefly report five patients treated with barbiturate anaesthesia for 4–13 days (two thiopentone, two pentobarbitone, one not stated). Monitoring of the EEG was recommended to guide the level of anaesthesia, targeted to obtain burst suppression with a 2–7 second interburst interval. In one of the patients, thiopentone was given as a bolus of 250 mg followed by an infusion of 80–120 mg/hour for 4 days. Unconsciousness occurred, and assisted ventilation was necessary, without muscle relaxants. Orlowski *et al.* (1984) successfully treated status in three children with hypothermia and thiopentone coma at infusion rates of 5–55 mg/kg per hour for 48–120 hours.

Treatment with thiopentone is usually required for several days, and too early a cessation of therapy results in recurrence. Feneck (1981) reported a patient in whom approximately 25 g of thiopentone were infused over 114 hours without accumulation. Thiopentone anaesthesia should not be given without assisted ventilation and full ITU support, and EEG monitoring is necessary on prolonged therapy.

On theoretical grounds barbiturates have a number of advantages over other agents. All barbiturates reduce membrane damage from free radicals, lower lactate, reduce cerebral oxygen uptake and cerebral energy production, and lower body temperature, properties which might be expected to reduce the propensity for seizure-induced cerebral damage. This proposition has not been formally studied, and indeed recently the cerebral-protective potential of barbiturates in other clinical situations has been disputed.

Toxic effects in status epilepticus

Dose-related sedation and respiratory depression are invariable with thiopentone, and at higher levels profound. As a result of acute tolerance effects, however, the levels at which coma supervenes vary. In status all patients should be electively intubated and ventilated on initiation of thiopentone therapy. Hypotension is very common with thiopentone therapy, is occasionally severe, and often limits the dose or the infusion rate. An infusion of dopamine is commonly required to control blood pressure. Thiopentone can cause painful spasm at the injection site, and tissue necrosis can occur; for this reason, the concentration of the infusion solution should not exceed 2.5%, and bolus injections are best given into a side arm of tube with a fast-flowing intravenous 0.9% sodium chloride (normal saline) or 5% dextrose drip. Cerebral blood flow and the cerebral metabolic rate are signficantly reduced and intracranial pressure lowered with thiopentone anaesthesia. Cough, laryngeal spasm and bronchospasm may occur, which may pose a problem in raised intracranial pressure if the airway has not been secured. The drug may diminish splanchnic blood flow, resulting in pancreatitis and hepatic disturbance. Thiopentone has a particularly strong propensity to precipitate attacks in variegate or acute intermittent porphyria, and should never be used in these conditions. An acute hypersensitivity reaction (with laryngeal oedema, bronchospasm, hypotension and erythema) occurs in about 1 in 30 000 administrations, and, although rare, carries a 50% mortality. The drug should be used with caution in patients with hepatic, cardiac or renal disease, and also in those with myxoedema, dystrophia myotonica, myasthenia gravis or familial periodic paralysis. The risks of toxicity are greater in the elderly.

Administration and dosage in status epilepticus

Thiopentone can react with polyvinyl infusion bags or plastic giving sets. The bolus injection is usually prepared from a 2.5g bottle with 100 ml of diluent to produce a 2.5% solution. The continuous infusion should be made up in 0.9% sodium chloride (normal saline). The intravenous solution has a pH of 10.2–11.2 and is incompatable with a large number of acidic or oxidising substances, and therefore no other drugs should be added. The solution is unstable if exposed to air, and thiopentone is highly irritant if injected outside a vein.

A commonly used regimen for administration of thiopentone is as follows. Thiopentone is given as a 100–250 mg bolus over 20 seconds into the side arm of a fast-running drip, with further 50 mg boluses every 2–3 minutes until seizures are controlled, with intubation and artifical ventilation. It is then given by intravenous infusion at the minimum dose required to control seizure activity (burst suppression on the EEG), which is usually 3–5 mg/kg per hour, although higher doses are not uncommonly needed. After 24 hours, the dose should be controlled by blood level monitoring of thiopentone and its metabolite pentobarbitone. After about 2–3 days, metabolism may be near saturation, and daily or twice-daily blood level estimations should be made to ensure than they do not rise excessively. The dosage should be lowered if systolic blood pressure falls below 90 mmHg, or if vital functions are impaired. The thiopentone should be continued for at least 12 hours after seizure activity has ceased, and then slowly discontinued. Thiopentone has a strong tendency to accumulate, and after stopping prolonged administration, it may take many hours or days for levels to fall. A full range of ITU facilities are required. Central venous pressure should be monitored, and continuous blood pressure measurements taken via an arterial line. Swan–Ganz monitoring is sometimes advisable, and EEG or cerebral function monitoring is essential if thiopentone infusions are prolonged. A dopamine infusion is frequently needed to maintain blood pressure.

Summary of use in status epilepticus (table 5.18)

Thiopentone is the compound traditionally used, in Europe at least, for barbiturate anaesthesia in status. The rather insouciant attitude to its infusion which was previously adopted is to be deplored; nevertheless, it is reasonably safe, provided full ITU facilities are employed. It has strong antiepileptic properties, and possibly also additional cerebral-protective effects, although acute tolerance may occur on prolonged therapy, necessitating high doses. All patients require intubation and most artifical ventilation. ITU facilities should be employed. Central venous pressure and continuous blood pressure measurements via an arterial line are necessary on prolonged therapy, with Swan–Ganz monitoring in some patients. EEG (or

Table 5.18. *Thiopentone sodium (thiopental sodium)*

Indication (stage of status)
Refractory status

Usual preparations
Injection of thiopentone sodium (2.5 g and 5 g with 100 ml and 200 ml diluent to make
   100 ml and 200 ml of a 2.5% solution)
500 mg and 1 g vials to make 2.5% solutions

Usual dosage
100–250 mg i.v. bolus given over 20 s, with further 50 mg boluses every 2–3 minutes
   until seizures are controlled, followed by a continuous i.v. infusion (in 0.9% sodium
   chloride[a]) to maintain burst suppression (usually 3–5 mg/kg per h)

Advantages
Greater intrinsic antileptic action than other barbiturate or nonbarbiturate anaesthetics
Less sedation than pentobarbitone
Potential cerebral-protective action
Reduces intracranial pressure and reduces cerebral blood flow
Very rapid onset of action

Disadvantages
Saturable kinetics
Strong tendency to accumulate
Long recovery time, compared with nonbarbiturate anaesthetics
Acute tolerance
Active metabolite
Requires blood level monitoring (parent drug and metabolite)
Requires intensive care, artificial ventilatory support and intensive EEG and
   cardiovascular monitoring
Respiratory depression and sedation inevitable, and hypotension common
Pancreatitis, hepatic dysfunction, spasm at injection site
Reacts with co-medication, and with plastic giving sets, is unstable when exposed to air
Autoinduction
Hepatic disease prolongs elimination

i.v., intravenous.
[a] Normal saline.

cerebral function) monitoring is essential on prolonged therapy. Hypotension can
be a troublesome side-effect, often requiring a concomitant dopamine infusion.
Other toxic effects on prolonged therapy include pancreatitis and hepatic disturbance, and thiopentone may cause acute hypersensitivity. It should be administered
cautiously in the elderly, and in those with cardiac, hepatic or renal disease.
Thiopentone can react with co-medication, and also polyvinyl infusion bags or
plastic giving sets. Thiopentone pharmacokinetics are saturable at conventional
doses, and the drug also has a strong tendency to accumulate. Recovery times
may therefore be very protracted, if large doses have been given. On prolonged
therapy, at least daily measurements of blood levels are recommended. Although
thiopentone has been used in the treatment of status for 30 years, published

evidence of its safety and effectiveness is sparse in both adults and children. Whether nonbarbiturate anaesthetics, with their much more satisfactory pharmacokinetic properties but less antiepileptic action, will prove as effective as barbiturate anaesthesia in refractory status is not yet established. Until then, thiopentone still has an important place in the management of status.

Pentobarbitone sodium (pentobarbital sodium)

Pentobarbitone (sodium 5-ethyl-5-(1-methylbutyl)barbiturate; $C_{11}H_{17}N_2NaO_3$; molecular weight 248.3) is a barbiturate, produced by the desulphuration of thiopentone. It is a hygroscopic crystalline powder, very soluble in water, and with a pK_a of 8.1. The solution of the sodium salt has a pH of 9.1–11. It has a strong antiepileptic action, and as a primary metabolite of thiopentone is indeed responsible for some of the parent drug's anticonvulsant effect in status. It has theoretical advantages over thiopentone, including a shorter elimination half-life, first-order kinetics at doses at which thiopentone exhibits zero-order kinetics, apparently lesser propensity to cause hypotension, a GABAergic activity which might enhance the barbiturate's cerebral protective effect, and less cardiotoxicity in overdose. As will become plain, however, pentobarbitone has trenchant drawbacks which limit its usefulness. A commonly used commercial preparation of pentobarbitone is Nembutal sodium.

Pharmacokinetics

Pentobarbitone has a slightly slower onset of action than thiopentone, as its distribution from blood to brain takes longer. However, cerebral concentrations are maintained longer, and there is less of a first-pass effect than with thiopentone. The mean elimination half-life of pentobarbitone is 27 hours (range usually 20–30 hours), which is shorter than that of phenobarbitone or thiopentone. The half-life is prolonged in hepatic disease, but not in renal disease, and is shorter in children and on prolonged dosing (due to autoinduction). The volume of distribution is 1 l/kg, and it is about 59–63% protein bound. It is extensively metab-

269

olised in the liver by hydroxylation, oxidation and carboxylation. The clearance of pentobarbitone in adults is approximately 0.026 l/kg per hour.

Clinical and toxic effects in status epilepticus

Animal experimentation has shown pentobarbitone to have an antiepileptic action, with peak effects after 15 minutes (Raines *et al.* 1979). Young *et al.* (1983) first mentioned the successful use of pentobarbitone in two patients in status. Rashkin *et al.* (1987) then described in detail nine patients with refractory status treated with intravenous pentobarbitone. Bolus loading doses of 5 mg/kg were followed by bolus doses of 25–50 mg/kg given every 2–5 minutes until EEG burst suppression intervals of 15 seconds were achieved. This loading phase usually lasted less than 1 hour, and was then followed by a continuous infusion of 5 mg/kg per hour for 12–24 hours. In the first five patients this was followed by a tapering of 1 mg/kg per hour every 6 hours. The dose was increased to the previous level if seizure activity returned. In the later four patients, the drug was discontinued without tapering, which had been found to be unnecessary because of persisting high pentobarbitone levels. Seizures stopped on pentobarbitone loading in all nine patients, in eight within 1 hour. Of these, seven patients died, and one of the the survivors died 3 weeks later in respiratory failure. All patients developed hypotension during the loading phase. Persisting pentobarbitone levels were found up to 8 days after cessation of therapy, and detectable barbiturate levels complicated the declaration of brain death in several cases. In the next clinical report, Lowenstein *et al.* (1988) devised a new protocol for refractory status based on their experience with eight patients, in all of whom seizures were successfully aborted. Pentobarbitone was given as a bolus (or repeated boluses of 15 mg/kg) followed by an infusion at a dose sufficient to produce burst suppression (usually between 0.3 and 4 mg/kg per hour). EEG was vital to record the depth of anaesthesia and monitor seizure activity, which was not possible to detect clinically in the unconscious patients who had become entirely unresponsive, uniformly flaccid, and had lost brain stem reflexes (other than pupillary responses). Hypotension was common but could be controlled with dopamine infusion. Pentobarbitone infusion was continued for between 11 hours and 14 days in all the patients, but the drug could be detected in the blood for up to 80 hours after discontinuation of even short infusions (fig. 5.14). Two patients died. In the survivors, recovery of brain stem reflexes occurred within 6–24 hours of stopping the infusion, motor function 1–72 hours, and simple cognitive function 2–18 days. Two patients experienced flaccid weakness of all four limbs for several weeks, which seems to be a side-effect peculiar to pentobarbitone, and both had received the highest cumulative barbiturate dose. Blood levels at burst suppression ranged from 17–93 µmol/l. In this and other series, the relationship between blood level and effect seemed unreliable, and tolerance to the effect of the barbiturate, even at stable levels, was often found. In a subsequent report of 17 patients, six recovered fully, two with severe sequelae and nine died (Yaffe & Lowenstein 1992). Van Ness (1990) gave pentobarbitone to seven patients with severe complex partial or generalised status epilepticus, refractory to diazepam and phenytoin, in whom status had persisted for between

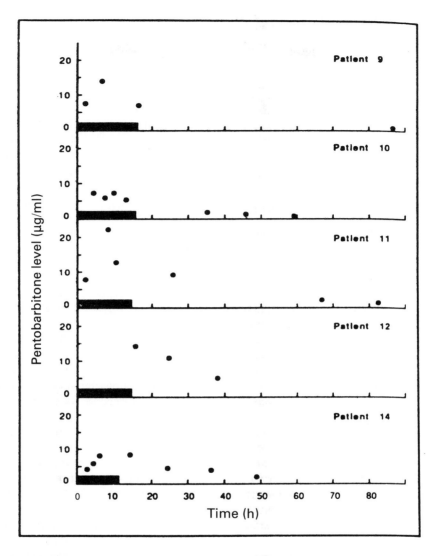

Fig. 5.14. Pentobarbitone levels in five patients following a continuous infusion for 10–17 hours. Pentobarbitone was given at a dose of 15 mg/kg in the first hour, and then 1–2 mg/kg/hour, with additional loading doses of 5 mg/kg as required. Note that persisting pentobarbitone levels were recorded for up to 80 hours, and recovery from the infusion was often very delayed (see the text for clinical details). (From Lowenstein *et al.* 1988, with kind permission.)

271

2 hours and 24 days before pentobarbitone therapy was started. The pentobarbitone was administered in 0.9% sodium chloride (normal saline) via an infusion pump, according to the following scheme. A loading dose of about 6–8 mg/kg (one case required 20 mg/kg to achieve burst suppression) was given over 40–60 minutes to avoid hypotension, the infusion was then continued at a rate of 1–4 mg/kg per hour for up to 24 hours, and stopped without tapering. The infusion rate was reduced if systolic blood pressure fell below 90 mmHg, and in one patient additional fluid was required to bolster blood pressure. The infusion rate was varied to achieve a burst suppression rate of between 3 and 9 bursts/minute. If, on stopping therapy, either clinical or EEG seizures recurred, the infusion was restarted using the same protocol; this was done in two of the seven patients, both of whom died. Decerebrate posturing was noted in six of the seven patients at about the time that burst suppression occurred, and is a direct pharmacological effect which should not be misinterpreted as seizure activity. Seizures stopped in all cases, four patients recovered, but two patients died after a vegetative state with recurring seizures after withdrawal of the drug and one died in asystole after 7 hours of therapy. The results are disappointing, and the outcome does not seem to justify the conclusion drawn by Van Ness (1990) that pentobarbitone should become the drug of choice in refractory status epilepticus! In a meta-analysis of 37 patients treated with high dose pentobarbitone therapy 12 (32%) died, in 4 of whom the pentobarbitone was considered to have contributed to death (Bleck 1992). Hypotension is as common with pentobarbitone as with thiopentone, and the persisting high pentobarbitone levels after therapy is stopped suggest that elimination half-lives are longer in status than is usually recorded. The putative cerebral-protective and GABAergic effects of pentobarbitone have not shown in these cases an actual improvement in mortality. Osorio & Reed (1989), however, reported better results in 12 patients treated for a median of 38 hours (range 7–244 hours), at somewhat higher doses (median 3.5 mg/kg per hour, range 2.5–9.0; median pentobarbitone level was 28.5/µmol/l, range 10–101). Seizures were initially rapidly controlled, but control was not sustained for hours or days. There was a marked tendency for breakthrough seizures if the drug was tapered too quickly. Of the 12 patients, 10 survived, one with irreversible neurological impairment. Two died, one during and one after anaesthesia. One further patient was severely neurologically impaired. EEG monitoring of seizure activity is essential in pentobarbitone coma, but problems arise in the interpretation of muscular twitching without EEG correlate; drug dose should be increased if these are taken as evidence of subtle status (see p. 54). Although the burst suppression pattern is often said to be a useful target in barbiturate coma, it bears an unreliable relationship to blood level or to seizure control in my experience, and this seems particularly to be so in the case of pentobarbitone (see Osorio & Reed 1989).

With pentobarbitone therapy, haemodynamic and respiratory complications are frequent and dose dependent. Hypotension is common but easily controlled with an infusion of dopamine. Drug-induced muscle weakness is a prominent feature, and may contribute to the difficulty in weaning patients from the ventilator. Skin oedema and mild ileus are common. Particular attention should be paid to

Table 5.19. *Pentobarbitone sodium (pentobarbital sodium)*

Indications (stage of status)
Refractory status

Usual preparation
100 mg in a 2 ml injection vial, in propylene glycol (40%) and ethyl alcohol (10%)

Usual dosage
i.v. loading dose of 5–20 mg/kg, at a rate not exceeding 25 mg/min, followed by a
continuous infusion of 0.5–1.0 mg/kg per h, increasing if necessary to 1–3 mg/kg/h.
Additional 5–20 mg/kg boluses can be given if breakthrough seizures occur.

Advantages over thiopentone
Shorter elimination half-life than thiopentone
Nonsaturable kinetics
No active metabolites
Longer duration of action than thiopentone
GABAergic action may enhance cerebral-protective effects
Stable compound, unreactive with plastic

Disadvantages
Very limited clinical experience, and published trials have uniformly poor outcome
Respiratory depression and sedation invariable
Hypotension and cardiorespiratory dysfunction common
Decerebrate posturing and flaccid paralysis during anaesthesia, and flaccid weakness may
persist for weeks in survivors
Tendency for seizures to recur when drug withdrawn
Requires blood level monitoring
Requires intensive care, artificial ventilatory support and intensive EEG and
cardiovascular monitoring
Inconsistent relationship between serum level and seizure control
Longer recovery time than other barbiturate or nonbarbiturate anaesthetics

decreases in pulmonary artery wedge pressure, which signals impending haemodynamic instability; Swan–Ganz monitoring is recommended (Osorio & Reed 1989).
Pentobarbitone has a negative inotropic effect, and may cause a precipitous fall
in blood pressure in patients with congestive cardiac failure. Pulmonary oedema
is also common. Because of the toxicity of pentobarbitone, and the poor outcome
of reported series, the exact place of pentobarbitone in the therapy of status
must be considered quite unclear, despite the enthusiastic endorsement by some
observers. The drug should not be used in acute intermittent porphyria.

Administration and dosage in status epilepticus

Pentobarbitone is stable for 12 hours in either 0.9% sodium cloride (normal
saline) or 5% dextrose, up to a concentration of 12.5 mg/ml. Unlike thiopentone,
it is not sorbed by plastic. On the initiation of therapy, all patients should be
intubated and artificially ventilated, central venous pressure should be continuously monitored, and continuous blood pressure measurements should be insti-

tuted via an arterial line. Swan–Ganz monitoring is also advisable, a dopamine infusion line should be prepared, and EEG or cerebral function monitoring is essential. Intravenous loading of pentobarbitone (5–20 mg/kg) is given at an infusion rate not exceeding 25 mg/minute, followed by a continuous infusion of 0.5–1 mg/kg per hour, increasing if necessary to 1–3 mg/kg per hour. The dose should be titrated to produce burst suppression on the EEG, although lessened if hypotension develops. If breakthrough seizures occur, bolus doses of 5–20 mg/kg can be given, and the continuous infusion rate slightly increased (to a maximum of 3 mg/kg per hour). When 12 hours have elapsed after the last EEG epileptic paroxysm, the infusion rate should be tapered by 1 mg/kg per hour every 4–6 hours if the blood pentobarbitone level is greater than 50 mg/l, or by 0.5 mg/kg per hour if the level is less than 50 mg/l.

Summary of use in status epilepticus (table 5.19)

The roles of pentobarbitone and thiopentone in status are very similar. Both drugs are closely chemically related, but pentobarbitone has important theoretical advantages over thiopentone, including its shorter elimination half-life, GABA-mimetic effect, a longer duration of action, and non-saturable kinetics. It has no active metabolites and is a stable compound unreactive with plastic. Both drugs cause severe respiratory and cerebral depression, and hypotension. In practice, however, the outcome in published series is not strikingly better; indeed it seems somewhat worse. Pentobarbitone has unique side-effects, and the overall condition of the reported patients treated by pentobarbitone coma seems particularly ominous. The drug has potentially fatal haemodynamic side-effects, tolerance is common, complete seizure control seems to take some time to achieve, and the relationship between effect and blood level is inconsistent. There is a tendency for seizures to recur on weaning. Published experience in children or the newborn is very limited. Further research work is needed before pentobarbitone can be endorsed as the anaesthetic of choice for barbiturate anaesthesia in status.

Isoflurane

Isoflurane (1-chloro-2,2,2-trifluroroethyl difluoromethyl ether; $C_3H_2ClF_5O$; molecular weight 184.5) is in theory a potentially useful drug for inducing anaesthesia in status. It is a volatile liquid that was introduced into clinical practice as an inhalational nonbarbiturate anaesthetic. It has properties similar to its isomer enflurane and to halothane. Discovered in 1965, isoflurane was not widely used until the mid 1970s because of unfounded anxieties about its carcinogenicity (Eger 1981*a,b*). Its role in status has been explored in recent years. It has pharmacological properties which confer advantages over other inhalational agents (e.g. enflurane and halothane), and on these grounds is undoubtedly the inhalational anaesthetic of choice in status. Isoflurane also exhibits anticonvulsant properties, at least in experimental animal work, distinct from its anaesthetic actions, perhaps mediated by the depression of transmission of seizure discharges rather than by an effect on the active focus (Langmoen, Hegstad & Berg-Johnsen 1992). It is a stable compound (Eger 1981*a,b*), resistant to degradation, not oxidised on exposure to light, not absorbed by rubber or plastic tubing, and is nonflammable. A commonly used commercial preparation of isoflurane is Florane.

Pharmacokinetics

Isoflurane is less soluble in blood than is halothane or enflurane, and it is absorbed and excreted rapidly and accumulated less. The volume of distribution and clearance of the drug are not known. There is a linear relationship between alveolar and blood concentration (Cromwell *et al.* 1971). Induction of anaesthesia requires minimum alveolar concentrations of 1.5–3.5% and maintenance of anaesthesia of 0.7–2.1%. Most of the drug is excreted by inhalation, only 0.2% is metabolised in the liver, and less than 0.2% is excreted unchanged by the kidneys (Holaday *et al.* 1975). Inorganic fluoride and trifluoroacetic acid are its principal metabolic products (Hitt *et al.* 1974), and are pharmacologically inactive. In contrast to halothane, there is no risk of liver injury during prolonged exposure. The recovery after cessation of anaesthesia is very rapid (faster than after halothane or enflurane), and is a great advantage of inhalational compared with barbiturate anaesthetics. In a study of 896 patients anaesthetised with isoflurane, recovery (to eye opening) occurred 7.3 minutes after cessation of anaesthesia in those anaesthetised for less than 1 hour, and 11.2 minutes for those anaesthetised for 5–6 hours. In the patient with status reported by Hughes, Sharpe & McLachlan (1992) consciousness returned within 15 minutes after 48 hours of drug administration. Pharmacological experience with the prolonged use of isoflurane needed in status is sparse. There is a danger of accumulation, as the drug is highly concentrated in muscle and fat, and half-life values can exceed 40 hours.

Clinical effect in status epilepticus

The potential of isoflurane for treating status was first suggested by Ropper *et al.* (1986), but there have been few published clinical reports. Kofke *et al.* (1989) described 11 episodes (in nine patients) with protracted generalised or subtle status treated with isoflurane. The EEG and clinical seizure activity were abolished in all patients, with treatment of between 1 and 55 hours. Anaesthesia was administered to produce burst suppression with interburst intervals of 15–30 seconds, full electrical silence being considered too dangerous in view of the haemodynamic consequences of the dose of isoflurane required. All the patients were given vasopressor and/or fluid infusions to maintain acceptable arterial pressure, and one patient required an infusion of adrenaline, but the hypotensive effect of isoflurane is generally mild and readily reversed. In this respect isoflurane is a good choice in patients with existing cardiovascular disease. In two patients multi-organ failure complicated the course of the status. One patient required inspired isoflurane concentrations of 4–5% for several hours, which is a potentially toxic dose. Only three patients survived, one after 48 hours of isoflurane therapy, and in eight of the 11 episodes, seizures recurred after stopping the isoflurane. Although these were poor risk patients, the results appear worse than those expected with barbiturate anaesthesia. The authors concluded that isoflurane did not reverse the underlying mechanisms of status, and it is interesting to speculate whether or not barbiturate anaesthesia is superior in this regard. Hilz *et al.* (1992) reported a patient, refractory to thiopentone, who was then treated successfully with isoflurane (up to 1.5%) for two periods of 3 hours. The EEG showed severe slowing of background activity (1–2 Hz) at 1.0% inhalation, and seizure activity was abolished at 1.0–1.5%, without adverse haemodynamic effects. A detailed report is also given by Hughes *et al.* (1992) of a patient with chronic encephalitis who had epilepsia partialis continua for 2 months and 3–5 generalised seizures an hour before treatment, and was unresponsive to other therapy including phenytoin, phenobarbitone, diazepam and paraldehyde. Anaesthesia was achieved immediately using isoflurane, with an end tidal concentration of 0.5%. Seizures ceased immediately, and the drug was maintained at constant dosage for 24 hours. Then following a focal seizure, the dose was increased to 0.7%, which was continued for a further 48 hours without seizures. The anaesthetic was then withdrawn, and the patient awoke within 15 minutes, with a measured end tidal volume of between 0% and 0.2%. She was extubated 6 hours later, and although the focal seizures continued, the generalised seizures were much improved. Sakaki *et al.* (1992) reported the successful treatment of four patients in status after surgery to lesions in the motor area of the brain, using relatively low doses of isoflurane. The drug can be safely used in acute intermittent porphyria.

Toxic effects in status epilepticus

Isoflurane has the toxic side-effects common to all inhalational anaesthetics, but has some advantages. Respiratory depression is less than with enflurane, although more profound than with halothane (Eger 1981*b*). Isoflurane causes a fall in respiratory rate, but no decrease in tidal volume. The effect of isoflurane on cardiac function is less than that of enflurane or halothane (Graves, McDermott & Bidwai 1974; Tarnow *et al.* 1977), which is a great advantage. Dose-related hypotension does occur, due mainly to a reduction of peripheral resistance, but is less marked than with other inhalational agents where reduced cardiac output contributes to hypotension; nevertheless, a dopamine infusion is sometimes required to maintain blood pressure (Sakaki *et al.* 1992). Isoflurane depresses cardiac contractility, and stroke volume, cardiac work and oxygen consumption are also reduced. Right atrial pressure and central venous pressure are maintained and there is no clinical effect on cardiac output. At the doses required to produce burst suppression, halothane will produce strong negative inotropic effects and an increase in intra-cranial pressure. In contrast to halothane, isoflurane does not often cause cardiac arrhythmia (Pauca & Dripps 1973). Isoflurane causes less increase in intracranial pressure and less impairment of autoregulation or cerebral blood flow than halo-thane or enflurane (Adams *et al.* 1981; Eger 1981*b*). Seizures or EEG activation have been only occasionally reported with isoflurane anaesthesia, in contrast to the appreciable convulsant effects of enflurane (Clark, Hosick & Adam 1973; Clark & Rosner 1973; Fariello 1980; Poulton & Ellington 1984; Hymes 1985; Nicoll 1986). The pupils are small during anaesthesia. Isoflurane has a stronger muscle relaxant effect than either halothane or enflurane. The lack of involvement of hepatic or renal mechanisms in the handling of isoflurane make it highly suitable for use in hepatic or renal disease. Moreover, isoflurane does not cause hepato-toxicity (in contrast to halothane) or nephrotoxicity (in contrast to enflurane) nor does it have metabolic side-effects. Initial fears that the drug was carcinogenic have been refuted (Eger *et al.* 1978). As with all forms of prolonged anaesthesia, risks include pressure sores, infection, hypothermia and venous thrombosis.

Administration and dosage in status epilepticus

Facilities for administering inhalational anaesthesia and scavenging are required, together with artifical ventilation. EEG monitoring is mandatory. Muscle relaxants are usually not necessary. Hughes *et al.* (1992) also recommend the monitoring of end tidal drug concentrations, inspired oxygen, intra-arterial blood pressure, capnography and oximetry, continuous monitoring of vital signs and ECG, and the use of high pressure and disconnect alarms on the ventilator. Isoflurane is presented as a nearly pure liquid, and is administered from a vaporiser via an anaesthetic system with scavenging capability. It seems reasonable to give isoflur-ane at a concentration which produces burst suppression with an interburst interval of about 15–30 seconds. The dosages most commonly used by Kofke *et al.* (1989) were end tidal isoflurane concentrations of 0.8% initially, which could be increased to about 2%; 0.7% was the concentration used successfully in the patient described by Hughes *et al.* (1992). Apart from the use of suxamethonium (succinylcholine) with small doses of morphine, muscle relaxants should be avoided so that seizure activity can be judged clinically as well as by EEG.

Summary of use in status epilepticus (table 5.20)

The role of inhalational anaesthesia in status has not been defined. Anaesthesia and abolition of clinical and EEG seizure activity are rapidly obtained on isoflurane administration, but there are logistical problems and potentially serious side-effects. The need for an inhalational anaesthetic system, with facilities for scaveng-ing, in an ITU setting is a particular practical disadvantage. Side-effects include respiratory and cerebral depression, and hypotension, but adverse effects on car-diac, renal and hepatic function are rare. Isoflurane has only slight intrinsic anti-convulsant action, and seizures recurred in most of the reported cases when treatment was withdrawn. Experience in status is slight, especially in children,

Table 5.20. *Isoflurane*

Indication (stage of status)
Refractory status

Usual preparation
Nearly pure (99.9%) liquid, for use in a correctly calibrated vaporiser via an anaesthetic system

Usual dosage
Inhalation of isoflurane at dosages producing end tidal concentrations of 0.8–2%, dose titrated to maintain burst suppression

Advantages
Isoflurane has a number of advantages over other inhalational anaesthetics such as halothane or enflurane: e.g. less soluble, no hepatotoxicity or nephrotoxicity, less effect on cardiac output, fewer cardiac arrhythmias, less hypotension, less effect on cerebral blood flow and autoregulation, less increase in intracranial pressure, less convulsant effect, linear kinetics
Pharmacology extensively studied
No hepatic metabolism, and excreted by exhalation: unaffected by hepatic or renal disease
Very rapid onset of action and rapid recovery
No tendency to accumulate

Disadvantages
Very little published experience in status
Requires anaesthetic system with scavenging
Requires assisted ventilation, intensive care and intensive care monitoring, and exhaustive cardiorespiratory monitoring
No experience with long-term usage
Tendency for seizures to recur when withdrawn
Hypotension common (but generally mild)
Little intrinsic antiepileptic activity
Respiratory depression and sedation inevitable

and there is no published experience in the newborn. One specific role for the anaesthetic, for instance in the postoperative situation, is to produce rapid control, to provide time for other antiepileptic drugs with slower onsets of action to take effect. There is no doubt that isoflurane is the inhalational agent of choice, with clinical and pharmacokinetic advantages over halothane, enflurane and other agents, and it has excellent pharmacokinetic properties. The relative merits of barbiturate and nonbarbiturate anaesthetics are, however, not yet fully established. If nonbarbiturate anaesthesia is to be used, the newer nonbarbiturate intravenous anaesthetics are certainly more convenient than the inhalational agents, but experience with all these drugs is very limited.

Etomidate

$$CH_3-CH_2-O-\overset{\overset{\textstyle O}{\|}}{C}$$

Etomidate (D-ethyl-(R)-1-(1-phenylethyl)-1-H-imidazole-5-carboxylate: $C_{12}H_{16}N_2O_2$; molecular weight 244.3) was the first nonbarbiturate intravenous anaesthetic to be given to control status. It is a carboxylated imidazole derivative, extensively used in anaesthesia in Europe, and only recently licensed for anaesthetic use in the USA. It is soluble in lipid and water, with a pK_a of 4.1. A commonly used commercial preparation of etomidate is Hypnomidate.

Pharmacokinetics

Etomidate is very rapidly distributed, it has a biphasic distribution curve with α and β half-lives of 3 and 27 minutes, is highly lipophilic, and has a large volume of distribution (about 2.0–4.5 1/kg). It is metabolised in the liver, and only 2% is excreted in the urine unchanged. The mean elimination half-life is 5 hours (range 2–11 hours). It is about 75% bound to the plasma proteins, therefore low albumin states increase the free drug concentration. The clearance of etomidate in adults is approximately 0.55 1/kg per hour. An intravenous infusion of etomidate produces anaesthesia within 30–60 seconds. A standard induction dose of 0.3 mg/kg produces sleep for 4–8 minutes. There is a low incidence of apnoea, and in normal anaesthetic practice etomidate very rarely causes marked hypotension or respiratory difficulty, or affects cardiac rhythm or rate. Therapeutic concentrations are said to lie between 0.3 and 1.0 mg/l.

Clinical effect in status epilepticus

In animals, etomidate has been shown to have anticonvulsant and cerebral-protective properties, and a GABA-like action (Wauquier 1983; Milde & Milde 1986). There is a single well-documented report of the use of etomidate in eight patients with intractable status, treated in intensive care in Nottingham (Yeoman *et al.* 1989). The patients were anaesthetised with an intravenous bolus

279

of etomidate (dose 0.3 mg/kg), muscle relaxants, neuromuscular blocking drugs and controlled ventilation. EEG was monitored by using a cerebral activity monitor. This first bolus rapidly controlled seizures and, if they recurred, further bolus doses were given. After the initial bolus injections, a continuous infusion of etodimate (5 mg/ml in 5% dextrose) was given at a rate of 20 µg/kg per minute, subsequently adjusted to maintain mean cortical activity at 5 µV, with absence of burst suppression and seizure activity. Periodically a full 16 channel EEG was undertaken. After 24 hours, the patient was slowly weaned off etomidate. If seizures recurred, the infusion rate was increased to the minimum dose that would result in their abolition, and reduction was again attempted after a further 24 hours. Corticosteroid therapy was given at a dose of 100 mg every 6 hours, and continued for 72 hours after stopping the etomidate infusion. Seizures were rapidly controlled in all eight patients, usually after the first bolus. The drug was continued for between 48 and 280 hours (at initial infusion rates between 17 and 38 µg/kg per minute and maximum rates of 22–111 µg/kg per minute). Hypotension was observed in five of the eight patients, all more than 3 hours after induction of anaesthesia, but it was mild and easily controlled with fluid replacement without reducing the infusion rate; this is in marked contrast to experience with, for example, thiopentone. Weaning from the infusion was associated with a recurrence of seizure activity, which in two patients required alternative antiepileptic drug therapy. All patients survived the infusion, although one patient died from pneumonia 5 hours after the cessation of the drug infusion.

Toxic effects in status epilepticus

Etomidate has caused both myoclonus and seizures and can activate the EEG in epileptic subjects, properties shared by other anaesthetic agents. Muscle twitching without EEG changes occurs in about 50% of patients when etomidate is used in anaesthesia, and should not be confused with seizures. The antiepileptic effect occurs only with profound cerebral depression, and may reflect anaesthesia rather than specific antiepileptic properties. Etomidate produces a 30% decrease in regional cerebral blood flow and a greater reduction in cerebral metabolism, and also reduces intracranial pressure. Whether the reduction in cerebral blood flow is advisable in status, where high blood flow may be required to prevent regional hypoxia, is unknown, but presumably the effects on cerebral metabolism and intracranial pressure are potentially beneficial.

Long-term infusion of etomidate results in impaired adrenal activity, which can be fatal if overlooked. Cortisteroid replacement is therefore essential. There is a theoretical risk of accumulation, but clinical experience of long-term therapy is very limited, and the extent of this risk is unknown. Etomidate is, however, remarkably free from adverse cardiovascular or respiratory effects, does not cause severe hypotension, and is especially favoured in anaesthetic practice for patients with cardiovascular disease.

Table 5.21. *Etomidate*

Indication (stage of status)
Refractory status

Usual preparation
10 ml ampoule containing 20 mg etomidate (2 mg/ml), in propylene glycol (35%)
1 ml ampoule containing 125 mg etomidate for dilution

Usual dosage
i.v. bolus of 0.3 mg/kg, repeated if necessary, followed by a continuous infusion at an
  initial rate of about 20 µg/kg per min (5 mg/ml of etomidate in 5% dextrose), titrated
  up or down to maintain burst suppression. Corticosteroid co-medication is required

Advantages
Intrinsic antiepileptic properties (but slight) and cerebral-protective properties
Very rapid onset of effect and recovery
Low risk of respiratory depression
Low risk of cardiovascular toxicity

Disadvantages
Tendency for seizures to recur on weaning
Hypotension (but risk lower than with other anaesthetics)
Drug-induced myoclonus
Drug-induced muscular twitching without EEG change
Reduction in cerebral blood flow and metabolism and intracranial pressure
Very little published experience in status
Very little experience with long-term therapy
Requires assisted ventilation, ITU and intensive care monitoring, and exhaustive
  cardiorespiratory monitoring
Interferes with adrenocorticoid function, and so corticosteroid therapy required
Respiratory depression and sedation inevitable

Administration and dosage in status epilepticus

Etomidate is dissolved in 35% propylene glycol (which can be allergenic), and is
presented as a solution containing 20 mg in a 10 ml ampoule (2 mg/ml). A more
concentrated solution of 125 mg/ml in 1 ml ampoules is also available for dilution
as a continuous infusion. A suggested dosage regimen is as follows. First, an
intravenous bolus of etomidate (0.3 mg/kg) is given with neuromuscular blocking
drugs where necessary and controlled ventilation. This can be succeeded by
further bolus doses if seizures recur. Then a continuous infusion of etomidate
(5 mg/ml in 5% dextrose) is given at a rate of 20 µg/kg per minute, subsequently
adjusted to maintain mean cortical activity at 5 µV on the cerebral activity monitor,
with absence of burst suppression. After 24 hours, the drug is slowly tapered, and
the infusion reinstituted if seizures recur, for a further 24 hours. Corticosteroid
co-medication must be given in a dose of 100 mg every 6 hours and continued
for 72 hours after cessation of the etomidate infusion.

Summary of use in status epilepticus (table 5.21)

The place of etomidate in the therapy of status is uncertain. It is a highly effective anaesthetic, with low toxicity, and is particularly safe in patients with cardiovascular disease. It may well have anticonvulsant properties in addition (this is controversial), but, paradoxically, convulsions and myoclonus have also been precipitated, especially in patients with pre-existing epilepsy. It requires full ITU monitoring and obligatory corticosteroid co-medication, as etomidate interferes with adrenocortical function. There is a low risk of respiratory and cardiovascular toxicity, but hypotension is common, and seizures tend to recur when the patient is weaned from the drug. It reduces cerebral blood flow and metabolism, which is of uncertain benefit in status. There is little experience of prolonged etomidate usage, and few reports of its use in status. Preliminary studies have been promising, and in view of the its potential clinical advantages in status, further investigation is warranted.

Propofol

Propofol

Propofol (2,6-diisopropylphenol; $C_{12}H_{18}O$; molecular weight 178) is another short-acting intravenous anaesthetic which can be administered by intravenous bolus or infusion. Propofol is highly lipid soluble and slightly soluble in water; it is formulated as an isotonic emulsion. The pK_a is 11. It is a very effective anaesthetic, relatively nontoxic, and, as with etomidate, has been used recently in refractory status to great effect. Blood concentrations of propofol of 1.6–6.4 mg/l have been associated with sleep in volunteers, and 1.0–2.2 mg/l with recovery from anaesthesia. Blood concentrations at the time of recovery from anaesthesia are higher in those who have been treated by infusion with higher doses on a longer-term basis, perhaps due to acute tolerance (Cockshott *et al.* 1990). A commonly used commercial preparation of propofol is Diprivan.

Pharmacokinetics

The distribution half-life of propofol is 2–4 minutes and the elimination half-life 30–60 minutes. It is extremely lipid soluble and its volume of distribution is very large indeed (297–1100 l/kg). Because of its high lipid solubility, the rate of entry of propofol into brain is solely dependent on cerebral blood flow. It is 97–98% bound to plasma proteins, and extensively metabolised in the liver, to the glucuronide and 4-sulphate quinol derivative. The total body clearance of propofol is very high (1.5–2 l/minute). This is higher than hepatic blood flow, implying extrahepatic clearance, although the mechanism is unclear. The induction characteristics of propofol are similar to those of thiopentone, with dose-related depression of conscious level, cardiovascular and respiratory function. In the unpremedicated patient, the dose of propofol of 2–2.5 mg/kg is usually sufficient to induce anaesthesia, and infusion rates of 6–12 mg/kg per hour are required to maintain anaesthesia in surgery. The pH of the 1% emulsion is 7.8.

Clinical effect in status epilepticus

Propofol has been shown to be effective in generalised pentylenetetrazol-induced status in rabbits and less so in partial status due to cortically applied penicillin (De Riu *et al.* 1992). It has been the subject of only seven published clinical case reports, but is nevertheless now quite widely used in ITUs, at least in the UK. Yanny & Christmas (1988) reported one refractory patient successfully treated by propofol with a loading dose of 120 mg with suxamethonium, followed by an infusion of propofol at a rate of 6 mg/kg per hour for 24 hours. Seizures were monitored with a cerebral function monitor, and the patient was artificially ventilated. MacKenzie, Kapadia & Grant (1990) reported two patients with subtle status in acute encephalopathy, treated successfully with propofol. Artificial ventilation, intensive cardiovascular and EEG monitoring were employed in both cases. Seizure activity was abolished by an initial bolus of 2 mg/kg followed by an infusion of 7 mg/kg per hour for 5 days in one patient, and an infusion of 6–10 mg/kg per hour for 12 hours in the second patient, which was then reduced and withdrawn after 12 days (this patient had responded to a thiopentone infusion, but it had been discontinued because of hypotension and oliguria). De Maria *et al.* (1991) reported similar success in a patient with adversive status given propofol as a bolus dose of 100 mg, followed by an infusion of 3 mg/kg per hour, reduced after 20 hours to 1.5 mg/kg per hour and then stopped 1 hour later. Alia *et al.* (1991) described two refractory patients successfully treated with a bolus of 100 mg followed by an infusion of 500 mg over 2 hours. Wood, Browne & Pugh (1988) reported a patient with acute encephalitis treated with a single bolus dose of 100 mg followed by a continuous infusion at an initial rate of 5–7 mg/kg per hour; she received the infusion for 18 days before she died of encephalitis, disseminated intravascular coagulation and acute renal failure.

Toxic effects in status epilepticus

Propofol commonly causes involuntary movements that may be mistaken for convulsions and can also precipitate convulsions. One patient, 20 minutes after cessation of a short propofol anaesthesia for a minor operation, developed status requiring thiopentone infusion (Mäkelä *et al.* 1993). Propofol is otherwise an essentially nontoxic anaesthetic, and causes relatively few haemodynamic side-effects. Unlike etomidate, it does not affect adrenocortical function. A prolonged infusion in the large doses required in status will result in marked lipaemia, an accumulation of inactive glucuronide metabolites and a metabolic acidosis, especi-

Table 5.22. *Propofol*

Indication (stage of status)
Refractory status

Usual preparation
20 ml ampoule containing 10 mg/ml (i.e. 200 mg) as an emulsion

Usual dosage
2 mg/kg bolus, repeated if necessary, followed by a continuous infusion of 5–10 mg/kg
   per h initially, reducing to 1–3 mg/kg per h, guided by EEG.

Advantages
Very rapid onset of action and recovery
Few haemodynamic side-effects
Weak intrinsic antiepileptic activity
Pharmacology studied extensively
Easier to administer than inhalational anaesthetics

Disadvantages
Involuntary movements (without EEG change)
Very little published experience in status, or of prolonged infusions in children
Occasionally reported to cause seizures
Metabolised in the liver
Very little experience with long-term therapy
Requires assisted ventilation, ITU and intensive care monitoring, and exhaustive
   cardiorespiratory monitoring
Lipaemia, acidosis
Respiratory depression and sedation inevitable

---

ally in children. There is indeed limited experience of prolonged infusions in young children, in whom large doses of propofol are usually required (infusions of 9–15 mg/kg per hour in children over 3 years of age), and, in a recent report of five deaths in critically ill babies treated with prolonged propofol infusions, it was suggested that the metabolic disturbance caused by propofol might have contributed to the demise of the infants (Parke *et al.* 1992).

Administration and dosage in status epilepticus

Propofol is presented as a 1% solution in 20 ml ampoule containing 10 mg/ml of an emulsion, with soya bean oil and purified egg phosphatide. In status, a sensible though essentially untried regimen would be as follows: initially 2 mg/kg bolus doses are given, which can be repeated if seizures continue, followed by an infusion of about 5–10 mg/kg per hour with the dose guided by EEG. The dose should be gradually reduced, and the infusion tapered 12 hours after seizure activity is halted. Propofol of course requires the same ITU facilities, assisted respiration and EEG or cerebral activity monitoring as do thiopentone or pentobarbitone anaesthesia. Doses should be lower in the elderly.

Summary of use in status epilepticus (table 5.22)

Experience of the use of propofol in status is very limited, as indeed it is of the prolonged administration of propofol in any clinical circumstance. Propofol, is however, a highly effective and nontoxic intravenous anaesthetic. In experimental models, it has intrinsic anticonvulsant properties, but in anaesthetic practice it has also caused seizures and even status, and to what extent it exhibits specific antiepileptic properties at the doses used in status is unknown. It requires the full panoply of ITU care and intensive monitoring. Propofol acts very rapidly indeed, and recovery is also very quick. It causes profound respiratory and cerebral depression, but hypotension is mild and it has few other cardiovascular side-effects. It may cause involuntary movements which should not be mistaken for seizures. Experience of propofol infusions in young children is very limited, and the drug has been implicated, albeit on flimsy evidence, in five deaths in critically ill children. It causes lipaemia and may cause acidosis. Propofol is extraordinarily soluble in lipids, and has an enormous volume of distribution; there is a potential risk of accumulation, although this has not proved to be a problem in clinical practice. It is metabolised in the liver, and cleared very rapidly at a rate which exceeds hepatic blood flow, suggesting additional extrahepatic clearance. It is safe and easy to use, and is potentially superior to etomidate in long-term use in status. Although propofol has been the subject of few case reports, its use in status is promising and warrants further study.

Other drugs used in status epilepticus

It was only in the mid nineteenth century that the treatment of status was distinguished from the treatment of epilepsy in general. What specific remedies were employed before then is not certain – presumably there was none. The value of bromides for status was soon established, but even as early as 1880 it was recognised that massive sedation or anaesthesia was sometimes more effective in this desperate situation. Gowers in 1888, noting that bromide therapy often failed, commended chloroform inhalation (although he recognised this too often provided only transient amelioration), chloral and morphia. He was pessimistic about the outcome of status, and this pessimism permeated all subsequent thought. Clark & Prout (1903/4) proposed the following curious mixture: tinc. opii. desdor. gtt. 5, pot. brom. 1.5, chloral hdr. 1.2, liq. morph. sulph. 30, and while this was taking effect ether anaesthesia. Various nonpharmacological measures were also employed at the time, including the application of ice to the spine (Gowers 1888) and lumbar puncture (Jardine 1907, cited by Muskens 1928). Muskens (1928) found prolonged anaesthesia with ether or chloroform to be 'of great value', also the placing of the patient in a quiet darkened room (how unlike the modern ITU!), enemata to empty the colon and rectum, and the administration of bromide, chloral, dormiol or amylene hydrate. Kinnier Wilson (1940) in his definitive textbook also recommended bromides and opiates and Clark & Prout's concoction, and was the first to note that if status was due to sedative withdrawal, the withdrawn drug should be immediately replaced, per rectum if necessary. Also recommended were the hypodermic injection of phenobarbitone at a dose of 1–3 grains (approximately equivalent to 60–200 mg), bromide (10%), or hyoscine, rectal paraldehyde (doses up to 24 ml), repeated lumbar puncture, intrathecal bromide, chloroform, oxygen, venusection and saline injections.

Before the introduction of the benzodiazepine drugs, *chloral* was widely given, and latterly intrarectal chloral (30 mg/kg) has been successfully used without side-effects in five patients resistant to diazepam + phenytoin, valproate and phenobarbitone, an enthusiastic endorsement of an ancient therapy (Lampl *et al.* 1990). During the past 50 years other barbiturate and nonbarbiturate sedatives have also been used, including *bromethol, hexobarbitone, methohexital, butallylonal, secobarbital, amylobarbitone, diethylamine barbiturate* and *nitrazepam* (Roger *et al.* 1974).

More recently, there has been a steady trickle of anecdotal reports of other new drugs. Althesin was a steroidal anaesthetic (now withdrawn) used occasionally in status (Munari *et al.* 1979). *Fosphenytoin* is a phenytoin pro-drug which is water soluble and has the great advantage of almost complete absorption after an intramuscular injection. On entry into blood, the phosphate group is removed and fosphenytoin is converted into the parent drug, and effective levels are said to be achieved within 20–30 minutes of an intramuscular loading dose (Ramsey 1993). The dose equivalent of fosphenytoin to phenytoin is 3:2, and the drug is currently undergoing clinical trials (Smith *et al.* 1989). *Magnesium sulphate* was first recommended in the treatment of status in 1901, and since then has retained a small band of enthusiasts, especially for the treatment of eclamptic convulsions (Storchheim 1933; Taylor 1981; Dinsdale 1988; Goldman & Finkbeiner 1988). Magnesium sulphate has been formally compared with phenytoin and diazepam, but recent experimental and clinical studies provide conflicting evidence of whether magnesium has useful antiepileptic action (Fisher *et al.* 1988; Link, Anderson & Meyer 1991; Cotton, Janusz & Berman 1992). Magnesium is very insoluble in lipid, and does not diffuse freely to brain; quite how it exerts an antiepileptic action is unclear. It paralyses skeletal muscle, may interfere with afferent input to the brain and reduces cerebral oedema, and these properties may contribute to its action. There are sporadic reports of success with *sodium valproate* by a nasogastric tube, rectal and oral administration in status (Manhire & Espir 1974; Vadja, Symington & Bladin 1977; Snead & Miles 1985; Giroud & Dumas 1988), and recently sodium valproate has become available in an intravenous preparation for patients who are temporarily unable to tolerate oral therapy. Although, a regimen composed of an intravenous bolus dose of 10 mg/kg followed by infusions of 0.6 mg/kg per hour for 24 hours has been suggested (Brown & Hussain 1991*b*), this has not been sufficiently evaluated in status. A single case report suggests lamotrigine might be effective in status (Pisani, Gallitto & Di Perri 1991). *Clorazepate* is a pro-drug of *N*-desmethyldiazepam, which can be given orally (being converted in the stomach to the active compound) or by intravenous infusion. It has been in clinical use since the mid 1960s as an anxiolytic, and more recently as adjunctive therapy in refractory epilepsy. There are sporadic reports of efficacy in status (Van der Kleijn *et al.* 1983). *Flunitrazepam* is another benzodiazepine which has been used in place of lorazepam or diazepam. There is a single report of the use of verapamil (15 mg) given intrathecally to two patients in status without effect (Besser & Kramer 1992). The use of *tiagabine hydrochloride*, a potent inhibitor of GABA uptake, has been reported in experimental status (Walton & Treiman 1992). In addition to their use in infantile spasms, *adrenocorticotrophic hormone* and the *adrenocortical steroids* have a time-honoured place in the adjunctive treatment of refractory status. Personal experience suggests that corticosteroids are particularly effective in epilepsia partialis continua and in nonconvulsive status, although whether this is a primary or secondary effect, for example by reducing cerebral oedema, is uncertain. Nevertheless, corticosteroid therapy is worth trying in a crisis setting in any truly refractory case. For adults, a daily dose of 12–16 mg of *dexamethasone* given for several days would seem reasonable.

Occasionally, resective neurosurgical therapy has been attempted to control status. I am aware of a patient with prolonged tonic–clonic status, due to Rasmussen's chronic encephalitis, whose seizures were halted (temporarily) by emergency temporal lobectomy, and Gorman *et al.* (1992) have reported the successful treatment of a 9 year old child with continuous focal motor seizures by cortical resection of heterotopic tissue in the frontal lobe. Whether neurosurgery should be more frequently employed in status is quite unclear. The mortality of status in lesional cases refractory to drug therapy is high, and emergency neurosurgery should probably be at least considered in such patients. Magnetic resonance imaging will prove a particularly valuable investigation in this situation, as surgery in status will almost certainly have to be confined to resection of imaged cortical abnormalities.

Finally, the exciting prospect should be mentioned of adjunctive therapy with antagonists of glutamate, other excitatory neurotransmitters, or calcium receptor blockers. These drugs have antiepileptic properties and also the potential to prevent status-induced cellular damage. This latter property is a therapeutic approach of great potential importance, but one which has not as yet been formally studied in human status.

Emergency treatment of other forms of status epilepticus

This chapter has been concerned, to this point, with the emergency treatment of tonic–clonic status. Urgent therapy is needed to reverse the physiological (especially cardiovascular and metabolic) changes induced by the seizures, as these carry substantial morbidity and mortality. In general terms, the homoeostatic perturbations are less severe in other forms of status, and the same degree of urgency is therefore not required (exceptions include neonatal and febrile status). When immediate anticonvulsant action is not required, oral therapy is sufficient, and the principles of medical and surgical treatment are broadly similar to those of ordinary epilepsy, a detailed description of which is beyond the scope of this book. Here, an outline only is given of therapy of the other types of status.

Neonatal status epilepticus

Neonatal status requires urgent intravenous treatment, both to terminate seizures rapidly and to prevent recurrence. Phenobarbitone is often recommended as the drug of first choice (see Lockman 1989; Lockman *et al.* 1979), although phenytoin, clonazepam, paraldehyde and sodium valproate have also been used (Kellaway & Mizrahi 1987; Anonymous 1989). Details of the pharmacology and therapeutics of the individual drugs in the neonatal period are given in the earlier sections of this book. The cause of the status may also require specific treatment (e.g. calcium, glucose, pyridoxine, antibiotics, electrolyte correction, etc.). The convulsing neonate should be urgently transferred to the neonatal ITU, and requires specialised medical, paediatric and anaesthetic care. EEG monitoring is mandatory, and assisted ventilation often required. For details of the ITU measures necessary, the reader is referred to the standard neonatology texts (e.g. Volpe 1981, 1987; Fenichel 1985).

Status epilepticus in neonatal epilepsy syndromes

Overt status requires the same emergency antiepileptic treatment as other forms of neonatal status. Early infantile epileptic encephalopathy (Ohtahara syndrome) and neonatal myoclonic encephalopathy are often treated with corticosteroids in addition, although prognosis is poor, and evidence demonstrating any clear-cut benefit from steroids is rather lacking.

Infantile spasm (West syndrome)

Appropriate therapy directed against the underlying cause may be needed and should be given urgently including treatment of infection, hypoglycaemia, metabolic disorders, and treatment of endocrine disorders, and enzyme defects. Symptomatic therapy of the spasms is usually with intramuscular ACTH at a dose of 150 IU per day (in two divided doses) for 1 week, halving the dose in the second week, and then lowering the dose gradually according to response. Usual short-term therapy is continued for 5–8 weeks. Higher steroid doses may be required for resistant spasms in some children, and therapy for longer periods (4–6 months). The relative merits of ACTH and oral prednisone have been much debated, but it seems that most paediatricians prefer the former despite the inconvenience of injection. Recently, vigabatrin has been shown to be an effective alternative (Chiron *et al.* 1991), and may well become the treatment of choice. Other remedies which have been show to be effective include benzodiazepine drugs, valproate, pyridoxine phosphate and gammaglobulins. Long-term antiepileptic drug therapy is usually also required. Resective neurosurgery has also been carried out in refractory cases in whom focal lesions are demonstrable (Chugani *et al.* 1990).

Febrile status epilepticus

Urgent therapy is required. It is usual to administer diazepam intravenously as a single bolus of 0.2–0.3 mg/kg, or, if the weight of the infant is not known,

288

according to the formula 1 mg per year of age + 1 mg (i.e. 3 mg for a 2 year old child). An alternative which is often easier to accomplish in a convulsing infant is the rectal instillation of diazepam solution (or the convenient Stesolid disposable rectal tube) at a dose of 0.6–0.8 mg/kg (approximately 5–7.5 mg in children under 3 years and 7.5–10 mg in children over 3 years of age). Although diazepam is generally recommended as first-line therapy, rectal or intravenous clonazepam or paraldehyde can also be given. If first-line therapy fails, intravenous pheno-barbitone, phenytoin, valproate, chlormethiazole, lignocaine or general anaesthesia have been tried. The child should be admitted to hospital, and the cause of the febrile status ascertained and treated appropriately. Febrile seizures can be averted by steps to lower body temperature; for example, stripping the child, tepid sponging, fanning, and giving paracetamol orally or by rectal suppository at a dose of 10–20 mg/kg. In susceptible children, rectal diazepam can also be given prophylactically.

Status epilepticus in childhood myoclonic syndromes

Treatment of the syndrome of severe myoclonic epilepsy in infants and status is difficult. The conventional anticonvulsants, corticosteroids and immunotherapy may improve the epilepsy somewhat, although seizure control is not obtained. Urgent treatment of fever or infection must be given to prevent the precipitation of status. The status is highly resistant to therapy. *Myoclonic status in nonprogressive encephalopathy* is also often refractory to therapy, including ACTH, although a combination of valproate and ethosuximide may be effective (Dalla Bernardina *et al.* 1992). If the status can be controlled, the child's intellectual abilities may be improved. The response to treatment of status in *myoclonic–astatic epilepsy* is unpredictable. Valproate is usually given first, and other effective therapies include acetazolamide, nitrazepam, ethosuximide and corticosteroids (Doose 1985). Bromides were recently recommended in patients with severe tonic–clonic seizures (Doose 1992) in refractory cases at a dose of 40–60 mg/kg, achieving blood levels of 140–190 mg/100 ml.

Status epilepticus in benign childhood epilepsy syndromes

Status in these conditions is treated in the same way as in other childhood epilepsies. Fejerman & Di Blasi (1987) reported a rapid response to corticosteroids in two children with benign partial epilepsy who were refractory to conventional antiepileptic therapy.

Electrical status epilepticus during slow wave sleep and the syndrome of acquired epileptic aphasia

The electrographic status in these conditions does not generally require urgent therapy. Indeed, it is not clear to what extent it is worth while attempting to abolish the electrographic activity by oral antiepileptics, which is anyway often not possible. When antiepileptic drug therapy is given, clonazepam or valproate therapy are usually tried initially (Yasuhara *et al.* 1991), and ACTH and steroids

289

have been given. Occasionally, overt convulsive or nonconvulsive status occurs, which should be treated in the conventional manner, as should coexisting chronic epilepsy. In the Landau–Kleffner syndrome, early corticosteroid therapy has been advocated (Mantovani & Landau 1980; Ravnik 1985; Lerman, Lerman-Sagie & Kivity 1991).

Absence status epilepticus, and de novo *absence status epilepticus of late onset*

Both typical absence status and absence status of late onset are usually rapidly terminated by intravenous benzodiazepine. It is usual to give diazepam at a dose of 0.2–0.3 mg/kg, clonazepam 1 mg/kg (0.5 mg in children) or lorazepam 0.07 mg/kg (children 0.1 mg/kg), repeated as required. In the rare cases in which this is ineffectual, and when intravenous therapy is required, valproate, phenytoin or chlormethiazole can be given. The more atypical is the absence status, the less responsive it is to benzodiazepine (or other) therapy. In most cases of primary generalised epilepsy, long-term valproate or ethosuximide therapy are also recommended (Porter & Penry 1983; Berkovic *et al.* 1989*a*), although lamotrigine may be equally effective. In cases without a prior history of epilepsy, and in whom a treatable precipitating cause is identified, long-term maintenance therapy in patients with late-onset absence status may not be necessary.

Epilepsia partialis continua

In acute cases, the seizures can remit spontaneously. In a well-established case, emergency treatment of the condition is usually unnecessary and is often ineffective. Intravenous therapy, even to the point of general anaesthesia, may produce temporary respite, but the seizures usually recur. Any of the conventional oral antiepileptics can be tried, with phenytoin, carbamazepine or phenobarbitone being the drugs of first choice. Oral corticosteroid or gammaglobulin therapy may be helpful in resistant cases. There is a single uncontrolled report of the successful use of intravenous nimodipine (2 mg/hour for 1–2 days) in two patients with epilepsia partialis continua in the setting of an acute cerebral event (Brandt *et al.* 1988). Resective neurosurgical therapy should be considered in refractory cases (see Olivier 1991; Lüders 1992; Engel 1993).

Myoclonic status epilepticus in coma

Although anticonvulsant therapy is often administered (usually intravenous phenytoin or phenobarbitone), there is no clear evidence that attempts to treat the myoclonus will improve outcome. Corticosteroid therapy can also be tried, although clear evidence of efficacy is lacking. Myoclonic status in this situation is almost always the signature of diffuse and severe cerebral damage, and the prognosis is accordingly poor whatever treatment regimen is employed. The only exception is myoclonic status in coma occurring in patients with a history of generalised epilepsy where prognosis is better, and the principles of treatment are similar to those of tonic–clonic status.

Specific forms of status epilepticus in mental retardation

Seizures in the Lennox–Gastaut syndrome are often highly resistant to treatment. In acute atypical absence status, intravenous benzodiazepine therapy can be given, although the response is less satisfactory than in typical absence status. Paraldehyde, chlormethiazole, phenobarbitone or steroid therapy can also be helpful. Usually, oral rather than intravenous treatment is more appropriate, and any of the conventional anticonvulsant drugs can be tried, those of first choice being valproate, lamotrigine, clonazepam and clobazam. Carbamazepine has been said to worsen seizures in some cases (Snead & Hosey 1985), although evidence on this point is is unconvincing. *Tonic status* is also highly resistant to therapy (Bladin, Vajda & Symington 1977). Conventional antiepileptics may be tried, although occasionally benzodiazepines may worsen the status (Tassinari *et al.* 1972; Livingston & Brown 1987). An alternative approach is to administer methylphenidate, the stimulating effect of which can inhibit seizures. In all types of status, high dose ACTH (80 IU/day) or corticosteroids (dexamethasone 0.3–1.0 mg/kg per day) may be helpful in the emergency situation. Generally speaking, heavy medication should be avoided in the Lennox–Gastaut syndrome, as sedation may worsen almost all seizure types in these patients. Corpus callosectomy or resective neurosurgery can be tried in severe drug-resistant cases, although the results are unpredictable.

Other forms of myoclonic status epilepticus

In myoclonic status in primary generalised epilepsy or the progressive myoclonic epilepsies, intravenous therapy is usually not required, but benzodiazepine infusion can be tried or occasionally valproate or tryptophan. For oral therapy, valproate, benzodiazepines (e.g. diazepam, clobazam or clonazepam) or piracetam are the drugs of choice.

Nonconvulsive simple partial status epilepticus

This form of status seldom requires intravenous therapy, and the principles of medical and surgical treatment are similar to those of ordinary partial epilepsy. In many patients, the seizures are relatively refractory to conventional treatment.

Complex partial status epilepticus and boundary syndromes

The relative indications for intravenous or oral therapy in complex partial status are uncertain. In most acute cases, intravenous benzodiazepine (as above, for absence status) should be given, with oral maintenance therapy, and is effective (see, for instance, Markand *et al.* 1978; Tomson *et al.* 1986; Dunne *et al.* 1987). The response to such intravenous therapy is often less rapid or complete than in typical absence status, and higher dosages may be required. Intravenous phenytoin or phenobarbitone can also be given. The drugs of choice for oral therapy are carbamazepine, phenytoin or phenobarbitone. Valproate, benzodiazepines (including clobazam), acetazolamide, vigabatrin, lamotrigine and corticosteroids can also be used. If the status is due to anticonvulsant withdrawal, the withdrawn drug

291

should be rapidly reinstated. Acute intravenous and longer-term oral therapy in the boundary syndromes should follow similar principles. The therapy of chronic epileptic psychosis is well described elsewhere (see Trimble 1991).

Prologue to therapy in status epilepticus

I have attempted in this chapter to lay out the merits of a wide range of therapies, fairly and comprehensively, but not, I hope, in too relentless a manner. If any single conclusion jumps out from these pages, it is the profound lack of useful comparative data. The relative effectiveness or hazard of conventional therapy has been very poorly evaluated, and almost none of the newer or less conventional alternative treatments have been subjected to anything more than cursory analysis; some have not even received adequate pharmacological or pharmacokinetic study. This is a quite unsatisfactory state of affairs, rendering it impossible to make more than what are essentially informed guesses at appropriate therapeutic regimens. Until the assessment of therapy in status is placed on a more exacting basis, treatment will remain empirical and subject to whimsy; the correction of this deficiency must be an urgent priority in epilepsy research.

CHAPTER 6

Prognosis and outcome of status epilepticus

Status is . . . a true climax of the disease [epilepsy] and less a chance termination which by proper treatment could be avoided; certainly chance plays no part as agent in the production of status. An epileptic is foredoomed to die of the status as a maximum development of the disease.

(Clark & Prout 1903/4)

Thus Clark & Prout, in true *fin de siècle* mood, saw the outcome of status; an apocalyptic view which sets the scene for our sombre reflections on prognosis. Neurological thought is often traced back (in Anglo-Saxon if not Gallic texts!) to Hughlings Jackson or Gowers, matchless theoreticians of nineteenth century epilepsy. On the subject of status epilepticus, though, both were almost silent. Jackson gives one case report of a female patient with recurrent status who survived the repeated episodes unharmed, and Gowers commented that he had not personally seen a case. In regard to prognosis in epilepsy, Gowers considered 'the danger to life in epilepsy is not great. Alarming as is the aspect of a severe epileptic fit – imminent as the danger to life appears when the patient is lying senseless, with livid, swollen and distorted features, and convulsions which almost asphyxiate him, looking "as if strangled by the bow of an invisible executioner" (Radcliffe), it is extremely rare for a patient to die in a fit' (Gowers 1881). As noted in chapter 1, status had been equally unrecorded by others at the time, and it fell to the new alienist physicians to describe the condition, which undoubtedly was relatively more common in asylums than in the general population. Hunter's observation that status was rare until the late nineteenth century may be correct, and certainly death due to epilepsy was considered rare by all writers on the subject in that century. As status began to be more widely recognised, however, its grim nature was quickly appreciated.

Outcome of tonic–clonic status epilepticus (including generic studies of status epilepticus)

Mortality and morbidity statistics from early series

The early studies of status were confined largely to tonic–clonic status, and have the predictable problems of case ascertainment, definition and selection bias. They are worth reviewing, however, as they help to define the natural history of the

293

condition at a time when treatment was rudimentary, and set the context for assessing the effectiveness of modern treatment. There is no doubt that the seriousness of status was well recognised from its earliest mention (indeed, the reader is referred to the very first sentence of this book), but as was frequently emphasised, the condition was by no means universally fatal. Binswanger (cited by Turner 1907) recorded a 50% mortality. Lorenz (1880, cited by Clark & Prout 1903/4) recorded death due to status in 36 (45%) of 80 cases. Crichton Browne (cited by Hunter 1959/60) reported that of 22 epileptic deaths at the West Riding Asylum, 7 (32%) were due to status: 'a considerable number of epileptics die in status – indeed, in this asylum, it is perhaps the most common mode of death in epileptics'. Although Bourneville (1876) himself noted that the longer the status proceeded and the higher the temperature, the worse the outcome, Clark & Prout (1903/4) observed recoveries from status of 12 days' duration and from patients with hyperpyrexia reaching 107 °F. Amongst their 52 cases, 100 status episodes were observed, with a 14% mortality. Turner (1907), too, in his 'statistical' study of epilepsy, recorded status in 15 (5%) of the 280 cases under his observation, with 29 attacks of status, and only 3 (10%) deaths. Hunter (1959/60) suggested that the condition was rare before the anticonvulsant era, and that most cases were due to sudden anticonvulsant withdrawal (a suggestion first made by Muskens (1928)) or intercurrent infection in patients taking anticonvulsant drugs. Using death certification figures (a notoriously unreliable tool!), he found that annual death rates from status accounted for 37–51% of deaths in epilepsy between 1949 and 1956. Death from status was particularly common in children, both in overall terms and as a proportion of all epilepsy-related deaths. About a quarter of deaths due to epilepsy occurred in mentally retarded patients or mental hospitals, and of these 42–64% were due to status, compared with 35–46% of epileptic deaths outside institutions. The fact that institutionalised patients die more often in status was also well recognised by Clark and Prout, Turner, and Browne, physicians to the Craig epileptic colony, the Chalfont colony and the West Riding Asylum, respectively. Gowers (1901), in a note added to the second edition of his textbook, records that Farquhar Buzzard ascertained the numbers and causes of death amongst the 2828 cases of epilepsy at the National Hospital in the 34.5 years in which records had been kept. Of the 38 deaths, only 12 were related to epilepsy and 7 were due to status. The morbidity of status was unrecorded in most early investigations, although sporadic mention of post-status hemiplegia and mental deterioration was made.

Recent studies of mortality

Hunter (1959/60) was perhaps the first to attempt a modern scrutiny of mortality data, and his paper spawned a further set of studies. A representative selection are shown in table 6.1, but before accepting these figures, several points must be stressed.

1. Although, at about this time, nonconvulsive status and other syndromes were being recognised, most studies are confined to convulsive status (exceptions include: Aicardi & Chevrie 1970; Goulon *et al.* 1985; Sung & Chu 1989*b*).

2. All were from specialised hospital settings. It is a remarkable indictment of our statistical age to admit that there are no trustworthy population-based data on death rates from status. Death certification figures for status will be highly unreliable, because of the tendency to ascribe the syndrome of sudden death in epilepsy to status, simply because no other suitable category exists (Brown *et al.* 1990). Specialist hospital-based studies overestimate the risk of death in status by overrepresenting severe cases or those persisting for long periods of time.

3. Death rates from status in existing epileptic cases may underestimate the risk, as many cases of status occur in people without a previous history of epilepsy (see pp. 28–9; in 76% of children and 12–60% of adults with status, it is the presenting feature of the epilepsy).

4. The problems of definition, rehearsed at length in chapter 2, pose further obstacles to accurate risk assessment. The case ascertainment of status, particularly if retrospective, can easily miss mild or short lived cases, the ones least likely to succumb. Furthermore, in symptomatic cases the relative contributions of the underlying cause and status to mortality or morbidity are often impossible to disentangle.

5. The results of treatment in early status are so good (i.e. 79% and 88% rendered immediately seizure free by diazepam or diazepam + phenytoin respectively, see pp. 207–9, 251) that many cases will indeed be short lived. Furthermore, effective early treatment will be given in many more patients who would otherwise have progressed to status without therapy; such cases too will be excluded from status statistics.

These sources of bias magnify the apparent overall mortality of status, and published figures must be considered maximum estimates. Treatment has improved and is applied earlier (this may be particularly important), and current mortality rates should now be considerably lower than those cited above; indeed, on the balance of the evidence, admittedly slight, presented below, mortality seems to have particularly improved in the past three decades. In table 6.1 are shown overall published mortality rates in 12 recent investigations, in which death occurred in 18% of the 1686 episodes. Eighty-nine per cent of deaths were considered due to the underlying cause of the status, and death was attributed directly to the epilepsy or its complications in only 2% of status episodes. Such figures must be considered rough estimates, as the attribution of cause of death is an often difficult and subjective judgement, with epilepsy contributing to a death which might be primarily due to the underlying lesion (see below). Death rates seem higher in adults (where status is anyway less common), probably reflecting the greater severity of underlying disease necessary to precipitate status.

The first important study of outcome in status in adults was that of Oxbury & Whitty (1971*a*) of 86 cases. Six (11%) of the 54 patients with known cerebral pathology died in status, and a further five (9%) died within the next 6 months. Only one of the 32 cases without known pathology died in status, and there were no deaths in the subsequent 6 months (an overall 6-monthly mortality of 14%). Of those who died in the acute phase, all but one had acute or progressive

Table 6.1. *Reported mortality in 1686 cases of status epilepticus from 12 case-series published after 1970*

Source	n	Deaths (overall)		Deaths directly due to status[a]	
		n	(%)	n	(%)
Children					
Aicardi & Chevrie 1970	239	27	(11)	14[b]	(6)
Cavazzuti *et al.* 1984	66	2	(3)	—	(–)
Maytal *et al.* 1989	193	7	(4)	0	(0)
Yager *et al.* 1988	52	3	(6)	1[b]	(2)
Phillips & Shanahan 1989	218	13	(6)	2	(1)
Subtotal	768	52	(7)	17	(2)
Adults					
Rowan & Scott 1970	42	9	(21)	4	(10)
Oxbury & Whitty 1971*a*	86	12	(14)	2	(2)
Heintel 1972	83	20	(25)	1	(1)
Celesia *et al.* 1972	17	10	(59)	—	(–)
Aminoff & Simon 1980	98	16	(16)	2	(2)
Goulon *et al.* 1985	282	100	(35)	2	(1)
Sung & Chu 1989*b*	98	34	(35)	5	(5)
Subtotal	710	201	(28)	16	(2)
Total	1686	308	(18)	33	(2)

[a] In this column are the number of deaths which occurred acutely, and were considered to be directly due to status or its treatment rather than to the underlying cause or late deaths. This can be considered a rough approximation only, as there is often a combination of factors influencing mortality (see the text).
[b] Approximate estimate.

disease (cases of pulmonary embolus, subarachnoid haemorrhage, glioblastoma, pneumococcal meningitis, carcinomatosis (two), and alcoholism), which no doubt contributed to death. The next influential report was that of Aminoff & Simon (1980): of 98 adult patients admitted to hospital with status, 16 (16%) died, but in only two was death directly attributable to status. In the other 14, death was considered to be due to the underlying disease or medical complications (cardiac arrest two, drug overdose two, cerebrovascular disease four, trauma one, tumour one, meningitis one and metabolic causes three). In the series of 154 patients with status from the same hospital but in the subsequent decade, the death rate was very similar (22 cases, 13%), and again in only two cases was status considered to be directly responsible; an interesting lack of improvement over time despite improvements in medical care. Other cited mortality figures are 21% of 42 patients (Rowan & Scott 1970), 7% of 68 cases (Janz 1961), 25% of 83 cases (Heintel 1972), 7% of 60 cases (of all types of status; Celesia 1976). In 342 patients with epilepsy developing after the age of 60 years, 102 (30%) experienced status with a mortality rate of 35% compared to 16% of those without a history of status, although status was a direct cause of death in only 5% (Sung & Chu 1989*b*).

The best recent investigation was a study of 282 consecutive admissions in adult status to two intensive care units (Goulon *et al.* 1985). One hundred (35%) died, but in only two was the death attributable to status (and in one of these the result of cardiac arrest before admission to hospital). In the rest, death was due to the underlying cause of the status. Of the 81 patients with pre-existing epilepsy, six (7%) died; and in those presenting in status *de novo* 47% died. Status may contribute to death, however, even where this is primarily due to the underlying neurological process, and this risk can be difficult to quantify. Goulon and colleagues noticed, for instance, that the prognosis of the underlying condition worsened if status occurred; thus, the mortality of bacterial meningitis admissions to the ITUs was 33% of 87 cases without status, compared to 82% of the 11 cases complicated by status. It is often not possible to ascertain to what extent excess mortality was due to the status, or whether the presence of status simply reflected a greater severity of underlying disease.

Status in children has been the subject of particular interest, not least because of its greater frequency, and greater severity. In a classic paper, Aicardi & Chevrie (1970) reported the outcome of status in 239 infants and children. Of these 27 (11%) died, 10 in the acute phase and 17 in the months or years after the event. In about half of these cases, death could be attributed to status itself. Follow-up was short in some cases, and the longer-term mortality might have been higher, as many children were left with severe neurological or mental handicaps. This was an influential report, providing statistical evidence of the gravity of childhood status for the first time: 85% of the patients were younger than 5 years, and 67 episodes of status were associated with fever. Aicardi & Chevrie noted that prolonged convulsions could be particularly devastating in febrile seizures in young babies, and that in all cases the duration of status was a critical factor. The importance of rapid therapy in young children was first stressed at this time. A much better prognosis was found by Cavazzuti, Ferrari & Lalla (1984) following up 482 children with seizures starting between 1 and 12 months of life: 66 had status, of whom only 3% died in the follow-up period.

Maytal *et al.* (1989) then described 193 children of whom only seven died, all of whom had acute or progressive cerebral insults. This report prompted an editorial arguing that 'status was now not as dangerous as once taught' (Freeman 1989), and a retort from Aicardi & Chevrie (1989), who, whilst agreeing that mortality and morbidity had fallen, attributed this to earlier and better therapy, and warned against complacency. This caveat should be well heeded, as, although childhood status is now less common and the outcome less devastating (at least in industrialised societies), there is indubitable clinical and experimental evidence of its potential dangers.

The most recent comprehensive investigation of outcome in childhood status was a study designed to revisit the ground laid by Aicardi & Chevrie, to see to what extent diagnostic and therapeutic advances had improved outcome in the subsequent two decades (Phillips & Shanahan 1989). A total of 218 episodes of childhood status admitted to a paediatric ITU over a 5 year period was studied, of which 13 (6%) ended fatally. Three children died within 24 hours of presentation and the other 10 in the subsequent days or weeks. In 11 there was an acute cerebral insult (meningitis in six, severe hypoxia in four, and fulminant hepatic failure in one), and one died with an unidentified cerebral encephalopathy. There was only one death amongst the 99 episodes of idiopathic status.

Recent studies of morbidity

It was only in 1970, following the publication of the paper by Aicardi & Chevrie, that attention moved to the subject of the residual morbidity of status. This paediatric paper had a great impact, and the neurological and mental sequelae of status in children became subjects of intensive scrutiny. There then followed the publication of several adult series, where deficits following status were also noted, albeit at a lesser frequency. The problems of disentangling the effects of status and of the underlying condition were early recognised, and although animal experimentation has shown quite clearly that status-like electrographic activity can result in cerebral damage, in human status this has been less easy to quantify. There is little doubt that children have a much greater risk of status-induced damage, and the younger the child the higher the risk. The duration of status is also an important factor in determining prognosis, and the longer the attack the more serious the outcome, although to what extent this simply reflects the severity of the underlying condition is not always possible to assess.

Oxbury & Whitty (1971a) were the first to report neurological outcome in adult cases. Of their 86 cases of status, five were found to be *undoubtedly deteriorated* after the attack. Three had had encephalitis but in two (2%) no reason other than status could be found for their serious impairment. Rowan & Scott (1970) recorded a rate of 26% 'neurological sequelae' but did not provide any further details. Of the 98 cases reported by Aminoff & Simon (1980), eight were left with permanent neurological deficits, six with varying degrees of intellectual impairment, and two with atrophy identified by computed tomography associated with spastic quadraparesis. Lowenstein & Alldredge (1993) compared outcome in the same hospital in the decade subsequent to the report of Aminoff & Simon (1980). Of 154 cases of status, 22 died and 15 (10%) had a poor outcome (defined as severe neurological deficit requiring long-term hospitalisation or full supportive care), figures which were disappointingly similar to the earlier series. In neither series was it clear to what extent these deficits could have been caused by the underlying aetiology of status. I have observed children and adults with motor impairment, movement disorders, intellectual and memory disturbance, and persisting vegetative states after status, but rarely can the status itself be conclusively blamed for these deficits. Underlying encephalitis seems particularly likely to result in persisting mental deficits and, in many cases of status with poor outcome, encephalitis is suspected even if not confirmed virologically. Nevertheless, it is clinical experience that mental and personality deterioration does occur in the wake of status in many patients, although these often improve. Formal evidence of psychological damage is lacking. There is only one published study of the

298

results of psychometric tests applied to patients before and after status (Dodrill & Wilensky 1990). In this rather inconclusive investigation, 143 adult epileptic patients were tested 5 years apart. Status occurred in the intervening period in nine cases. When these nine cases were compared with the other 144 on the WAIS and the WISC tests, somewhat deteriorated scores were found in the status group; however, the changes did not reach statistical significance. The fact that patients who experienced status had markedly lower scores than did the controls even at the first evaluation was only one of a number of confounding factors (Dodrill & Wilensky 1990).

In children, the risk of morbidity from status is greater than in adults. The younger the child, the more likely to occur are both motor or cognitive deficits. The important study of Aicardi & Chevrie (1970, 1983) was the first to explore the extent of the problem. Of the 239 cases of status between the ages of 1 month and 15 years, 47 (20%) previously well children developed motor deficits and 78 (33%) mental impairment, which could be directly attributable to the episode of status. The motor problems were hemiplegia in 28 (12%) of the type conforming to the HH syndrome (see below) and diplegia, extrapyramidal and cerebellar disturbance. Motor and mental sequelae often coexisted and overall 82 (34%) children were affected. Indeed, 21% continued to have epilepsy. Fujikawa *et al.* (1989*a,b*) recorded poststatus deficits in 40 (51%) of 79 children, of whom 25 (32%) were of the HH type, and 37% mental deficits. Yager *et al.* (1988) found a 28% morbidity amongst 52 children, and a proportion was attributable to the underlying cause. Maytal *et al.* (1989) recorded a lower morbidity amongst 193 children in status. New neurological signs were found in only 17 (9.1%) of 186 survivors, of whom 15 had underlying diseases which could have contributed to the new deficits. It was suggested that selection bias was partly responsible for the apparently worse outcome in the older studies, a point disputed by Aicardi & Chevrie (1983, 1989). A more likely reason is that treatment has both improved and is administered earlier. Whatever the reasons, catastrophic status in children does now seem less common.

Epilepsy frequently follows status in subjects who have previously not suffered from epileptic seizures. Amongst the 184 cases without prior epilepsy in the series of Aicardi & Chevrie (1970), epilepsy followed in 143 (77%), most commonly partial in nature, but unilateral seizures, infantile spasms (West syndrome), Lennox–Gastaut syndrome, and further episodes of status were also recorded. Tonic–clonic seizures occurred after status in five fewer patients than before. The development of epilepsy is usually associated with cerebral damage, often related to underlying pathology. About three quarters of those children with poststatus hemiplegia will also develop seizures (Gastaut *et al.* 1967; Aicardi, Amsili & Chevrie 1969 Aicardi & Chevrie 1970, 1983; Roger *et al.* 1972, 1974). Between about 40% and 70% of adult cases of status occur in non epileptics (see pp. 28–9), and in about 12% it is the initial manifestation of continuing seizures (Janz 1983). Although epilepsy is a common sequel to initial status, it is often impossible to decide whether this is due to status-induced cerebral damage or to the underlying cause. Further attacks of status are also common after a first episode. As

299

mentioned above, most forms of nonconvulsive status have a strong tendency to recur, as does status in the childhood epilepsy and boundary syndromes. The risk of recurrence of convulsive status in children has been studied by Shinnar *et al.* (1992), who recorded second attacks of status in 16 (17%) of a cohort of 95 children and further attacks in 5 (5%). The risk of recurrent status was particularly high in children with prior neurological abnormalities (about 50% in this group) and low in children who were neurologically normal at the time of the first status episode (about 3%). Similar risks of recurrence were recorded by Aicardi & Chevrie (1970, 1983) and Cavazutti *et al.* (1984).

Unilateral or bilateral ventricular enlargement on air encephalography was demonstrated in 15 children examined immediately after status and again several months later (Aicardi & Baraton 1971). The enlargement was related to the predominant localisation of the epileptic seizures, and usually was attributable to the epilepsy rather than to the underlying cause (Aicardi & Baraton 1971; Aicardi & Chevrie 1983). CT has also demonstrated this atrophy (Aicardi & Chevrie 1983; Labate *et al.* 1991). Magnetic resonance imaging (MRI) is of course ideally suited to investigation of this phenomenon, but no MRI studies have been yet published.

Factors influencing outcome

The most important is undoubtedly the underlying aetiology. As mentioned above, about nine out of ten deaths in status can be directly attributed to the underlying cause. This is especially so in adults, and in those not previously epileptic, where an acute brain lesion sufficient to precipitate status will often also cause severe cerebral damage. Particularly damaging are acute vascular events, encephalitis, trauma or a rapidly expanding cerebral mass lesion. The severity and course of such cerebral injuries will primarily determine outcome, both in terms of morbidity and mortality. For example, amongst the 118 children with acute status reported by Aicardi & Chevrie (1983), neurological sequelae occurred in 64% of those with symptomatic compared to 25% of those with cryptogenic status. In the series of 154 patients reported by Lowenstein & Alldredge (1993), 90% of patients with status due to alcohol abuse, drug withdrawal or trauma had a good outcome, compared with only 33% of those with stroke, metabolic abnormalities or anoxia. Similar findings are reported by others (Janz 1964; Aicardi & Chevrie 1970; Rowan & Scott 1970; Oxbury & Whitty 1971*a*; Heintel 1972; Aminoff & Simon 1980; Goulon *et al.* 1985; Yager *et al.* 1988; Maytal *et al.* 1989; Phillips & Shanahan 1989).

A second important prognostic factor is the duration of status. This was well shown by Barois *et al.* (1985), who studied 90 cases of short status, of whom only 4% died, and 29 cases of status lasting more than 24 hours, of whom 24% died and 24% were left with residual deficits or in a persisting vegetative state. The duration of status is longer in symptomatic cases, and it is difficult to differentiate the independent effects on outcome of underlying aetiology and duration of status. Lowenstein & Alldredge (1993) found a trend to poorer outcome within aetiological groups in their series of 154 patients, but stressed that the major determinant of overall outcome was underlying aetiology. Nevertheless, the importance of duration in determining both mortality and morbidity has been confirmed repeatedly in adults and in children (Whitty & Taylor 1949; Aicardi & Chevrie 1970; Rowan & Scott 1970; Oxbury & Whitty 1971a). The status-induced hemiconvulsion–hemiplezia (HH) and hemiconvulsion–hemiplezia–epilepsy (HHE) syndromes in children hardly ever occur in short-duration status (Aicardi & Chevrie 1970; Roger *et al.* 1974). It is because of this direct relationship between the duration of convulsive status and its outcome that it is essential to control seizures as rapidly as possible.

The presence of cardiorespiratory failure, autonomic disturbance, hyperthermia, hypoxia, and medical and systemic complications also worsen prognosis. Many such complications are directly due to therapy, and the risk of complications rises the longer the duration of the status. The extent to which such factors have influenced outcome in published series has not been investigated.

Finally, the age of the patient may influence outcome. Highest mortality rates are experienced in infancy and the neonatal period (see below) and in the elderly (Sung & Chu 1989b). In one large series of childhood cases, morbidity fell from 29% in those less than one year of age 1 to 11% in those between 1 and 3 years and 6% in those over 3 years (Maytal *et al.* 1989). The range of causes of status in children and adults is strongly age dependent, and how much of the influence of age on outcome is due simply to aetiological differences is unclear.

To study the influence on outcome of factors independently, Yager *et al.* (1988) used a stepwise regression procedure in their series of 52 children with status. The probability of adverse outcome was increased if seizure duration was long (>60 minutes; odds ratio 5.5), in encephalopathic as opposed to idiopathic cases (odds ratio 5.6 and 9.2 for acute and chronic encephalopathies), and reduced if there was a history of prior epilepsy (odds ratio 0.12).

Outcome of other syndromes of status epilepticus

Neonatal status epilepticus

The outcome of seizures in the neonatal period has been accurately established because of the ease in which selection bias can be avoided, and full case ascertainment and follow-up can be achieved. There are no studies of neonatal status alone, but as isolated seizures and status in the neonatal period commonly coexist, prognostic data on neonatal epilepsy can be taken accurately to refer also to neonatal status. Prognosis has been the subject of a series of excellent reviews, from which this section borrows heavily (Dennis 1978; Volpe 1981, 1987; Lombroso 1983; Kellaway & Mizrahi 1987; Mizrahi & Kellaway 1987). The overall mortality of neonatal seizures in six studies of 574 infants reported between 1970 and 1988 was 15%; neurological deficits were found in 37%, and only 48% were entirely normal. Improvements in neonatal care have reduced the mortality of status in the past two decades, although improvement in morbidity has been less obvious because of the larger number of preterm infants who now survive. A number of interrelated factors affect outcome in neonatal seizures.

Table 6.2. *Outcome of various causes of neonatal seizures in six case-series from 1970 to 1988*

	Total no.	Dead		Neurological deficit		Normal	
		n	(%)	*n*	(%)	*n*	(%)
Asphyxia/HIE/infarction	162	23	(14)	78	(48)	61	(38)
Haemorrhage (incl. IVH)	60	12	(20)	24	(40)	24	(40)
Infection	71	24	(34)	16	(22)	31	(44)
Congenital anomaly	42	15	(36)	26	(62)	1	(2)
Hypocalcaemia	74	11	(15)	16	(22)	47	(64)
Hypoglycaemia	34	1	(3)	9	(26)	24	(71)
Idiopathic/unknown	132	9	(7)	38	(29)	85	(65)
Total	575	95	(15)	207	(37)	273	(48)

HIE, hypoxic–ischaemic encephalopathy; IVH, intraventricular haemorrhage.
From Rose & Lombroso 1970; Bergman *et al.* 1983; Lombroso 1983; Mizrahi & Kellaway 1987; Dulac *et al.* 1985: Andre *et al.* 1988.

GESTATIONAL AGE: The gestational age of the infant has a considerable bearing on outcome. In a careful recent study of 71 neonates with seizures (45 term and 26 preterm), 18% of the term and 27% of the preterm infants died. Infants with status fared less well than the infants with isolated seizures (normal outcome in 53% and 78%, respectively). There is a particularly high mortality in infants with a gestational age of less than 31 weeks, although this was equally true for the infants with or without seizures (Bergman *et al.* 1983).

CAUSE: This perhaps is the most important factor determining outcome, and in table 6.2 are shown published mortality and morbidity data for different causes from the six studies published between 1970 and 1988. As can be seen, status due to congenital anomaly, haemorrhage and infection carry a poorer prognosis than those with seizures due to hypocalcaemia, hypoglycaemia or idiopathic cases. Aetiology is related to gestational age, and this factor is partly responsible for the worsened outcome in preterm infants.

SEIZURE TYPE AND EEG: It has been said that the more clinically obvious the seizure manifestation, the better the outcome (Lombroso 1983). Certainly, infants with subtle or tonic status fare particularly badly (see Bergman *et al.* 1983; Volpe 1987). Again the type of neonatal seizure reflects aetiology, and the poor outcome of tonic or subtle seizures may simply reflect the influences of gestational age and aetiology. Isoelectric, low voltage or burst suppression EEG patterns carry a very poor prognosis, focal or multifocal spikes a moderately poor and normal EEG a relatively good prognosis (see Lombroso 1983).

In view of the extensive prognostic data available, neonatal seizure disorders lend themselves to multifactorial predictive modelling. This would allow prognosis to be gauged in individual cases on the basis of the kind of prognostic factors listed above; to date no such models have been devised.

Status epilepticus in neonatal epilepsy syndromes

The outcome in the epilepsy syndromes depends on the nature of the underlying encephalopathy, and it is intuitively unlikely (there are no formal studies) that the presence or absence of status has any direct influence on prognosis. The prognosis in *early infantile epileptic encephalopathy* (Ohtahara syndrome) is lamentable, with death within the first 5 years in about 25% of children. Survivors are left with severe neurological impairment (usually bedridden with spastic quadraplegia), cerebral palsy and epilepsy (Ohtahara *et al.* 1987, 1992; Aicardi 1990; Brett 1991). The subsequent epilepsy is often severe, with a strong tendency to evolve into West or Lennox–Gastaut syndromes. In one series of 14 infants with Ohtahara syndrome, all ten of the survivors after infancy developed the clinical features of West syndrome between 2 and 6 months of life, and in two the epilepsy subsequently evolved into the Lennox–Gastaut pattern (Brett 1991). The prognosis of *neonatal myoclonic encephalopathy* is equally poor; 50% of infants die in the first 2 years of life, and the survivors remain in a vegetative state, or at best develop severe epilepsy and mental retardation (Brett 1991). The time course of an individual case depends to an extent on the underlying cause. In contrast, in children who exhibit the features of *benign familial neonatal convulsions* or *benign neonatal seizures*, the status usually remits without obvious neurological or epileptic sequel. It is assumed that the longer-term prognosis is also good, although there have been few follow-up studies and neurological abnormalities have been reported in up to 33% of non-familial cases and persistent epilepsy in 11% of familial cases (Plouin 1992); to what extent (if any) residual epilepsy-induced cerebral damage occurs is unknown.

Infantile spasm (West syndrome)

Sorel & Dusaucy-Bauloye (1958) were the first to report a dramatic response to steroid treatment (given on the mistaken suspicion of an underlying immunologically related encephalitis). Since then, this observation has been repeatedly confirmed. About 60–70% of infants respond to adrenocorticotrophic hormone (ACTH) or prednisone treatment, requiring only a short course in most cases. Once in remission, the spasms do not usually recur when treatment is withdrawn. Different dosage regimens are used, with experienced paediatricians giving up to 60–80 IU per day when lower doses have failed. Some patients who fail to respond to ACTH appear to remit on prednisone therapy and vice versa, for reasons which are quite obscure. About one third of cases relapse, but may respond to a second course of therapy. The response to steroid therapy is unpredictable, and although a good response has been said to be less likely the longer the duration of spasms or in symptomatic cases, evidence on both points is conflicting (Lacey & Penry 1976; Hrachovy & Frost 1990). About 5% of infants with infantile spasms die.

The long-term outcome of infantile spasm is dependent on the underlying cause. Although the spasms are usually eventually controlled, with few children having attacks after the age of 3 years, 70–96% of survivors develop mental retardation, in most cases severe, and 35–60% chronic epilepsy. As Brett (1991) recorded, the impairment is most marked in social and personal abilities, whilst motor skills develop more normally. Severe subnormality, absence of speech, hyperactivity, and autistic and manneristic traits may result, and the subsequent epilepsy is often of the Lennox–Gastaut type. Jeavons, Bower & Dimitrakoudi (1973) reported the long-term outcome of 150 cases. Twenty-two died, 67% had subsequent seizures, 24% were severely subnormal, and 47% exhibited neurological abnormalities. Only 16% appeared to have made a complete recovery, defined as attendance at a normal school. The best outcome was in the idiopathic or immunisation groups, of whom about 33% attended normal school. O'Donohoe (1979) followed 100 cases for 5–15 years, by which time 21% were normal physically and intellectually, 19% moderately or mildly subnormal, 46% severely subnormal, and 27% had cerebral palsy (often with subnormality). At follow-up, 19% of the children had died, one third during ACTH therapy. In another prospective study of 64 infants, only 5% had a normal outcome, 69% were severely impaired without any striking difference in outcome amongst those who did or did not respond to ACTH, and 53% developed subsequent epilepsy. The only factor found reliably to influence outcome was aetiology; 38% of the cryptogenic compared with 5% of the symptomatic group were categorised as normal or only mildly impaired at follow-up (Hrachovy & Frost 1990). The mortality rate of infantile spasms has ranged from 5% to 23% (Lacey & Penry 1976; Hrachovy & Frost 1990), and was approximately 30% before the introduction of effective therapy. The greatest mortality is before the age of 4 years. The small group of infants who make a complete recovery and who have no obvious cause were considered by Dulac *et al.* (1986) to constitute a idiopathic epilepsy syndrome (*benign epileptic infantile spasms*).

Febrile status epilepticus

Until recently, the outcome of childhood febrile convulsive status had been felt to be poor. Amongst the 239 children with status lasting 1 hour reported by Aicardi & Chevrie (1970), 67 were febrile status, and these cases had a particularly bad outcome. In a subsequent study, 131 children with febrile seizures with sequelae (epilepsy in 114 cases) were compared with 86 with uncomplicated febrile seizures (Aicardi & Chevrie 1983). Febrile status (seizures of 30 minutes or more duration), unilateral seizures and young age of onset were factors which were strongly associated with adverse outcome. About 50% of the children had febrile status, of whom only 17% recovered without neurological sequel.

Permanent hemiplegia after status was first recorded by Turner (1907), and is now designated the HH or HHE syndrome. This catastrophe occurs almost exclusively in children under the age of 3 years, and three quarters of cases occur after febrile status (Gastaut *et al.* 1967; Aicardi *et al.* 1969; Aicardi & Chevrie 1970, 1983; Roger *et al.* 1972, 1974; Maytal *et al.* 1989). With the more rapid and effective treatment of status, HH and HHE are now rare sequels to febrile status in developed countries, although sadly still common in the developing world. The clinical features of the syndromes are permanent hemiplegia or hemiparesis, mental retardation and chronic epilepsy (in about three quarters), deficits which follow prolonged asymmetrical or unilateral febrile convulsions (Aicardi *et al.* 1969). The affected children often have neurological signs or epilepsy before the episode of status, but the severe deficits develop directly in its wake. The duration of status is a critical factor, with hemiplegia likely to result only after very prolonged episodes. Roger *et al.* (1972) found no case due to a status of less than 2 hours' duration, and Aicardi *et al.* (1969) noted that the status exceeded 90 minutes' duration in all their 73 cases. In the latter series, in 20 (27%) seizure durations were between 6 and 24 hours, and in 31 (42%) in excess of 24 hours. The pathological findings in the acute phase are severe venous congestion and thrombosis, and massive cerebral oedema, which can cause arterial occlusion. CT scanning at the time of the convulsion will show unilateral oedema and brain swelling, which later results in progressive atrophy of the whole hemisphere and unilateral ventricular enlargement (postconvulsive hemiatrophia cerebri). Angiography will usually be normal, and the evidence that the cerebral damage is caused by arterial or venous infarction is slight. It is difficult not to accept the view of Aicardi & Chevrie (1983), that postconvulsive hemiplegia is now rare because of early and urgent therapy in febrile status, and too insouciant an attitude to the emergency treatment of febrile seizures must be deprecated. Febrile or nonfebrile status is not uncommon in the Sturge–Weber syndrome, and can precipitate the permanent hemiparesis characteristic of the syndrome.

More recent studies of febrile status have painted a much brighter picture of long-term outcome than these earlier case series. It was recognised that much of the conflicting statistical data were due to patient selection bias, and for this reason several large-scale population-based investigations of febrile seizures were carried out. No deaths from febrile seizures or status were recorded amongst the 2740 children in three prospective large-scale investigations (the National Co-operative Perinatal Project (NCPP); Nelson & Ellenberg 1981; Annegers *et al.* 1987; Berg *et al.* 1992), and permanent neurological damage was also rare. In the NCPP, a focal paresis occurred after the febrile seizure in only 0.4%, and no child developed the HHE syndrome. The risk of subsequent epilepsy has also been the subject of several long-term studies, with estimates ranging between 2% and 7%. In the NCPP, 74 of the 1706 children (4.3%) had a first seizure lasting longer than 30 minutes (i.e. febrile status), and only 3 (4%) developed subsequent epilepsy (and indeed, 90% of those in the cohort who did develop epilepsy had not had a prolonged febrile convulsion). The risk of subsequent complex partial seizures has been of particular interest, because of the pathological work (reviewed on pp. 152–4) suggesting that mesial temporal sclerosis is often caused by a complex febrile seizure. The NCPP found a 4-fold increased risk of epilepsy in children who had had a febrile convulsion, but only a 2-fold increase in complex partial epilepsy. Again the overall risk is very small, about 1 in 200 children developing subsequent complex partial seizures after a febrile convulsion. Furthermore, only 15% of children with complex partial seizures had a history of febrile convulsions. Whilst there is no reasonable doubt that a prolonged febrile seizure

305

may damage the mesial temporal structures, it must therefore be a rare event. Amongst a cohort of 16 004 neonatal survivors (98.5% of all infants born in the UK in 1 week in April 1970), 14 676 were studied at 10 years of life: 2.7% (398 cases) had at least one febrile seizure, and of these who were neurologically normal before the first febrile seizure (382 cases), only 2.4% (9 cases) developed subsequent epilepsy (Verity & Golding 1991). In all studies, the risk of subsequent epilepsy is higher after complex febrile seizures (prolonged, focal or multiple), possibly partly a reflection of a pre-existing disposition to epilepsy. Thus, only when the status is severe or prolonged is cerebral damage likely to result.

Status epilepticus in the childhood myoclonic epilepsies

Symptomatic cases fare generally less well than those with cryptogenic myoclonic epilepsy, and the outcome depends largley on the underlying syndrome or cause. The syndrome of *severe myoclonic epilepsy in infants* is poor. Severe polymorphic epilepsy usually develops, although the incidence of myoclonus and myoclonic status usually diminishes. All patients become mentally retarded, dependent and many do not develop speech. All of the 37 survivors over the age of 10 years reported by Dravet *et al.* (1982) were institutionalised. In *myoclonic status in non-progressive encephalopathy*, after the infantile period, the epilepsy improves markedly in all subjects, with status resolving, although absence seizures and isolated myoclonias persist. All children remain mentally retarded, however, about 30% profoundly retarded, and about half do not develop speech. In contrast, the prognosis of children showing the features of myoclonic astatic epilepsy is not uniformly grim. Spontaneous remission occurs in some patients, and up to 50% of patients make a complete recovery. In others generalised epilepsy develops, and a poorer prognosis is observed, particularly in young onset cases and in those with a history of status, although evidence on this latter point is conflicting (Doose *et al.* 1970; Doose & Völzke 1979; Völzke & Doose 1979). Case definition is contentious, and the wide variation in reported outcomes may reflect differing inclusion criteria of what is a rather heterogeneous 'syndrome'. Intellectual impairment or dementia may develop in some children, possibly due to prolonged episodes of status; this is the view of Doose & Völzke (1979), who observed marked debility or imbecility in 49.5% of their selected series of 95 patients. In other series, a better prognosis is recorded. Amongst the 13 children reported by Todt & Eysold (1988), the outcome was particularly good (these cases can best be categorised as myoclonic–astatic epilepsy, although differentiation from 'idiopathic' Lennox–Gastaut is contentious). All patients were seizure free on follow-up, six without therapy, in nine the EEG was normal and was improved in the rest with the disappearance of paroxysmal changes. Mental development was normal in five, the other eight cases showed mild mental retardation only, and no permanent neurological deficits occurred.

Status epilepticus in benign childhood epilepsy syndromes

The prognosis in *benign rolandic epilepsy*, in which status is anyway rare (Colamaria *et al.* 1991), is excellent. Seizures are usually easily controlled, and the epilepsy remits in adolescence in all cases. Neither intellectual nor neurological deterioration occurs. Even in patients in whom steroid therapy appears to be necessary to contain the status, long-term prognosis is excellent (Fejerman & Di Blasi 1987). The status and the isolated seizures in the syndrome of *benign occipital epilepsy* are also usually easy to control and the longer-term prognosis is good. Although seizures often persist in childhood, the epilepsy remits in most cases by the mid-teens (Panayiotopoulos 1989; Kivity & Lerman 1992). Intellectual or neurological deterioration does not usually occur.

Electrical status epilepticus during slow wave sleep

There is little satisfactory information about the outcome of ESES. Yasuhara *et al.* (1991) claimed that the EEG disturbance usually improves, although seizures, mental retardation and deterioration can persist. Tassinari *et al.* (1985) suggested that antiepileptic drug treatment improves the EEG appearances only temporarily, and that relapse is common after therapy is stopped. The seizures and the ESES tend to remit by the age of 15 years, but adults with similar EEG findings are encountered. The intellectual deficit that develops during the phase of ESES may improve but seldom returns to premorbid levels; indeed, many patients are left with profound mental deterioration or psychological deficits (Dalla Bernardina *et al.* 1989; Morikawa *et al.* 1989; Jayakar & Seshia 1991). There have been no formal comprehensive studies of outcome, however, and the long-term effect of the continuous EEG activity on cerebral function is not known.

Syndrome of acquired epileptic aphasia

Landau & Kleffner (1957) defined the condition in a report of six patients in 1957. The long-term outcome of these six cases (and three others) was then described by Mantovani & Landau (1980), at an interval of 10–28 years after the onset of aphasia. Four patients had recovered completely, four had moderate language problems, and one mild language dysfunction. The EEG had also recovered. In 17 other children, four recovered completely, nine were left with moderate language dysfunction and four were left severely dysphasic (Worster-Drought 1971; Shoumaker *et al.* 1974; Deonna *et al.* 1977; Cooper & Ferry 1978; Paquier *et al.* 1992). The EEG usually recovers, although ESES may persist in some patients. Overt seizures occur in only a proportion of cases, and usually but not always improve over time. The presence or absence of seizures does not seem to influence language outcome. In the short term at least, antiepileptic therapy has a variable effect on the electrographic status and overt seizures, but little effect on language function. It has been suggested that the outcome is worse in younger-onset patients (Bishop 1985), or in those with ESES, or persisting EEG abnormalities or seizures (Paquier *et al.* 1992). The proposition that cerebral damage is directly due to the continuous electrographic activity has not been tested. Nevertheless, aggressive anticonvulsant therapy is usually recommended to try to abolish the electrographic changes in the hope that this will ameliorate language problems (Mantovani & Landau 1980; Ravnik 1985; Sawhney *et al.* 1988; Lermann *et al.* 1991).

307

Absence status epilepticus

It is common clinical experience that the acute administration of benzodiazepine drugs in typical absence status will terminate the great majority if not all of the attacks. There is, however, little information about long-term outcome. Some evidence can be gathered from studies carried out before effective antiepileptic drugs were available, in which some very long attacks of absence status had been reported. In such cases, remission usually eventually occurred, even when attacks lasted weeks or months, with notably little mention of adverse consequences. Recurrent attacks are, however, extremely common. In one recent series, for instance, recurrent episodes of absence status occurred in 23 of 25 patients, at a pretreatment rate of over five attacks per year. Subsequent prophylactic therapy with valproate prevented recurrence in 14 of the 18 patients with primary generalised epilepsy, with a mean follow-up of over 4 years, and in the other four cases, recurrence was attributed to poor compliance or poor drug absorption (Berkovic *et al.* 1989*a*). No deaths or long-term morbidity have been reported due to absence status, although there have been no formal follow-up studies. This excellent prognosis is in marked contrast to that of atypical absence status, described below. As discussed on pp. 76–8, some patients with absence status have intermediate forms with features of both typical and atypical status, and others have focal features blurring the distinction between absence and complex partial status; it is likely that the prognosis is less good in both these circumstances, although the literature is confused on this point. Further prognostic studies in these conditions are badly needed.

Epilepsia partialis continua

The partial status is often refractory to normal therapy, the course of the seizures depending largely upon the underlying cause. In addition to conventional antiepileptic drug therapy, steroid administration is indicated in some cases, and the EPC in Rasmussen's encephalitis has been said to respond to treatment with gammaglobulin, although this has not been the case in my limited experience.

The long-term outcome of this condition also depends upon the underlying aetiology. Thus, the convulsive movements continue relentlessly in cases of Russian spring–summer encephalitis over many years, uninfluenced by medical therapy, and surgical excision seems to offer the only hope of remission (see pp. 25 and 290, and Omorokov 1927). On the other hand, in cases of Rasmussen's chronic encephalitis, there is typically a progressive phase (mean of 5.3 years in one series of 48 patients; Oguni *et al.* 1991) and the condition then becomes static. In the progressive phase, EPC can continue for hours, weeks, months or years, is usually recurrent if not continuous, and is accompanied by other seizures and progressing focal deficits. Death is exceptional, as eventually the condition stabilises, although always with severe disability. In the series of 48 patients from Montreal (Oguni *et al.* 1991), 96% developed a severe unilateral weakness, 85% mild to severe mental retardation, 49% a homonymous field defect, 29% a cortical sensory loss, 23% dysarthria and 18% dysphasia. Antiepileptic drugs are usually ineffective in controlling the EPC, and resective surgery offers the only hope of inducing a remission (Andermann 1991). In the retrospective series of Thomas *et al.* (1977) of 26 patients with EPC of various causes, 11 patients were alive and 15 had died after a follow-up of 1–18 years. Outcome was largely determined by the underlying cause, and seizures were more likely to remit in patients with stroke or other acute insults than in encephalitic cases.

Myoclonic status epilepticus in coma

Myoclonic status epilepticus in coma occurs usually in the setting of profound cerebral damage, and the prognosis is very gloomy. The majority of cases end fatally (77% of the 108 cases from the following series: Simon & Aminoff 1986; Celesia *et al.* 1988; Krumholz *et al.* 1988; Jumao-as & Brenner 1990; Lowenstein & Aminoff 1992) and survivors are left with severe neurological deficits. It is not known whether or not patients in coma with status do worse than those without, although this seems likely, or whether anticonvulsant therapy improves prognosis. Myoclonic status can occasionally develop in patients with pre-exisiting generalised epilepsy, especially after tonic–clonic status. In these cases, the underlying cerebral damage is not necessarily severe, and prognosis is somewhat better.

Specific forms of status epilepticus in mental retardation

Atypical absence status may persist for long periods of time, uninfluenced by treatment. As emphasised earlier (pp. 104–5), it is sometimes difficult to differentiate interictal and ictal states, or to assess the impact of the drugs on either the electrographic activity or the mental state. The overall outcome of the status is probably dependent upon the underlying aetiology, the age of onset (the earlier the onset, the worse the outcome), the severity and frequency of seizures and the background EEG abnormalities (for a discussion of these points, see Dravet *et al.* 1985*b*; Beaumanoir *et al.* 1988; Weiermann & Jacobi 1988). The same comments apply with greater force to the subclinical status so common in mentally retarded children and adults, and to minor motor status. Tonic status is also highly resistant to treatment, and may persist for hours, days or even months. The status may recur, and some patients die in status. It is not clear whether or not cerebral damage results from tonic status, and, as with other status syndromes, the most important factor influencing outcome is the underlying aetiology. There are no long-term or comprehensive outcome studies.

The *Lennox–Gastaut syndrome* in childhood also has a poor prognosis. Seizures are extremely resistant to therapy, although a trial of therapy with ACTH, corticosteroids or a ketogenic diet may be worth while. The long-term outcome for control is very poor, mental retardation usually progresses, as does the motor slowness. Whether or not the status causes cerebral damage (the view, for instance, of Doose & Völzke 1979) or whether both are due to the underlying encephalopathy is undetermined. Oller-Daurella & Oller (1988) reported briefly on 163 Lennox–Gastaut patients followed for more than 5 years, of whom 15% achieved long remission periods and 17% showed intellectual recovery. The condition is heterogeneous, and in those earlier reports, case definitions were seldom given.

Todt & Eysold (1988) followed 87 children for 6–31 years. Of the 37 children with the features of the full-blown syndrome prognosis was poor, none became seizure free, 49% were prone to episodes of overt status, focal neurological signs developed in 27%, and all developed mental retardation, which became severe in 76%. In contrast, the outcome in the 13 patients with only certain features of the syndrome was much better, with remission from seizures in all cases. These were the children who exhibited predominantly or exclusively myoclonic–astatic seizures, had a normal prior development, a response to therapy and primary generalised EEG changes, and would probably be best categorised as myoclonic–astatic epilepsy. In adults with the clinical and EEG features of the Lennox–Gastaut syndrome, the intellectual deterioration stabilises and the seizure disorder usually slowly improves over time. Rarely do seizures continue with either the frequency or ferocity observed in the childhood period.

Other syndromes of myoclonic status epilepticus

The outcome of myoclonic status depends on the underlying cause. In *cryptogenic* myoclonic syndromes, prognosis is variable and difficult to forecast in any individual case. In *primary generalised epilepsy*, myoclonic status has a good prognosis, and in only a few cases is the epilepsy difficult to control. Long-term antiepileptic therapy is required, however, and the status may be recurrent. There is usually no intellectual deterioration, nor evidence of status-induced cerebral damage. This is in marked contrast to the outcome of the status in the *progressive myoclonic epilepsies*, which may be severe and refractory to therapy. Overall outcome depends on the underlying syndrome (for a review, see Berkovic *et al.* 1986), and is probably not influenced by the presence or absence of status or its severity. Most of the inherited metabolic disorders have a poor prognosis. In Lafora body disease, for instance, there is relentless and rapid deterioration, with a mean survival of only 2–10 years after diagnosis and a mean age of death of 20 years. Mitochondrial disease producing myoclonic epilepsy has a much more variable progression and some cases survive into late adult life. Most patients with Unverricht–Lundborg disease are disabled within 10 years of the onset of the condition, and death is common by the third decade; however, mild cases do survive into the sixth decade as was originally observed by Lundborg. In all the myoclonic syndromes, the status is usually recurrent.

Nonconvulsive simple partial status epilepticus

Usually, the attacks are self-limiting and the prolonged attacks so typical of convulsive simple partial status (epilepsia partialis continua) are rare. The status often recurs, however, and the final outcome is variable, depending largely upon underlying aetiology. Thus, in acute disorders, the epilepsy usually remits with antiepileptic drug treatment (De Pasquet *et al.* 1976; Racy *et al.* 1980; Barry *et al.* 1985; Knight & Cooper 1986; Primavera *et al.* 1988; Sowa & Pituck 1989), or without (Dinner *et al.* 1981). Some cases are refractory to therapy (e.g. case 3 of Manford & Shorvon 1992), and recurrence in some cases is only prevented by resective surgical therapy (e.g. case 1 of Manford & Shorvon 1992).

There is no convincing human evidence that continuing simple partial seizures (convulsive or nonconvulsive) results in secondary damage, although experimental paradigms would be difficult to devise. Distant cerebral damage (say to the hippocampus) has been observed in animals after neocortical epilepsy (p. 141), and serial *in vivo* MRI studies would be a useful way of investigating this process in humans.

Complex partial status epilepticus

Untreated individual attacks of complex partial status have a widely varying duration, some lasting for weeks or even months. Most but not all episodes can be controlled with emergency antiepileptic therapy.

The long-term prognosis has not been formally studied, although experience suggests it to be surprisingly good, even in prolonged attacks. Death does not occur, nor do the episodes of status usually result in any neurological deterioration. This is in striking and unexplained contrast to the cerebral damage, which is frequently encountered after tonic–clonic status. Quite why cerebral damage is so rarely caused by complex partial status is unclear, but this implies, in adults at least, that persisting focal electrographic activity may not itself be unduly hazardous. Three patients have been reported with permanent memory disturbance following complex partial status (Engel *et al.* 1978; Treiman *et al.* 1981), although one had also had tonic–clonic status, and the follow up in another was very short. In contrast, in animal experimentation, limbic status has been repeatedly shown to result in neuronal damage (see pp. 161–5). The reason for this apparent species difference is unclear. There is, however, one brief report of pathological damage after nonconclusive status in three cases (the type and aetiology of the status is not given), in which neuronal loss was found with a distribution very similar to that seen in experimental limbic status (e.g. in hippocampus (CA1, CA3), amygdala, piriform cortex, dorsomedial thalamic nucleus, cerebellum and cerebral cortex) (Wasterlain *et al.* 1993). An episode of complex partial status will not necessarily worsen the course of the underlying epilepsy, but it is noticeable how commonly complex partial status recurs. Though there are no published statistical data concerning frequency of attacks, few if any patients encountered in my own clinical practice are without a history of previous episodes.

De novo *absence status epilepticus of late onset*

In patients with late-onset absence status and a prior history of primary generalised absence epilepsy, the prognosis is probably similar to that of typical absence status. Acute benzodiazepine administration will halt the status in almost every case, and long-term antiepileptic therapy is advisable and will prevent recurrence in most cases. Few are subsequently troubled by severe continuing seizures.

In patients without a prior history of epilepsy and in whom there are obvious precipitating factors, the long-term prognosis is equally good once the precipitants are removed. This is particularly true of cases due to benzodiazepine withdrawal, and the overall outcome is determined essentially by the underlying psychiatric condition. In such cases, long-term antiepileptic therapy may not be needed. In some patients, episodes of status recur, occasionally frequently (Andermann & Robb 1972; Guberman *et al.* 1986), but long-term epilepsy is not a common sequel. There are no reported deaths from late-onset absence status. Intellect, memory or behaviour do not deteriorate, even after severe or recurrent attacks, and there is little to suggest that the status results in significant cerebral damage.

References

Aaltonen, L., Kanto, J. & Salo, M. (1980). Cerebrospinal fluid concentrations and serum protein binding of lorazepam and its conjugate. *Acta Pharmacologica et Toxicologica*, **46**, 156–158.

Abernethy, D.G., Greenblatt, D.J., Divoli, M., Harmatz, J.S. & Shader, R.I. (1981). Alterations in drug distribution and clearance due to obesity. *Journal of Pharmacology and Experimental Therapeutics*, **217**, 681–685.

Adams, R.W., Cucchiara, R.F., Gronert, G.A., Messick, J.M. & Michenfelder, J.D (1981). Isoflurane and cerebrospinal fluid pressure in neurosurgical patients. *Anesthesiology*, **54**, 97–99.

Adebimpe, V.R. (1977). Complex partial seizures simulating schizophrenia. *Journal of the American Medical Association*, **237**, 1339–1341.

Agranat, A.L. & Trubshaw, W.H.D. (1955). The danger of decomposed paraldehyde. *South African Medical Journal*, **29**, 1021–1022.

Aguglia, U., Tinuper, P. & Farnarier, G. (1983). Etat confusionnel critique prolongé à point de départ frontal chez un sujet âgé. *Revue d'Electroencéphalographie et de Neurophysiologie Clinique*, **13**, 174–179.

Aguglia, U., Tinuper, P., Farnarier, G. & Gastaut, H. (1984). Etat d'absence à prédominance EEG unilatérale (à propos d'une observation privilégiée). *Revue d'Electroencéphalographie et de Neurophysiologie Clinique*, **14**, 213–215.

Agurell, S., Berlin, A., Ferngren, H. & Hellström, B. (1975). Plasma levels of diazepam after parenteral and rectal administration in children. *Epilepsia*, **16**, 277–283.

Aicardi, J. (1973). The problem of the Lennox syndrome. *Developmental Medicine and Child Neurology*, **15**, 77–81.

Aicardi, J. (1990). Neonatal myoclonic encephalopathy and early infantile epileptic encephalopathy. In *Neonatal seizures*, ed. C.G. Wasterlain & P. Vert, pp. 41–49. New York: Raven Press.

Aicardi, J. (1992*a*). *Diseases of the nervous system in childhood*. Clinics in Developmental Medicine, no. 115/118. Oxford: Blackwell Scientific Publications.

Aicardi, J. (1992*b*). Early myoclonic encephalopathy (neonatal myoclonic encephalopathy). In *Epileptic syndromes in infancy, childhood and adolescence*, 2nd edn, ed. J. Roger, M. Bureau, C. Dravet, F.E. Dreifuss, A. Perret & P. Wolf, pp. 13–23. London: John Libbey.

Aicardi, J., Amsili, J. & Chevrie, J.-J. (1969). Acute hemiplegia in infancy and childhood. *Developmental Medicine and Child Neurology*, **11**, 162–173.

Aicardi, J. & Baraton, J. (1971). A pneumoencephalographic demonstration of brain atrophy following status epilepticus. *Developmental Medicine and Child Neurology*, **13**, 660–667.

Aicardi, J. & Chevrie, J.-J. (1970). Convulsive status epilepticus in infants and children. *Epilepsia*, **11**, 187–197.

Aicardi, J. & Chevrie, J.-J. (1982). Atypical benign partial epilepsy of childhood. *Developmental Medicine and Child Neurology*, **24**, 281–292.

Aicardi, J. & Chevrie, J.-J. (1983). Consequences of status epilepticus in infants and children. In *Status epilepticus. Mechanisms of brain damage and treatment*. Advances in Neurology, vol. 34, ed. A.V. Delgado-Escueta, C.G. Wasterlain, D.M. Treiman & R.J. Porter, pp. 115–128. New York: Raven Press.

Aicardi, J. & Chevrie, J.-J. (1989). Status epilepticus. *Pediatrics*, **84**, 939–40.

Aicardi, J. & Gomes, A.L. (1988). The Lennox–Gastaut syndrome: clinical and electroencephalographic features. In *The Lennox–Gastaut syndrome*. Neurology and neurobiology, vol. 45, ed. E. Niedermeyer & R. Degen, pp. 25–46. New York: Alan R. Liss.

Aicardi, J. & Goutières, F. (1978). Encéphalopathie myoclonique néonatale. *Revue d'Electroencéphalographie et de Neurophysiologie Clinique*, **8**, 99–101.

Alia, G., Natale, E., Mattaliano, A. & Daniele, O. (1991). On two cases of status epilepticus treated with propofol. *Epilepsia*, **32** (suppl. 1), 77.

Altafullah, I., Asaikar, S. & Torres, F. (1991). Status epilepticus: clinical experience with two special devices for continuous cerebral monitoring. *Acta Neurologica Scandinavica*, **84**, 374–381.

Alzheimer, A. (1898). Ein Beitrag zur pathologischen Aanatomie der Epilepsie. *Monatsschrift für Psychiatrie und Neurologie*, **4**, 345–369.

Amand, G. (1971). Etats d'absence et états confusionnels prolongés au delà de 60 ans. *Revue d'Electroencéphalographie et de Neurophysiologie Clinique*, **1**, 221–223.

Amand, G. & Evrard, P. (1976). Le lorazepam injectable dans états de mal épileptiques. *Revue d'Electroencéphalographie et de Neurophysiologie Clinique*, **6**, 532–533.

Aminoff, M.J. & Simon, R.P. (1980). Status epilepticus: causes, clinical features and consequences in 98 patients. *American Journal of Medicine*, **69**, 657–666.

Andermann, F. (ed.) (1991). *Chronic encephalitis and epilepsy: Rasmussen's syndrome*. London: Butterworth-Heinemann.

Andermann, F., Cendes, F., Reiher, J., Palmini, A., Sherwin, A., Leduc, B., St Hilaire, J.-M., Guberman, A., McLachlan, R., Pillay, N., Purves, S., Goodman, L. & Bruni, J. (1992). A prospective double-blind study of the effects of intravenously administered lorazepam and diazepam in the treatment of status epilepticus. *Epilepsia*, **33** (suppl. 3), 3.

Andermann, F. & Robb, J.P. (1972). Absence status: a reappraisal following a review of thirty-eight cases. *Epilepsia*, **13**, 177–187.

Andersen, B.B., Mller, A., Gram, L., Jensen, N.O. & Dam, M. (1992). Phenytoin-loading: pharmacokinetic comparison between an intravenous bolus injection and a diluted standard solution. *Acta Neurologica Scandinavica*, **85**, 174–176.

André, M., Matisse, N., Vert, P. & Debruille, C. (1988). Neonatal seizures: recent aspects. *Neuropediatrics*, **19**, 201–207.

Andreasen, P.B., Hendel, J., Greisen, G. & Hvidberg, E.F. (1976). Pharmacokinetics of diazepam in disordered liver function. *European Journal of Clinical Pharmacology*, **10**, 115–120.

Annegers, J.F., Hauser, W.A., Shirts, S.B. & Kurland, L.T. (1987). Factors prognostic of unprovoked seizures after febrile convulsions. *New England Journal of Medicine*, **316**, 493–498.

Anonymous (1954). Death from decomposed paraldehyde. *British Medical Journal*, **2**, 1114–1115.

Anonymous (1989). Neonatal seizures. *Lancet*, **ii**, 135–137.

Anonymous (1992). Case records of the Massachusetts General Hospital. Case 22–1992. *New England Journal of Medicine*, 1480–1489.

314

Ansink, B.J., Sarphatie, H. & van Dongen, H.R. (1989). The Landau–Kleffner syndrome: case report and theoretical considerations. *Neuropediatrics*, **20**, 170–172.

Anthony, R.M., Andorn, A.C., Sunshine, I. & Thompson, W.L. (1977). Paraldehyde pharmacokinetics in ethanol abusers. *Federation Proceedings*, **36**, 285.

Anton, A. H., Uy, D. S. & Redderson, C. L. (1977). Autonomic blockade and the cardio-vascular and catecholamine response to electroshock. *Anesthesia and Analgesia, Current Researches*, **56**, 46–54.

Asher, D.M. & Gajdusek, D.C. (1991). Virologic studies in chronic encephalitis. In *Chronic encephalitis and epilepsy: Rasmussen's syndrome*, ed. F. Andermann, pp. 147–158. Boston, MA: Butterworth-Heinemann.

Auer, R.N. & Siesjö, B.K. (1988). Biological differences between ischemia, hypoglycemia, and epilepsy. *Annals of Neurology*, **24**, 699–707.

Ayala, G. (1929). Status epilepticus amauroticus. *Bollettino del'Academia Medica, Roma*, **55**, 288–290.

Babb, T.L. & Brown, W.J. (1986). Neuronal, dendritic and vascular profiles of human temporal lobe epilepsy corresponding with cellular physiology in vivo. In *Basic mechanisms of the epilepsies: molecular and cellular approaches*. Advances in Neurology, vol. 44, ed. A.V. Delgado-Escueta, A.A. Ward Jr, D.M. Woodbury & R.J. Porter, pp. 949–966. New York: Raven Press.

Bachelard, H.S., Badar-Goffer, R.S., Ben-Yoseph, O. & Morris, P.G. (1994). Use of combined ^{13}C-, ^{19}F- and ^{31}P-NMR spectroscopy in research on brain metabolism. In *Magnetic resonance scanning and epilepsy*, ed. S.D., Shorvon, D.R. Fish, F. Andermann, G. Bydder & H. Stefan. London: Plenum Press, in press.

Bailey, D.W. & Fenichel, G.M.0 (1968). The treatment of prolonged seizure activity with intravenous diazepam. *Journal of Pediatrics*, **73**, 923–927.

Baird, E.S. & Hailey, D.M. (1972). Delayed recovery from a sedative: correlation of the plasma levels of diazepam with clinical effects after oral and intravenous administration. *British Journal of Anaesthesia*, **44**, 803–808.

Balcar, V.J., Mark, J., Borg, J. & Mandel, P. (1978). Gaba-mediated inhibition of the epileptogenic focus, a process which may be involved in the mechanism of the cobalt-induced epilepsy. *Brain Research*, **154**, 182–185.

Ballenger, C.E., King, D.W. & Gallagher, B.B. (1983). Partial complex status epilepticus. *Neurology*, **33**, 1545–1552.

Bancaud, J. (1967). Origine focale multiple de certaines épilepsies corticales. *Revue Neurologique*, **117**, 222–243.

Bancaud, J. (1985). Kojewnikow's syndrome (epilepsia partialis continua) in children. In *Epileptic syndromes in infancy, childhood and adolescence*, ed. J. Roger, C. Dravet, M. Bureau, F.E. Dreifuss & P. Wolf, pp. 286–298. London: John Libbey.

Bancaud, J., Bonis, A., Talairach J., Bordas-Ferrar, M. & Buser, P. (1970). Syndrome de Kojewnikow et accès somato-moteurs. *Encéphale*, **59**, 391–493.

Bancaud, J. & Talairach, J. (1992). Clinical semiology of frontal lobe seizures. In *Frontal lobe seizures and epilepsies*. Advances in Neurology, vol. 57, ed. P. Chauvel, A.V. Delgado-Escueta, E. Halgren & J. Bancaud, pp. 3–58. New York: Raven Press.

Bancaud, J., Talairach, J., Morel, P., Bresson, M., Bonis, A., Geier, S., Hernon, E. & Buser, P. (1974). 'Generalised' epileptic seizures elicited by electrical stimulation of the frontal lobe in man. *Electroencephalography and Clinical Neurophysiology*, **37**, 275–282.

Barkovich, A.J., Gressens, P. & Evrard, P. (1992). Formation, maturation, and disorders of brain neocortex. *American Journal of Neuroradiology*, **13**, 423–446.

Barois, A., Estournet, B., Baron, S. & Levy-Alcover, M. (1985). Pronostic à long terme

315

des états de mal convulsifs prolongés. A propos de vingt-neuf observations d'états de mal convulsifs de plus du vingt-quatre heures. *Annales de Pédiatrie*, **32**, 621–626.

Barry, E., Sussman, N.M., Bosley, T.M. & Harner, R.N. (1985). Ictal blindness and status epilepticus amauroticus. *Epilepsia*, **26**, 577–584.

Bateman, D.E. (1989). Pseudostatus epilepticus. *Lancet*, **ii**, 1278–1279.

Bateman, D.E., O'Grady, J.C., Willey, C.J., Longley, B.P. & Barwick, D.D. (1983). De novo minor status epilepticus of late onset presenting as stupor. *British Medical Journal*, **287**, 1673–1674.

Bauer, G., Aichner, F. & Mayr, U. (1982). Non-convulsive status epilepticus following generalized tonic–clonic seizures. *European Neurology*, **21**, 411–419.

Bauer, G., Aichner, F. & Mayr, U. (1983). Status atypischer Absencen im Jugend- und Erwachsenenalter. *Nervenarzt*, **54**, 100–105.

Bauer, J., Stefan, H., Huk, W.J., Feistel, H., Hiltz, M.-J., Brinkmann, H.-G., Druschky, K.-F. & Neundorfer, B. (1989). CT, MRI and SPECT neuroimaging in status epilepticus with simple partial and complex seizures: case report. *Journal of Neurology*, **236**, 296–299.

Bayne, L.L. & Simon, R.P. (1981). Systemic and pulmonary vascular pressures during generalised seizures in sheep. *Annals of Neurology*, **10**, 566–569.

Bazán, N.G., Rodríguez de Turco, E.B. & Morelli de Liberti, S.A. (1983). Free arachidonic acid and membrane lipids in the central nervous system during bicuculline-induced status epilepticus. In *Status epilepticus. Mechanisms of brain damage and treatment*. Advances in Neurology, vol. 34, ed. A.V. Delgado-Escueta, C.G. Wasterlain, D.M. Treiman & R.J. Porter, pp. 305–310. New York: Raven Press.

Beau, M. (1836). Recherches statistiques pour servir à l'histoire de l'épilepsie et de l'hystérie. *Archives Générales de Médicine*, **11**, séries 2, 328–352.

Beaumanoir, A. (1982). The Lennox–Gastaut syndrome: a personal study. *Revue d'Electroencéphalographie et de Neurophysiologie Clinique*, **12** (suppl. 35).

Beaumanoir, A. (1983). Continuous spike-and-wave discharges during sleep. Significance. *Electrocephalography and Clinical Neurophysiology*, **55**, 18–19.

Beaumanoir, A. (1985). The Landau–Kleffner syndrome. In *Epileptic syndromes in infancy, childhood and adolescence*, ed. J. Roger, C. Dravet, M. Bureau, F.E. Dreifuss & P. Wolf, pp. 181–191. London: John Libbey.

Beaumanoir, A. (1992). The Landau–Kleffner syndrome. In *Epileptic syndromes in infancy, childhood and adolescence*, 2nd edn., ed. J. Roger, M. Bureau, C. Dravet, F.E. Dreifuss, A. Perret & P. Wolf. pp. 231–244. London: John Libbey.

Beaumanoir, A., Foletti, G., Magistris, M. & Volanschi, D. (1988). Status epilepticus in the Lennox–Gastaut syndrome. In *The Lennox–Gastaut syndrome*. Neurology and neurobiology, vol. 45, ed. E. Niedermeyer & R. Degen, pp. 283–300. New York: Alan R. Liss.

Beaumanoir, A., Jenny, P. & Jekiel, M. (1980). Etude de quatre 'petit mal status' postpartum. *Revue d'Electroencéphalographie et de Neurophysiologie Clinique*, **10**, 381–385.

Beaussart, M. & Faou, R. (1978). Evolution of epilepsy with rolandic paroxysmal foci: a study of 324 cases. *Epilepsia*, **19**, 337–342.

Beck, H. & Tousch, C. (1973). Traitement des états de mal épileptiques par le clonazepam. *Semaine des Hôpitaux de Paris*, **49** (suppl.), 39.

Becker, K.E. (1978). Plasma levels of thiopental necessary for anesthesia. *Anesthesiology*, **49**, 192–196.

Behrens, J.M. (1980). Psychomotor status epilepticus masking as a stroke. *Postgraduate Medicine*, **68**, 223–224, 226.

316

Belafsky, M.A., Carwille, S., Miller, P., Waddell, G., Boxley–Johnson, J. & Delgado–Escueta, A.V. (1978). Prolonged epileptic twilight states: continuous recordings with nasopharyngeal electrodes and videotape analysis. *Neurology*, 28, 239–245.

Bell, D.S. (1969). Dangers of treatment of status epilepticus with diazepam. *British Medical Journal*, 1, 159–161.

Ben-Ari, Y. (1985). Limbic seizure and brain damage produced by kainic acid: mechanisms and relevance to human temporal lobe epilepsy. *Neuroscience*, 14, 375–403.

Ben-Ari, Y., Tremblay, E., Ottersen, O.P. & Meldrum, B.S. (1980). The role of epileptic activity in hippocampal and 'remote' cerebral lesions induced by kainic acid. *Brain Research*, 191, 79–97.

Ben-Ari, Y., Tremblay, E., Ottersen, O.P. & Naquet, R. (1979). Evidence suggesting secondary epileptogenic lesions after kainic acid: pretreatment with diazepam reduces distant but not local brain damage. *Brain Research*, 165, 362–365.

Ben-Ari, Y., Repressa, A., Tremblay, E. & Nitecka, L. (1986). Selective and non-selective seizure related brain damage produced by kainic acid. In *Excitatory amino acids and epilepsy*. Advances in Experimental Medicine and Biology, vol. 203, ed. R. Schwarcz & Y. Ben-Ari, pp. 647–658. New York: Plenum Press.

Bendix, T. (1964). Petit mal status. *Electroencephalography and Clinical Neurophysiology*, 17, 210–211.

Benowitz, N.L., Simon, R.P. & Copeland, J.R. (1986). Status epilepticus: divergence of sympathetic activity and cardiovascular response. *Annals of Neurology*, 19, 197–199.

Bentley, G. & Mellick, R (1975). Chlormethiazole in status epilepticus – three cases. *Medical Journal of Australia*, 1, 537–538.

Béquet, D., Bodiguel, E., Renard, J.-L. & Gosasguen, J. (1990). Etat de mal partiel complexe temporal. *Revue Neurologique*, 146, 147–150.

Berg, A.T., Shinnar, S., Hauser, W.A., Alemany, M., Shapiro, E.D., Salomon, M.E. & Crain, E.F. (1992). A prospective study of recurrent febrile seizures. *New England Journal of Medicine*, 327, 1122–1127.

Bergman, I., Painter, M.J., Hirsch, R.P., Crumrine, P.K. & David, R. (1983). Outcome in neonates with convulsions treated in an intensive care unit. *Annals of Neurology*, 14, 642–647.

Berkovic, S.F., Andermann, F., Andermann, E. & Gloor, P. (1987). Concepts of absence epilepsies: discrete syndromes or biological continuum? *Neurology*, 37, 993–1000.

Berkovic, S.F., Andermann, F., Carpenter, S. & Wolfe, L.S. (1986). Progressive myoclonic epilepsies: specific causes and diagnosis. *New England Journal of Medicine*, 315, 296–305.

Berkovic, S.F., Andermann, F., Guberman, A., Hipola, D. & Bladin, P.F. (1989*a*). Valproate prevents the recurrence of absence status. *Neurology*, 39, 1294–1297.

Berkovic, S.F., Andermann, F., Guberman, A., Hipola, D. & Bladin, P.F. (1990). Absence status. *Neurology*, 40, 1010.

Berkovic, S.F. & Bladin, P.F. (1982). Absence status in adults. *Clinical and Experimental Neurology*, 19, 198–207.

Berkovic, S.F., Carpenter, S., Evans, A., Karpati, G., Shoubridge, E.A., Andermann, F., Meyer, E., Tyler, J.L., Diksic, M., Arnold, D., Wolfe, L.S., Andermann, E. & Hakim, A.M. (1989*b*). Myoclonus epilepsy and ragged-red fibres (MERRF): 1. a clinical, pathological, biochemical, magnetic resonance spectrographic and positron emission tomographic study. *Brain*, 112, 1231–1260.

Bernhard, C.G., Bohm, E. & Hojeberg, S. (1955). A new treatment of status epilepticus:

317

intravenous injections of a local anaesthetic (lidocaine). *Archives of Neurology and Psychiatry*, **74**, 208–214.

Bertram, E.H. & Lothman, E.W. (1990). NMDA receptor antagonists and limbic status epilepticus: a comparison with standard anticonvulsants. *Epilepsy Research*, **5**, 177–184.

Bertram, E.H., Lothman, E.W. & Lenn, N. (1990). The hippocampus in experimental chronic epilepsy: a morphometric analysis. *Annals of Neurology*, **27**, 43–48.

Besser, R. & Kramer, G. (1992). No evidence for efficacy of intrathecal verapamil in the treatment of tonic–clonic status epilepticus. *Journal of Epilepsy*, **5**, 61–63.

Beydoun, A., Yen, C.E. & Drury, I. (1991). Variance of interburst intervals in burst suppression. *Electroencephalography and Clinical Neurophysiology*, **79**, 435–439.

Billard, C., Autret, A., Laffont, F., De Giovanni, E., Lucas, B., Santini, J.J., Dulac, O. & Plouin, P. (1981). Aphasie acquise de l'enfant avec épilepsie à propos de 4 observations avec état de mal électrique infraclinique du sommeil. *Revue d'Electroencéphalographie et de Neurophysiologie Clinique*, **11**, 457–467.

Billard C., Autret, A., Laffont, F., De Giovanni, E., Lucas, B., Santini, J.J., Dulac, O. & Plouin, P. (1982). Electrical status epilepticus during sleep in children: a reappraisal from eight new cases. In *Sleep and epilepsy*, ed. M. B. Sterman, P. Shouse & P. Passouart, pp. 481–494. San Diego: Academic Press.

Bishop, D.V.M. (1985). Age at onset and outcome in 'acquired aphasia with convulsive disorder' (Landau–Kleffner syndrome). *Developmental Medicine and Child Neurology*, **27**, 705–712.

Bittencourt, P.R.M. & Richens, A. (1981). An anticonvulsant-induced status epilepticus in Lennox–Gastaut syndrome. *Epilepsia*, **22**, 129–134.

Bladin, P.F. (1973). The use of clonazepam as an anticonvulsant – clinical evaluation. *Medical Journal of Australia*, **1**, 683–688.

Bladin, P.F., Vajda, F.J. & Symington, G.R. (1977). Therapeutic problems related to tonic status epilepticus. *Clinical and Experimental Neurology*, **14**, 203–207.

Blatt, I., Jackson, S. & Dasheiff, R.M. (1992). Aphasic status epilepticus with reversible left posterior contrast enhancement on CT. *Epilepsia*, **33** (suppl. 3), 4.

Bleck, T.P. (1991). Convulsive disorders: status epilepticus. *Clinical Neuropharmacology*, **14**, 191–198.

Bleck, T.P. (1992). High-dose pentobarbital therapy of refractory status epilepticus: a meta-analysis of published studies. *Epilepsia*, **33** (suppl. 3), 5.

Blennow, G., Brierley, J.B., Meldrum, B.S. & Siesjö, B.K. (1978). Epileptic brain damage: the role of systemic factors that modify cerebral energy metabolism. *Brain*, **101**, 687–700.

Blume, E. (1988). The EEG features of the Lennox Gastaut syndrome. In *The Lennox Gastaut syndrome*. Neurology and Neurobiology, vol. 45, ed. E. Neidermeyer & R. Degen, pp. 159–176. New York: Alan R. Liss.

Blume, W.T., David, R.B. & Gomez, M.R. (1973). Generalised sharp and slow wave complexes. Associated clinical features and long-term follow-up. *Brain*, **96**, 289–306.

Böhm, M. (1969). Status epilepticus petit-mal: further observation of an adult case. *Electroencephalography and Clinical Neurophysiology*, **26**, 229.

Bonduelle, M., Sallou, C., Guillard, J. & Gaussel, J.J. (1964). L'état de mal psycho-moteur: ses rapports avec les automatismes et les psychoses aiguës épileptiques. *Revue Neurologique*, **110**, 365–376.

Booker, H. (1983). Prologue. In *Status epilepticus. Mechanisms of brain damage and treatment.* Advances in Neurology, vol. 34, ed. A.V. Delgado-Escueta, C.G. Wasterlain, D.M. Treiman, & R.J. Porter, pp. xxv-xxvii. New York: Raven Press.

Booker, H.E. & Celesia, G.G. (1973). Serum concentrations of diazepam in subjects with epilepsy. *Archives of Neurology*, **29**, 191–194.

Boréus, L.O., Jalling, B. & Kållberg, N. (1978). Phenobarbital metabolism in adults and newborn infants. *Acta Paediatrica Scandinavia*, **67**, 193–200.

Bornstein, M., Coddon, D. & Song. S. (1956). Case report: prolonged alterations in behavior associated with a continuous electroencephalographic (spike and dome) abnormality. *Neurology*, **6**, 444–448.

Bortone, E., Bettoni, G., Giorgi, C., Murgese, A., Stocchetti, M. & Mancia, D. (1992). Adult postanoxic 'erratic' status epilepticus. *Epilepsia*, **33**, 1047–1050.

Bostrom, B. (1982). Paraldehyde toxicity during treatment of status epilepticus. *American Journal of Diseases of Children*, **136**, 414–415.

Bouchet et Cazauvieilh (1825/6). De l'épilepsie considérée dans ses rapports avec l'aliénation mentale. Recherches sur la nature et le siège de ces deux maladies. *Archives Générales de Médecine*, **9**, 510–542; **10**, 5–50.

Boudouresques, J., Khalil, R., Roger, J., Pellissier, J.F., Delpuech, F., Tafani, B., Ali Cherif, A. & Boudouresques, G. (1980). Etat de mal épileptique et sclérose en plaques. *Revue Neurologique*, **136**, 777–782.

Boudouresques, J., Roger, J. & Gastaut, H. (1962). Crises aphasiques subintrantes chez un épileptique temporal: étude électroclinique. *Revue Neurologique*, **106**, 381–393.

Boulloche, J., Husson, A., Le Luyer, B. & Le Roux, P. (1990). Dysphagie, troubles du langage et pointes ondes centro-temporales. *Archives Françaises de Pédiatrie*, **47**, 115–117.

Bour, F., Plouin, P., Jalin, C., Frenkel, A.L., Dulac, O. & Bonifas, P. (1983). Les états de mal unilatéraux au cours de la période néonatale. *Revue d'Eletroencéphalographie et de Neurophysiologie Clinique*, **13**, 162–167.

Bourgeois, M. & Aicardi, J. (1992). Progressive neuronal degeneration (PND) and liver failure: a familial case with demonstration of cytochrome *c* oxidase deficiency. *Journal of Neurology*, **293** (suppl. 2), S6.

Bourneville, D.M. (1876). L'état de mal épileptique. In *Recherches cliniques et thérapeutiques sur l'épilepsie et l'hystérie. Compte-rendu des observations recueillies à la Salpêtrière*. Paris: Delahaye.

Bourrat, C., Garde, P., Boucher, M. & Fournet, A. (1986). Etats d'absence prolongée chez des patients âgés sans passé épileptique. *Revue Neurologique*, **142**, 696–702.

Boyd, E.M. & Singh, J. (1967). Acute toxicity following rectal thiopental, phenobarbital and leptazol. *Anesthesia and Analgesia Current Research*, **46**, 395–400.

Brachet-Liermain, A., Goutières, F. & Aicardi, J. (1975). Absorption of phenobarbital after the intramuscular administration of single doses in infants. *Journal of Pediatrics*, **87**, 624–626.

Brandt, L., Saveland, H., Ljungren, B. & Andersonn, K.-E. (1988). Control of epilepsia partialis continua with intravenous nimodipine: report of two cases. *Journal of Neurosurgery*, **69**, 949–950.

Bratz, E. (1899). Ammonshornbefunde bei Epileptischen. *Archiv für Psychiatrie und Nervenkrankheiten*, **31**, 820–836.

Brenner, R.P. (1980). Absence status: case reports and review of the literature. *Encéphale*, **6**, 384–392.

Brett, E.M. (1966). Minor epileptic status. *Journal of the Neurological Sciences*, **3**, 52–75.

Brett, E.M. (ed.) (1991). *Paediatric neurology*. London: Churchill Livingstone.

Bright, R. (1831). *Reports of medical cases, selected with a view of illustrating the symptoms and cure of diseases by a reference to morbid anatomy*, vol. 2. London: Taylor.

319

Brown, A. & Brierley, J.B. (1973). The earliest alterations in rat neurones and astrocytes after anoxia-ischaemia. *Acta Neuropathologica*, **23**, 9–22.

Brown, A. & Horton, J.M. (1967). Status epilepticus treated by intravenous infusions of thiopentone sodium. *British Medical Journal*, **1**, 27–28.

Brown, C.R., Sarnquist, F.H., Canup, C.A. & Pedley, T.A. (1979). Clinical electroencephalographic and pharmacokinetic studies of a water-soluble benzodiazepine, midazolam maleate. *Anesthesiology*, **50**, 467–470.

Brown, J.K. & Hussain, I.H.M.I. (1991*a*). Status epilepticus. 1. Pathogenesis. *Developmental Medicine and Child Neurology*, **33**, 3–17.

Brown, J.K. & Hussain, I.H.M.I. (1991*b*). Status epilepticus. II. Treatment. *Developmental Medicine and Child Neurology*, **33**, 97–109.

Brown, S.W., Mawer, G.E., Lawler, W., Taylor, D.C., Shorvon, S.D., Betts, T.A., Noronha, M.J., Richens, A., Chadwick, D., Besag, F.M.C. & Fenwick, P.B.C (1990). Sudden death and epilepsy. *Lancet*, **335**, 606–607.

Browne, T.R. (1983). Paraldehyde, chlormethiazole, and lidocaine for treatment of status epilepticus. In *Status epilepticus. Mechanisms of brain damage and treatment*. Advances in Neurology, vol. 34, ed. A.V. Delgado-Escueta, C.G. Wasterlain, D.M. Treiman & R.J. Porter, pp. 509–517. New York: Raven Press.

Browne, T.R. & Chang, T. (1989). Phenytoin: biotransformation. In *Antiepileptic drugs*, 3rd edn, ed. R. Levy, F.E. Dreifuss, R. Mattson, B. Meldrum & J.K. Penry, pp. 197–213. New York: Raven Press.

Browne, T.R. & Penry, J.K. (1973). Benzodiazepines in the treatment of epilepsy: a review. *Epilepsia*, **14**, 277–310.

Buchman, A.S., Klawans, H.L. & Russell, E.J. (1987). Metrizamide and its neurologic complications. *Clinical Neuropharmacology*, **10**, 1–25.

Burstein, C.L. (1943). The hazard of paraldehyde administration: clinical and laboratory studies. *Journal of the American Medical Association*, **121**, 187–190.

Butler, T.C. (1950). The rate of penetration of barbituric acid derivatives into the brain. *Journal of Pharmacology and Experimental Therapeutics*, **100**, 219–226.

Calabrese, V.P., Gruemer, H.D., James, K., Hranowsky, N. & DeLorenzo, R.J. (1991). Cerebrospinal fluid lactate levels and prognosis in status epilepticus. *Epilepsia*, **32**, 816–821.

Callahan D.J. & Noetzel, M.J. (1992). Prolonged absence status epilepticus associated with cabamazepine therapy, increased intracranial pressure and transient MRI abnormalities. *Neurology*, **42**, 2198–2201.

Calmeil, L.F. (1824). De l'épilepsie, étudiée sous le rapport de son siège et de son influence sur la production de l'aliénation mentale. Paris: Thèse de Université de Paris.

Camfield, P.R. & Camfield, C.S. (1987). Neonatal seizures: a commentary on selected aspects. *Journal of Child Neurology*, **2**, 244–251.

Carmichael, R.R., Mahoney, C.D. & Jeffrey, L.P. (1980). Solubility and stability of phenytoin sodium when mixed with intravenous solutions. *American Journal of Hospital Pharmacy*, **37**, 95–98.

Carter, C. (1958). Use of parenteral diphenylhydantoin (Dilantin) sodium in control of status epilepticus. *Archives of Neurology and Psychiatry*, **79**, 136–137.

Carter, S. & Gold, A. (1970). Valium in management of status epilepticus: a correction. *Pediatrics*, **45**, 513.

Cavazzuti, G.B., Ferrari, P. & Lalla, M. (1984). Follow-up study of 482 cases with convulsive disorders in the first year of life. *Developmental Medicine and Child Neurology*, **26**, 425–437.

320

Celesia, G.G. (1976). Modern concepts of status epilepticus. *Journal of the American Medical Association*, **235**, 1571–1574.

Celesia, G.G., Booker, H.E. & Sato, S. (1974). Brain and serum concentrations of diazepam in experimental epilepsy. *Epilepsia*, **15**, 417–425.

Celesia, G.G., Grigg, M.M. & Ross, E. (1988). Generalized status myoclonicus in acute anoxic and toxic-metabolic encephalopathies. *Archives of Neurology*, **45**, 781–784.

Celesia, G.G., Messert, B. & Murphy, M.J. (1972). Status epilepticus of late adult onset. *Neurology*, **22**, 1047–1055.

Chang, T. & Glazko, A.J. (1972). Diphenylhydantoin: biotransformation. In *Antiepileptic drugs*, ed. D.M. Woodbury, J.K. Penry & R.P. Schmidt, pp. 149–162. New York: Raven Press.

Chapman, A.G. (1985). Cerebral energy metabolism and seizures. In *Recent advances of epilepsy*, vol. 2, ed. T.A. Pedley & B.S. Meldrum, pp. 19–64. Edinburgh: Churchill Livingstone.

Charcot, J.-M. (1889). [*Clinical lectures on the diseases of the nervous system*], transl. T. Savill. London: New Sydenham Society.

Chaslin, P. (1889). Note sur l'anatomie pathologique de l'épilepsie dite essentielle – la sclérose neurologique. *Comptes Rendus de la Société Biologique (Paris)*, pp. 169–171.

Chauvel, P., Liègeois-Chauvel, C., Marquis, P. & Bancaud, J. (1986). Distinction between the myoclonus-related potential and the epileptic spike in epilepsia partialis continua. *Electroencephalography and Clinical Neurophysiology*, **64**, 304–307.

Chauvel, P., Trottier, S., Vignal, J.P. & Bancaud, J. (1992). Somatomotor seizures of frontal lobe origin. In *Frontal lobe seizures and epilepsies*. Advances in Neurology, vol. 57, ed. P. Chauvel, A.V. Delgado-Escueta, E. Halgren & J. Bancaud, pp. 185–232. New York: Raven Press.

Chevrie, J.-J. (1991). Epileptic seizures and epilepsies in childhood. In *Clinical neurology*, ed. M. Swash & J. Oxbury, pp. 233–254. Edinburgh: Churchill Livingstone.

Chevrie, J.-J. & Aicardi, J. (1972). Childhood epileptic encephalopathy with slow spike-wave. A statistical study of 80 cases. *Epilepsia*, **13**, 259–271.

Chiron, C., Dulac, O., Beaumont, D., Palacios, L., Pajot, N. & Mumford, J. (1991). Therapeutic trial of vigabatrin in refractory infantile spasms. *Journal of Child Neurology*, **6** (suppl. 2), S52-S59.

Choi, D.W. (1987). Ionic dependence of glutamate neurotoxicity. *Journal of Neuroscience*, **7**, 369–379.

Chugani, H.T., Shields, W.D., Shewmon, D.A., Olson, D.M., Phelps, M.E. & Peacock, W.J. (1990). Infantile spasms. 1. PET identifies focal cortical dysgenesis in cryptogenic cases for surgical treatment. *Annals of Neurology*, **27**, 406–413.

Clancy, R.R., Legido, A. & Lewis, D. (1988). Occult neonatal seizures. *Epilepsia*, **29**, 256–261.

Clark, D.L., Hosick, E.C., Adam, N., Castro, A. D., Rosner, B.S. & Neigh, J.L. (1973). Neural effects of isoflurane (Forane) in man. *Anesthesiology*, **39**, 261–270.

Clark, D.L. & Rosner, B.S. (1973). Neurophysiologic effects of general anesthetics. 1. The electroencephalogram and sensory evoked resonses in man. *Anesthesiology*, **38**, 564–582.

Clark, L.P. & Prout, T.P. (1903/4). Status epilepticus: a clinical and pathological study in epilepsy. [An article in 3 parts.] *American Journal of Insanity*, **60**, 291–306; **60**, 645–675; **61**, 81–108.

Clifford, D.B., Olney, J.W., Benz, A.M., Fuller, T.A. & Zorumski, C.F. (1990). Ketamine, phencyclidine and MK-801 protect against kainic acid-induced seizure-related brain damage. *Epilepsia*, **31**, 382–390.

Clifford, D.B., Zorumski, C.F. & Olney, J.W. (1989). Ketamine and MK-801 prevent degeneration of thalamic neurons induced by focal cortical seizures. *Experimental Neurology*, **105**, 272–279.

Cloyd, J.C., Gumnit, R.J. & McLain, L.W. (1980). Status epilepticus: the role of intravenous phenytoin. *Journal of the American Medical Association*, **244**, 1479–1481.

Cocito, L., Favale, E. & Reni, L. (1982). Epileptic seizures in cerebral arterial occulsive disease. *Stroke*, **13**, 189–195.

Cockshott, I.D., Douglas, E.J., Prys Roberts, C., Turtle, M. & Coates, D.P. (1990). The pharmacokinetics of propofol during and after intravenous infusion in man. *European Journal of Anaesthesiology*, **7**, 265–275.

Colamaria, V., Plouin, P., Dulac, O., Cesaro, G. & Dalla Bernardina, B. (1988). Kojewnikow's epilepsia partialis continua: two cases associated with striatal necrosis. *Neurophysiological Clinics*, **18**, 525–530.

Colamaria, V., Sgrò, V., Caraballo, R., Simeone, M., Zullini, E., Fontana, E., Zanetti, R., Grimau-Merino, R. & Dalla Bernardina, B. (1991). Status epilepticus in benign rolandic epilepsy manifesting as anterior operculum syndrome. *Epilepsia*, **32**, 329–334.

Cole, A.J., Andermann, F., Taylor, L., Olivier, A., Rasmussen, T., Robitaille Y. & Spire, J.-P. (1988). The Landau–Kleffner syndrome of acquired epileptic aphasia: unusual clinical outcome, surgical experience, and absence of encephalitis. *Neurology*, **38**, 31–38.

Collins, R.C. & Olney, J.W. (1982). Focal cortical seizures cause distant thalamic lesions. *Science*, **218**, 177–179.

Collins, R.C., Olney, J.W. & Lothman, E.W. (1983). Metabolic and pathological consequences of focal seizures. In *Epilepsy*, ed. A.A. Ward Jr, J.K. Penry & D.P. Purpura, pp. 87–107. New York: Raven Press.

Colman, W.S. (1903). A case of automatic wandering lasting five days. *Lancet*, pp. 593–594.

Combes, J.G., Rufo, M., Vallade, M.J., Pinsard, N. & Bernard, R. (1975). Les convulsions néonatales, circonstances d'apparition et critères de pronostic. A propos de 129 observations. *Pédiatrie*, **30**, 477–492.

Comer, W.H., Elliott, H.W., Nomof, N., Navarro, G., Kokka, N., Ruelius, H.W. & Knowles, J.A. (1973). Pharmacology of parenterally administered lorazepam in man. *Journal of International Medical Research*, **1**, 216–225.

Commission on Classification and Terminology of the International League Against Epilepsy (1981). Proposal for revised clinical and electroencephalographic classification of epileptic seizures. *Epilepsia*, **22**, 489–501.

Commission on Classification and Terminology of the International League Against Epilepsy (1989). Proposal for revised classification of epilepsies and epileptic syndromes. *Epilepsia*, **30**, 389–399.

Congdon, P.J. & Forsythe, W.I. (1980). Intravenous clonazepam in the treatment of status epilepticus in children. *Epilepsia*, **21**, 97–102.

Cook, M.J., Free, S.L., Fish, D.R., Shorvon, S.D., Straughan, K. & Stevens, J.M. (1994*a*). Analysis of cortical patterns. In *Magnetic resonance scanning and epilepsy*, ed. S.D. Shorvon, D.R. Fish, F. Andermann, G. Bydder & H. Stefan. London: Plenum Press, in press.

Cook, M.J., Free, S.L., Fish, D.R., Shorvon, S.D., Straughan, K. & Stevens, J.M. (1994*b*). Volumetric MRI studies of the hippocampus. In *Magnetic resonance scanning and epilepsy*, ed. S.D. Shorvon, D.R. Fish, F. Andermann, G. Bydder & H. Stefan. London: Plenum Press, in press.

Cooper, J.A. & Ferry, P.C. (1978). Acquired auditory verbal agnosia and seizures in childhood. *Journal of Speech and Hearing Disorders*, **43**, 176–184.

Corsellis, J.A.N. & Bruton, C.J. (1983). Neuropathology of status epilepticus in humans. In *Status epilepticus. Mechanisms of brain damage and treatment.* Advances in Neurology, vol. 34, ed. A.V. Delgado-Escueta, C.G. Wasterlain, D.M. Treiman & R.J. Porter, pp. 129–139. New York: Raven Press.

Cotton, D.B., Janusz, C.A. & Berman, R.F. (1992). Anticonvulsant effects of magnesium sulfate on hippocampal seizures: therapeutic implications in preeclampsia-eclampsia. *American Journal of Obstetrics and Gynecology*, **166**, 1127–1136.

Coulter, D.L. (1986). Continuous infantile spasms as a form of status epilepticus. *Journal of Child Neurology*, **1**, 215–217.

Courjon, J., Fournier, M.H. & Mauguière, F. (1984). Les états de mal chez les épileptiques adultes suivis dans un hôpital neurologique. *Revue d'Electroencéphalographie et de Neurophysiologie Clinique*, **14**, 175–179.

Cowan, J.M.A., Rothwell, J.C., Rise, R.J.S. & Marsden, C.D. (1986). Electrophysiological positron emission studies in a patient with cortical myoclonus, epilepsia partialis continua and motor epilepsy. *Journal of Neurology, Neurosurgery and Psychiatry*, **49**, 796–807.

Cowan, L.D. & Hudson, L.S. (1991). The epidemiology and natural history of infantile spasms. *Journal of Child Neurology*, **6**, 355–364.

Coyle, J.T. (1987). Kainic acid: insights into excitatory mechanisms causing selective neuronal degeneration. *Ciba Foundation Symposium*, **126**, 186–280.

Craig, C.R. & Colasanti, B.K. (1986). GABA receptors, lipids, and gangliosides in cobalt epileptic focus. In *Basic mechanisms of the epilepsies: molecular and cellular approaches.* Advances in Neurology, vol. 44, ed. A.V. Delgado-Escueta, A.A. Ward Jr, D.M. Woodbury & R.J. Porter, pp. 379–391. New York: Raven Press.

Cranford, R.E., Leppik, I.E., Patrick, B., Anderson, C.B. & Kostick, B. (1978). Intravenous phenytoin: clinical and pharmacokinetic aspects. *Neurology*, **28**, 874–880.

Crawford, T.O. & Mitchell, W.G. (1989). Phenobarbital for status. *Neurology*, **39**, 609.

Crawford, T.O., Mitchell, W.G., Fishman, L.S. & Snodgrass, R. (1988). Very-high-dose phenobarbital for refractory status epilepticus in children. *Neurology*, **38**, 1035–1040.

Crawford, T.O., Mitchell, W.G. & Snodgrass, S.R. (1987). Lorazepam in childhood status epilepticus and serial seizures: effectiveness and tachyphylaxis. *Neurology*, **37**, 190–195.

Crisp, C.B., Gannon, R. & Knauft, F. (1988). Continuous infusion of midazolam hydrochloride to control status epilepticus. *Clinical Pharmacology*, **7**, 322–324.

Cromwell, T.H., Eger, E.I., Stevens, W.C. & Dolan, W.M. (1971). Forane uptake, excretion and blood solubility in man. *Anesthesiology*, **35**, 401–408.

Cukier, F., Sfaello, Z. & Dreyfus-Brisac, C. (1976). Les états de mal du nouveau-né à terme et du prématuré. *Gaslini*, **8**, 100–106.

Dalby, M.A. (1969). Epilepsy and 3 per second spike and wave rhythms; a clinical, electrographic, and prognostic analysis of 346 patients. *Acta Neurologica Scandinavica*, **45** (suppl. 40), 1–183.

Dalen, J.E., Evans, G.L., Banas, J.S., Brooks, H.L., Paraskos, J.A. & Dexter, L. (1969). The hemodynamic and respiratory effects of diazepam (valium). *Anesthesiology*, **30**, 259–263.

Dalla Bernardina B., Fontana, E., Michelizza, B., Colomaria, V., Capovilla, G. & Tassinari, C.A. (1989). Partial epilepsies of childhood bilateral synchronisation, continuous spike–wave during slow sleep. In *The eighth epilepsy international symposium*, ed. J. Manelis, E. Bental, J.N. Loeber & F.E. Dreifuss, pp. 295–302. New York: Raven Press.

Dalla Bernardina, B., Fontana, E., Sgro, V., Colamaria, V. & Elia, M. (1992). Myoclonic epilepsy ('myoclonic status') in non-progressive encephalopathies. In *Epileptic syndromes in infancy, childhood and adolescence*, 2nd edn, ed. J. Roger, M. Bureau, C. Dravet, F.E. Dreifuss, A. Perret & P. Wolf. pp. 89–96. London: John Libbey.

Dalla Bernardina, B., Tassinari, C.A., Druvet, C., Bureau, M., Beglini, G. & Roger, J. (1978). Epilepsie partielle bénigne et état de mal électroencéphalographique pendant le sommeil. *Revue d'Eléctroencéphalographie et de Neurophysiologie Clinique*, **a**, 19–22.

Danner, R., Shewmon, A. & Sherman, M.P. (1985). Seizures in an atelencephalic infant: is the cortex essential for neonatal seizures? *Archives of Neurology*, **42**, 1014–1016.

de Elió, F.J., de Jalón, P.G. & Obrador, S. (1949). Some experimental and clinical observations on the anticonvulsive action of paraldehyde. *Journal of Neurology, Neurosurgery and Psychiatry*, **12**, 19–24.

DeGiorgio, C.M., Rabinowicz, A.L., Bird, E.H. & Altman, K. (1991). Lidocaine in refractory nonconvulsive status epilepticus: confirmation of efficacy with continuous EEG monitoring. *Epilepsia*, **32** (suppl. 1), 77.

DeGiorgio, C.M., Tomiyasu, U., Gott, P.S. & Treiman, D.M. (1992). Hippocampal pyramidal cell loss in human status epilepticus. *Epilepsia*, **33**, 23–27.

de Jong, R.H. & Bonin, J.D. (1981). Benzodiazepines protect mice from local anesthetic convulsions and death. *Anesthesia and Analgesia*, **60**, 385–389.

de Lanerolle, N.C. & Spencer, D.D. (1991). Neurotransmitter markers in human seizure foci. In *Neurotransmitters and epilepsy*. Frontiers of Clinical Neuroscience, vol. 11, ed. R.S. Fisher & J.T. Coyle, pp. 201–218. New York: Wiley-Liss.

De Lorenzo, R.J. (1983). Calcium-calmodulin protein phosphorylation in neuronal transmission: a molecular approach to neuronal excitability and anticonvulsant drug action. In *Status epilepticus. Mechanisms of brain damage and treatment*. Advances in Neurology, vol. 34, ed. A.V. Delgado-Escueta, C.G. Wasterlain, D.M. Treiman & R.J. Porter, pp. 325–338. New York: Raven Press.

De Marco, P. (1988). Electrical status epilepticus during slow sleep: one case with sensory aphasia. *Clinical Electroencephalography*, **19**, 111–113.

De Marco, P. (1991). Habitual status epilepticus in children. *Bollettino di Lega Italiana Contro L'Epilessia*, **74**, 101–102.

De Maria, G., Guarneri, D., Pasolini, M.P. & Antonini, L. (1991). Stato di male versivo trattato con propofol. *Bollettino di Lega Italiana Contro L'Epilessia*, **74**, 191–192.

DeMoor, J. (1898). Le méchanisme et la signification de l'état moniliforme des neurones. *Annales de la Société Royale de la Médicine Naturelle de Bruxelles*, **7**, 205–250.

De Pasquet, E.G., Gaudín, E.S., Bianchi, A. & De Mendilauarsu, S.A. (1976). Prolonged and monosymptomatic dysphasic status epilepticus. *Neurology*, **26**, 244–247.

De Riu, P.L., Petruzzi, V., Testa, C., Mulas, M., Melis, F., Caria, M.A. & Mameli, O. (1992). Propofol anticonvulsant activity in experimental epileptic status. *British Journal of Anaesthesia*, **69**, 177–181.

Delgado-Escueta, A.V. & Enrile-Bacsal, F. (1983). Combination therapy for status epilepticus: intravenous diazepam and phenytoin. In *Status epilepticus. Mechanisms of brain damage and treatment*. Advances in Neurology, vol. 34, eds. A.V. Delgado-Escueta, C.G. Wasterlain, D.M. Treiman, & R.J. Porter, pp. 477–485. New York: Raven Press.

Delgado-Escueta, A.V. & Treiman, D.M. (1987). Focal status epilepticus: modern concepts. In *Epilepsy: electroclinical syndromes*, ed. H. Lüders & R.P. Lesser, pp. 347–392. London: Springer-Verlag.

Delgado-Escueta, A.V., Ward, A.A. Jr, Woodbury, D.M. & Porter, R.J. (eds.) (1986*a*). *Basic mechanisms of the epilepsies: molecular and cellular approaches*. Advances in Neurology, vol. 44. New York: Raven Press.

Delgado-Escueta, A.V., Ward, A.A. Jr, Woodbury, D.M. & Porter, R.J. (1986*b*). New wave of research in the epilepsies. In *Basic mechanisms of the epilepsies: molecular and cellular approaches*. Advances in Neurology, vol. 44, ed. A.V. Delgado-Escueta, A.A. Ward Jr, D.M. Woodbury & R.J. Porter, pp. 3–56. New York: Raven Press.

Delgado-Escueta, A.V., Wasterlain, C.G., Treiman, D.M. & Porter, R.J. (eds.) (1983). *Status epilepticus: mechanisms of brain damage and treatment*. Advances in Neurology, vol. 34. New York: Raven Press.

Dening, T.R., Berrios, G.E. & Walshe, J.M. (1988). Wilson's disease and epilepsy. *Brain*, 111, 1139–1155.

Dennis, J. (1978). Neonatal convulsions: aetiology, late neonatal status and long-term status. *Developmental Medicine and Child Neurology*, 20, 143–158.

Deonna, T.W. (1991). Acquired epileptiform aphasia in children (Landau–Kleffner Syndrome). *Journal of Clinical Neurophysiology*, 8, 288–298.

Deonna, T., Beaumanoir, A., Gaillard, F. & Assal, G. (1977). Acquired aphasia in childhood with seizure disorder: a heterogeneous syndrome. *Neuropädiatrie*, 8, 263–73.

Deonna, T., Peter, C. & Ziegler, A.L. (1989). Adult follow-up of the acquired aphasia-epilepsy syndrome in childhood: report of seven cases. *Neuropädiatrics*, 20, 132–138.

Deshmukh, A., Wittert, W., Schnitzler, E. & Mangurten, H.H. (1986). Lorazepam in the treatment of refractory neonatal seizures. *American Journal of Diseases of Children*, 140, 1042–1044.

Deuel, R.K. & Lenn, N.J. (1977). Treatment of acquired epileptic aphasia. *Journal of Pediatrics*, 90, 959–961.

Dinner, D.S., Lüders, H., Lederman, R. & Gretter, T.E. (1981). Aphasic status epilepticus: a case report. *Neurology*, 31, 888–890.

Dinsdale, H.B. (1988). Does magnesium sulfate treat eclamptic seizures? Yes. *Archives of Neurology*, 45, 1360–1361.

Dinsmore, W., Crane, J. & Callender, M.E. (1985). Status epilepticus and near hanging. *Postgraduate Medical Journal*, 61, 519–520.

Dodrill, C.B. & Wilensky, A.J. (1990). Intellectual impairment as an outcome of status epilepticus. *Neurology*, 40 (suppl. 2), 23–27.

Dollery, C. (ed.) (1991). *Therapeutic drugs*. Edinburgh, Churchill Livingstone.

Domek, N.S., Barlow, C.F. & Roth, L.J. (1960). An ontogenetic study of phenobarbital-C^{14} in cat brain. *Journal of Pharmacology and Experimental Therapeutics*, 130, 285–293.

Dongier, S. (1959/60). Statistical study of clinical and electroencephalographic manifestations of 536 psychotic episodes occurring in 516 epileptics between clinical seizures. *Epilepsia*, 1, 117–142.

Dongier, S. (1967). A propos des états de mal généralisés à expression confusionnelle. Etude psychologique de la destructuration de la conscience au cours de l'état de petit mal. In *Les états de mal épileptiques*, ed. H Gastaut, J. Roger & H. Lob, pp. 110–118. Paris: Masson.

Doose, H. (1983). Nonconvulsive status epilepticus in childhood: clinical aspects and classification. In *Status epilepticus. Mechanisms of brain damage and treatment*. Advances in Neurology, vol. 34, ed. A.V. Delgado-Escueta, C.G. Wasterlain, D.M. Treiman & R.J. Porter, pp. 83–92. New York: Raven Press.

Doose, H. (1985). Myoclonic–astatic epilepsy of early childhood In *Epileptic syndromes of infancy, childhood and adolescence*, ed. J. Roger, C. Dravet, M. Bureau, F.E. Dreifuss & P. Wolf, pp. 78–88. London: John Libbey.

Doose, H. (1992). Myoclonic astatic epilepsy of early childhood. In *Epileptic syndromes in infancy, childhood and adolescence*, 2nd edn, ed. J. Roger, M. Bureau, C. Dravet, F.E. Dreifuss, A. Perret, & P. Wolf. pp. 103–114. London: John Libbey.

Doose, H., Gerken, H., Leonhardt, R., Völzke, E. & Völz, C. (1970). Centrencephalic myoclonic-astatic petit mal. *Neuropädiatrie*, **2**, 59–78.

Doose, H. & Völzke, E. (1979). Petit mal status in early childhood and dementia. *Neuropädiatrie*, **10**, 10–14.

Drake, M.E. & Coffey, C.E. (1983). Complex partial status epilepticus simulating psychogenic unresponsiveness. *American Journal of Psychiatry*, **140**, 800–801.

Dravet, C. (1965). *Encéphalopathie épileptique de l'enfant avec pointe-onde lente diffuse ("petit mal variant")*. Marseilles: Thesis, University of Marseilles.

Dravet, C. & Bureau, M. (1981). L'épilepsie myoclonique bénigne du nourisson. *Revue d'Electroencéphalographie et de Neurophysiologie Clinique*, **11**, 438–444.

Dravet, C., Bureau, M., Guerrini, R., Giraud, N. & Roger, J. (1992). Severe myoclonic epilepsy in infants. In *Epileptic syndromes in infancy, childhood and adolescence*, 2nd edn, ed. J. Roger, M. Bureau, C. Dravet, F.E. Dreifuss, A. Perret & P. Wolf, pp. 75–88. London: John Libbey.

Dravet, C., Bureau, M. & Roger, J. (1985a). Severe myoclonic epilepsy in infants. In *Epileptic syndromes in infancy, childhood and adolescence*, ed. J. Roger, C. Dravet, M. Bureau, F.E. Dreifuss & P. Wolf, pp. 58–67. London: John Libbey.

Dravet, C., Natale, O., Magaudda, A., Larrieu, J.L., Bureau, M., Roger, J. & Tassinari, C.A. (1985b). Les états de mal dans le syndrome de Lennox–Gastaut. *Revue d'Electroencéphalographie et de Neurophysiologie Clinique*, **15**, 361–368.

Dravet, C., Roger, J., Bureau, M. & Dalla Bernardina, B. (1982). Myoclonic epilepsies in childhood. In *Advances in epileptology. The eighth epilepsy international symposium*, ed. H. Akimoto, H. Kazamatsuri, M. Seino & A.A. Ward Jr. New York: Raven Press, pp. 135–140.

Dreifuss, F.E., Penry, J.K., Rose, S.W., Kupferberg, H.J., Dyken, P. & Sato, S. (1975). Serum clonazepam concentrations in children with absence seizures. *Neurology*, **25**, 255–258.

Dreyer, R. (1965). Zur Frage des status epilepticus mit psychomotorischen Anfällen: ein Beitrag zum temporalen status epilepticus und zu atypischen Dämmerauständen und Verstimmungen. *Nervenarzt*, **36**, 221–223.

Dreyfus-Brisac, C. & Monod, N. (1972). Neonatal status epilepticus. *Electroencephalography and Clinical Neurophysiology*, **15**, 38–52.

Dreyfus-Brisac, C. & Monod, N. (1977). Neonatal status epilepticus. In *Handbook of electroencephalography and clinical neurophysiology*, vol. 15, ed. A. Remond, pp. 39–52. Amsterdam: Elsevier.

Dreyfus-Brisac, C., Peschanski, N., Radvanyi, M.F., Cukier-Hemeury, F. & Monod, N. (1981). Convulsions du nouveau-né: aspects clinique, électrographique, étiopathogénique et pronostique. *Revue d'Electroencéphalographie et de Neurophysiologie Clinique*, **11**, 367–378.

Dreyfus-Brisac, C., Radvanyi, M.F., Monod, N., Cukier-Hemeury, F. & Peschanski, N. (1981). Les convulsions du nouveau-né. *La Revue du Praticien*, **57**, 4119–4128

Dubinsky, J.M. & Rothman, S.M. (1990). Intracellular calcium concentrations during 'chemical hypoxia' and excitotoxic neuronal injury. *Journal of Neurosciences*, **11** 2545–2551.

Dudek, F.E., Snow, R.W. & Taylor, C.P. (1986). Role of electrical interactions in synchronization of epileptiform bursts. In: *Basic mechanisms of the epilepsies: molecular and cellular approaches*. Advances in Neurology, vol. 44, ed. A.V. Delgado-Escueta, A.A. Ward Jr, D.M. Woodbury & R.J. Porter, pp. 593–618. New York: Raven Press.

Dugas, M., Masson, M., Le Heuzey, M.F. & Regnier, N. (1982). Aphasie 'aquise' de l'enfant avec épilepsie (syndrome de Landau et Kleffner): douze observations person-nelles. *Revue Neurologique*, **138**, 755–780.

Dulac, O., Aubourg, P., Checoury, A., Devictor, D., Poulin, P. & Arthuis, M. (1985). Etats de mal convulsifs du nourrisson: aspects sémiologiques, étiologiques et pronos-tiques. *Revue d'Electroencéphalographie et de Neurophysiologie Clinique*, **15**, 255–262.

Dulac, O., Billard, C. & Arthuis, M. (1983). Aspects électro-cliniques et évolutifs de l'épilepsie dans le syndrome aphasie épilepsie. *Archives Françaises de Pédiatrie*, **40**, 299–308.

Dulac, O., Plouin, P., Jambaque, I. & Motte, J. (1986). Spasmes infantiles épileptiques bénins. *Revue d'Electroencéphalographie et de Neurophysiologie Clinique*, **16**, 371–382.

Dundee, J.W. & Gray, R.C. (1967). Thiopentone in status epilepticus. *British Medical Journal*, **1**, 362.

Dundee, J.W., Halliday, N.J., Harper, K.W. & Brogden, R.N. (1984). Midazolam: a review of its pharmacological properties and therapeutic use. *Drugs*, **28**, 519–543.

Dundee, J.W., Lilburn, J.K., Toner, W. & Howard, P.J. (1978). Plasma lorazepam levels. *Anaesthesia*, **33**, 15–19.

Dunn, D.W. (1988). Status epilepticus in children: etiology, clinical features and outcome. *Journal of Child Neurology*, **3**, 167–173.

Dunn, D.W. (1990). Status epilepticus in infancy and childhood. *Pediatric Neurology*, **8**, 647–657.

Dunne, J.W., Summers, Q.A. & Stewart-Wynne, E.G. (1987). Non-convulsive status epi-lepticus: a prospective study in an adult general hospital. *Quarterly Journal of Medicine*, **62**, 117–126.

Dwyer, B.E. & Wasterlain, C.G. (1983). Regulation of brain protein synthesis during status epilepticus. In *Status epilepticus. Mechanisms of brain damage and treatment*. Advances in Neurology, vol. 34, ed. A.V. Delgado-Escueta, C.G. Wasterlain, D.M. Treiman & R.J. Porter, pp. 297–304. New York: Raven Press.

Eadie, M.J. & Tyrer, J.H. (1989). *Anticonvulsant therapy: pharmacological basis and practice*. Edinburgh: Churchill Livingstone.

Eger, E.I. (1981*a*). Isoflurane: a review. *Anesthesiology*, **55**, 559–576.

Eger, E.I. (1981*b*). *Isoflurane (Forane): a compendium and reference*. Madison, OH: Ohio Medical Products.

Eger, E.I., White, A.E., Brown, C.L., Biava, C.G., Corbett, T.S. & Stevens, W.C. (1978). A test of the carcinogenicity of enflurane, isoflurane, halothane, methoxyflurane and nitrous oxide in mice. *Anesthesia and Analgesia*, **57**, 678–694.

Egli, M. & Albani, C. (1981). Relief of status epilepticus after im administration of the new short-acting benzodiazepine midazolam (Dormicum). *Excerpta Medica*, ICS (548), 44.

El-Ad, B. & Neufeld, M.Y. (1990). Periodic febrile confusion as a presentation of complex partial status epilepticus. *Acta Neurologica Scandinavica*, **82**, 350–352.

Elliott, H.W. (1976). Metabolism of lorazepam. *British Journal of Anaesthesia*, **48**, 1017–1023.

Ellis, J.M. & Lee, S.I. (1978). Acute prolonged confusion in later life as an ictal state. *Epilepsia*, **19**, 119–128.

Emre, M. (1992). Palatal myoclonus occurring during complex partial status epilepticus. *Journal of Neurology*, **239**, 228–230.

Engel, P. (ed.) (1993). *The surgical treatment of the epilepsies*, 2nd edn. New York: Raven Press.

Engel, J., Ludwig, B.I. & Fetell, M. (1978). Prolonged partial complex status epilepticus: EEG and behavioral observations. *Neurology*, **28**, 863–869.

Eriksson, M. & Zettersttöm, R. (1979). Neonatal convulsions. *Acta Paediatrica Scandinavica*, **68**, 807–811.

Escueta, A.V., Boxley, J., Stubbs, N., Waddell, G. & Wilson, W.A. (1974). Prolonged twilight state and automatisms: a case report. *Neurology*, **24**, 331–339.

Evrard, P., de Saint-Georges P., Kahhim, H. & Gadisseux J.-F., (1989). Pathology of prenatal encephalopathies. In *Child neurology and developmental disabilities*, ed. J. French, S. Harel & P. Casaer, pp. 153–176. Baltimore: Paul H. Brookes.

Eyre, J.A., Cozeer, R.C. & Wilkinson, A.R. (1983). Diagnosis of neonatal seizure by continuous recording and rapid analysis of the electroencephalogram. *Archives of Disease in Childhood*, **58**, 785–790.

Fagan, K.J. & Lee, S.I. (1990). Prolonged confusion following convulsions due to generalised nonconvulsive status epilepticus. *Neurology*, **40**, 1689–1694.

Fahn, S. & Cote, L.J. (1968). Regional distribution of gamma-aminobutyric acid (GABA) in the brain of the rhesus monkey. *Journal of Neurochemistry*, **15**, 209–213.

Falconer, M.A., Serafetinides, E.A. & Corsellis, J.A.N. (1964). Etiology and pathogenesis of temporal lobe epilepsy. *Archives of Neurology*, **10**, 233–248.

Farber, J.L. (1981). The role of calcium in cell death. *Life Science*, **29**, 1289–1295.

Fariello, R.G. (1980). Epileptogenic properties of enflurane and their clinical interpretation. *Electroencephalography and Clinical Neurophysiology*, **48**, 595–598.

Fariello, R.G., Forchetti, C.M. & Fisher, R.S. (1991). GABAergic function in relation to seizure phenomena. In *Frontiers of clinical neuroscience*, vol. 11 *Neurotransmitters and epilepsy*, ed. R.S. Fisher, & J.T. Coyle, pp. 77–94. New York: Wiley-Liss.

Fariello, R.G., Golden, G.T., Smith, G.G. & Reyes, P.F. (1989). Potentiation of kainic acid epileptogenicity and sparing from neuronal damage by an NMDA receptor antagonist. *Epilesy Research*, **3**, 206–213.

Fejerman, N. & Di Blasi, M. (1987). Status epilepticus of benign partial epilepsies in children: report of two cases. *Epilepsia*, **28**, 351–355.

Feneck, R.O. (1981). A case of status epilepticus: use of thiopentone and IPPV to control otherwise refractory convulsions. *Anaesthesia*, **36**, 691–695.

Fenichel, G.M. (1985). *Neonatal neurology*. New York: Churchill Livingstone.

Ferngren, H.G. (1974). Diazepam treatment in the development of tolerance to the anti-pentylenetetrazole effects of diazepam. *Neuroscience Letters*, **42**, 95–98.

Figot, P.P., Hine, C.H. & Way, E.L. (1952). The estimation and significance of paraldehyde levels in blood and brain. *Acta Pharmacologica et Toxicologica*, **8**, 290–304.

Fincham, R.W., Yamada, T., Schottelius, D.D., Hayreh, S.M.S. & Damasio, A. (1979). Electroencephalographic absence status with minimal behavior change. *Archives of Neurology*, **36**, 176–178.

Fischer, S.P., Lee, J., Zatuchni, J. & Greenberg, J. (1977). Disseminated intravascular coagulation in status epilepticus. *Thrombosis and Haemostasis*, **38**, 909–913.

Fischer-Williams, M. (1963). Burst-suppression activity as an indication of undercut cortex. *Electroencephalography and Clinical Neurophysiology*, **15**, 723–724.

Fisher, R.S. (1989). Animal models of the epilepsies. *Brain Research Reviews*, **14**, 245–278.

Fisher, R.S. (1991*a*). Animal models of the epilepsies. In *Frontiers of clinical neuroscience*, vol. 11 *Neurotransmitters and epilepsy*, ed. R.S. Fisher & J.T. Coyle, pp. 61–76. New York: Wiley-Liss.

Fisher, R.S. (1991*b*). Glutamate and epilepsy. In *Frontiers of clinical neuroscience*, vol. 11 *Neurotransmitters and epilepsy*, ed R.S. Fisher & J.T. Coyle, pp. 131–146. New York: Wiley-Liss.

Fisher, R.S. & Coyle, J.T. (eds.) (1991). *Frontiers of clinical neuroscience*, Vol. 11 *Neurotransmitters and epilepsy*. New York: Wiley-Liss.

Fisher, R.S., Kaplan, P.W., Krumholz, A., Lesser, R.P., Rosen, S.A. & Wolff, M.R. (1988). Failure of high-dose intravenous magnesium sulfate to control myoclonic status epilepticus. *Clinical Neuropharmacology*, **11**, 537–544.

Foerster, C. (1977). Aphasia and seizure disorder in childhood. In *Epilepsy. The eighth international symposium*, ed. J.K. Penry, pp. 305–306. New York: Raven Press.

Foerster, O. & Penfield, W. (1930). The structural basis of traumatic epilepsy and results of radical operations. *Brain*, **53**, 99–119.

Forsgren, L., Edvinsson, S.-O., Blomquist, H.K., Heijbel, J. & Sidenvall, R. (1990). Epilepsy in a population of mentally retarded children and adults. *Epilepsy Research*, **6**, 234–248.

Franck, G., Sadzot, B., Salmon, E., Depresseux, J.C., Grisar, T., Peters, J.M., Guillaume, M., Quaglia, L., Delfiore, G. & Lamotte, D. (1986*a*). Regional cerebral blood flow and metabolic rates in human focal epilepsy and status epilepticus. In *Basic mechanisms of the epilepsies: molecular and cellular approaches*. Advances in Neurology, vol. 44, ed. A.V. Delgado-Escueta, A.A. Ward Jr, D.M. Woodbury & R.J. Porter, pp. 935–948. Raven Press: New York.

Franck, G., Sadzot, B., Salmon, E., Maquet, P., Peter, J.M., Quaglia, L., Delfiore, G. & Lamotte, D. (1986*b*). Etude chez l'homme, par tomographie à émission de positrons, du métabolisme et du débit sanguin cérébral dans les épilepsies partielles complexes et dans différents états de mal. *Revue d'Electroencéphalographie et de Neurophysiologie Clinique*, **16**, 199–216.

Freeman, J.M. (1989). Status epilepticus: it's not what we've thought or taught. *Pediatrics*, **83**, 444–445.

Friedlander, W.J. & Feinstein, G.H. (1956). Petit mal status: epilepsia minoris continua. *Neurology*, **6**, 357–362.

Friedman, H., Ochs, H.R., Greenblatt, D.J. & Shader, R.I. (1985). Tissue distribution of diazepam and its metabolite desmethyldiazepam: a human autopsy study. *Journal of Clinical Pharmacology*, **25**, 613–615.

Fujikawa, D.G. (1988). Brain damage from pilocarpine-induced seizures is ameliorated by an N-methyl-D-aspartate antagonist. *Society of Neurosciences Abstract*, **14**, 472.

Fujikawa, D.G. & Cheung, M.C. (1989). Extracellular glutamate and aspartate concentrations in the amygdala are unchanged by pilocarpine seizures and microinjection of AP7. *Journal of Cerebral Blood Flow and Metabolism*, **11** (suppl. 2), S107.

Fujikawa, D.G., Soderfeldt, B. & Wasterlain, C.G. (1992). Neuropathological changes during generalized seizures in newborn monkeys. *Epilepsy Research*, **12**, 243–251.

Fujikawa, D.G., Dwyer, B.E., Lake, R.R. & Wasterlain, C.G. (1989*a*). Local cerebral glucose utilization during status epilepticus in newborn primates. *American Journal of Physiology*, **256** (*Cell Physiology*, **25**), C1160-C1167.

Fujikawa, D.G., Wasterlain, C.G., Yang. C. & Thompson, K. (1989*b*). Ketamine protects against brain damage from pilocarpine seizures in entorhinal-kindled rats. *Society of Neurosciences Abstracts*, **15**, 1215.

Fujiwara, T., Ishida, S., Miyakoshi, M., Sakuma, N., Mariyama, S., Morikawa, T., Seino, M. & Wada, T. (1979). Status epilepticus in childhood: a retrospective study of initial convulsive status and subsequent epilepsies. *Folia Psychiatrica et Neurologica Japonica*, **33**, 337–344.

Fujiwara, T., Watanabe, M., Matsuda, K., Senbongi, M., Yagi, K. & Seino, M. (1991). Complex partial status epilepticus provoked by ingestion of alcohol: a case report. *Epilepsia*, **32**, 650–656.

Fujiwara, T., Watanabe, M., Nakamura, H., Kudo, T., Yagi, K. & Seino, M. (1988). A comparative study of absence status epilepticus between children and adults. *Japanese Journal of Psychiatry and Neurology*, **42**, 497–508.

Gabor, A.J. (1990). Lorazepam versus phenobarbital: candidates for drug of choice for treatment of status epilepticus. *Journal of Epilepsy*, **3**, 3–6.

Gal, P., Toback, J., Boer, H.R., Erken, N.V. & Wells, T.J. (1982). Efficacy of phenobarbital monotherapy in the treatment of neonatal seizures – relationship to blood levels. *Neurology*, **32**, 1401–1404.

Galan, J.A., Anderson, A.E., Yeakley, J.W., Curtis, V.L., Wheless, J.W. & Willmore, L.J. (1992). MELAS-associated status epilepticus: metabolic intervention and treatment resistent seizures. *Epilepsia*, **33** Supplement 3, 5.

Gale, K. (1989). GABA in epilepsy: the pharmacological basis. *Epilepsia*, **30** (suppl. 3), S1-S11.

Gall, M., Scollo-Lavizzari, G. & Becker, H. (1978). Absence status in the adult. *European Neurology*, **17**, 121–128.

Galvin, G.M. & Jelinek, G.A. (1987). Midazolam: an effective intravenous agent for seizure control. *Archives of Emergency Medicine*, **4**, 169–172.

Gamble, J.A.S., Dundee, J.W. & Assaf, R.A.E. (1975). Plasma diazepam levels after single dose oral and intramuscular administration. *Anaesthesia*, **30**, 164–169.

Garcia, D.A., Malagon, V.J., Franco, D.J. & Ramos, P.J. (1987). Status epilepticus within the Lennox–Gastaut syndrome: clinical characteristics and management. *Clinical Electroencephalography*, **18**, 89–92.

Gardner, H.L., Levine, H. & Bodansky, M. (1940). Concentration of paraldehyde in the blood following its administration during labor. *American Journal of Obstetrics and Gynecology*, **40**, 435–439.

Gascon, G., Victor, D., Lombroso, C. & Goodglass, H. (1973). Language disorder, convulsive disorders and electroencephalographic abnormalities. *Archives of Neurology*, **28**, 151–162.

Gastaut, H. (1967). A propos d'une classification symptomatologique des états de mal épileptiques. In *Les états de mal épileptiques*, ed. H. Gastaut, J. Roger & H. Lob, pp. 1–8. Paris: Masson.

Gastaut, H. (1969). Clinical and electroencephalographical classification of epileptic seizures. *Epilepsia*, **10** (suppl.), S2-S13.

Gastaut, H. (1970). Clinical and electroencephalographical classification of epileptic seizures. *Epilepsia*, **11**, 102–113.

Gastaut, H. (ed.) (1973). *Dictionary of epilepsy*, Part 1 *Definitions*. Geneva: World Health Organization.

Gastaut, H. (1979). Aphasia: the sole manifestation of focal status epilepticus. *Neurology*, **29**, 1638.

Gastaut, H. (1982). The Lennox–Gastaut syndrome: comments on the syndrome's terminology and nosological position amongst the secondary generalised epilepsies of childhood.

In *Henri Gastaut and the Marseilles School's Contribution to the Neurosciences* (EEG suppl. no. 35), ed. R.J. Broughton, pp. 71–84. Amsterdam: Elsevier Biomedical Press.

Gastaut, H. (1983). Classification of status epilepticus. In *Status epilepticus. Mechanisms of brain damage and treatment*. Advances in Neurology, vol. 34, ed. A.V. Delgado-Escueta, C.G. Wasterlain, D.M. Treiman & R.J. Porter, pp. 15–35. New York: Raven Press.

Gastaut, H., Broughton, R., Roger, J. & Tassinari, C.A. (1974). Generalised convulsive seizures without local onset. In *Handbook of clinical neurology*, vol. 15. *The epilepsies*, ed. O. Magnus & A.M. Lorentz de Haas, pp. 107–129. Amsterdam: North Holland Publishing Company.

Gastaut, J., Courjon, J., Poiré, R. & Weber, M. (1971). Treatment of status epilepticus with a new benzodiazepine more active than diazepam. *Epilepsia*, **12**, 197–214.

Gastaut, H., Naquet, R., Poiré, R. & Tassinari, C.A. (1965). Treatment of status epilepticus with diazepam (valium). *Epilepsia*, **6**, 167–182.

Gastaut, H., Poirer, F., Payan, H., Salomon, G., Toga, M. & Vigouroux, M. (1960). H.H.E.-syndrome, hemiconvulsions-hemiplagia-epilepsy. *Epilepsia*, **1**, 418–447.

Gastaut, H., Roger, J. & Lob, H. (eds.) (1967). *Les états de mal épileptique: compte rendu de la réunion européenne d'information électroencéphalographique*, Xth Colloque de Marseille 1962. Paris: Masson.

Gastaut, H., Roger, J., Ouahchi, S., Timsit, M. & Broughton, R. (1963). An electroclinical study of generalised epileptic seizures of tonic expression. *Epilepsia*, **4**, 15–44

Gastaut, H., Roger, J. & Roger, A. (1956). Sur la signification de certaines fugues épileptiques: état de mal temporal. *Revue Neurologique*, **94**, 298–301.

Gastaut, H., Roger, J., Soulayrol, R., Tassinari, C., Regis, H., Dravet, C., Bernard, R., Pinsard, N. & Saint-Jean, M. (1966). Childhood epileptic encephalopathy with diffuse slow spike waves (otherwise known as 'petit mal variant') or Lennox syndrome. *Epilepsia*, **7**, 139–179.

Gastaut, H. & Tassinari, C. (1975). Status epilepticus. In *Handbook of electroencephalography and clinical neurophysiology*, vol. 13A, ed. A. Redmond, pp. 39–45. Amsterdam: Elsevier.

Gavassetti, M. (1586). *Alter de rebus praeter naturam: alter de indicationibus curativis*. Libri duo: Venice.

Geier, S. (1978). Prolonged psychic epileptic seizures: a study of the absence status. *Epilepsia*, **19**, 431–445.

Ghezzi, A., Montanini, R., Basso, P.F., Zaffaroni, M., Massimo, E. & Cazzullo, C.L. (1990). Epilepsy in multiple sclerosis. *European Neurology*, **30**, 218–223.

Ghilain, S., Van Rijckevorsel-Harmant, K., Harmant, J. & De Barsy, T.H. (1988). Midazolam in the treatment of epileptic seizures. *Journal of Neurology, Neurosurgery and Psychiatry*, **51**, 732.

Gibberd, F.B. (1972). Petit mal status presenting in middle age. *Lancet*, i, 269.

Gibbs, F. & Gibbs, E. (1952). *Atlas of electroencephalography*, vol. 2. Cambridge, MA: Addison-Wesley.

Gibbs, F.A., Gibbs, E.L. & Lennox, W.G. (1937). Epilepsy: a paroxysmal cerebral dysrhythmia. *Brain*, **60**, 377–389.

Gilliam, F., Simonian, N. & Chiappa, K. (1992). Complex partial status associated with ifosfamide infusion. *Epilepsia*, **33** (suppl. 3), 3.

Gilmore, H.E., Veale, L.A., Darras, B.T., Dionne, R.E., Rabe, E.F. & Singer, W.D. (1984). Lorazepam treatment of childhood status epilepticus. *Annals of Neurology*, **16**, 377.

331

Gimenez-Roldán, S., López Agreda, J.M. & Martin, F.J. (1972). Un nuevo medicamento eficaz en el tratamiento del status epilepticus – Ro 5–4023. *Medicina Clinica*, **58**, 133.

Giorgi, C., Stocchetti, N., Pavesi, G., Marchini, M., Parenti, R., Bortone, E. & Mancia, D. (1991). Myoclonic epileptic status in a case of post-anoxic coma. *Bollettino di Lega Italiana Contro L'Epilessia*, **74**, 107–109.

Giovanardi Rossi, P., Pazzaglia, P. & Frank, G. (1976). Afasia acquisita con anomalie convulsive nell'età evolutiva: studio clinico, neuropsicologico ed elettroencefalografico di un caso. *Rivista di Neurologia*, **46**, 130–162.

Giroud, M. & Dumas, R. (1988). Traitement des états de mal épileptique par le valproate de sodium. *Neurophysiologie Clinique*, **18**, 21–32.

Giuditta, A., Metafora, S., Popoli, M. & Perrone-Capano, C. (1983). Brain protein and DNA synthesis during seizures. In *Status epilepticus. Mechanisms of brain damage and treatment*. Advances in Neurology, vol. 34, ed. A.V. Delgado-Escueta, C.G. Wasterlain, D.M. Treiman & R.J. Porter, pp. 289–296. New York: Raven Press.

Gloor, P. (1979). Generalized epilepsy with spike-and-wave discharge: a reinterpretation of its electrographic and clinical manifestations. *Epilepsia*, **20**, 571–588.

Gloor, P. & Fariello, R.G. (1988). Generalised epilepsy: some of its cellular mechanisms differ from those of focal epilepsy. *Trends in Neurosciences*, **11**, 63–68.

Goetz, C.G. (1987). Charcot at the Salpêtrière: ambulatory automatisms. *Neurology*, **37**, 1084–1088.

Gökyiğit, A., Apak, S. & Çalişkan, A. (1986). Electrical status epilepticus lasting for 17 months without behavioural changes. *Electroencephalography and Clinical Neurophysiology*, **63**, 32–34.

Goldberg, M.A. & McIntyre, H.B. (1983). Barbiturates in the treatment of status epilepticus. In *Status epilepticus. Mechanisms of brain damage and treatment*. Advances in Neurology, vol. 34, ed. A.V. Delgado-Escueta, C.G. Wasterlain, D.M. Treiman & R.J. Porter, pp. 499–504. New York: Raven Press.

Goldensohn, E.S. & Gold, A.P. (1960). Prolonged behavioral disturbances as ictal phenomena. *Neurology*, **10**, 1–9.

Goldie, L. & Green, J.M. (1961). Observations on episodes of bewilderment seen during a study of petit mal. *Epilepsia*, **2**, 306–331.

Goldman, R.S. & Finkbeiner, S.M. (1988). Therapeutic use of magnesium sulfate in selected cases of cerebral ischemia and seizure. *New England Journal of Medicine*, **319**, 1224–1225.

Goldmann, J.W., Glastein, G. & Adams, A.H. (1981). Adult onset absence status: a report of six cases. *Clinical Electroencephalography*, **12**, 199–204.

Good, J.M. (1822). The study of medicine. London: Baldwin, Cradock and Joy.

Gorman, D.G., Shields, W.D., Shewmon, D.A., Chugani, H.T., Finkel, R., Comair, Y.G. & Peacock, W.J. (1992). Neurosurgical treatment of refractory status epilepticus. *Epilepsia*, **33**, 546–549.

Goulon, M., Lévy-Alcover, M.A. & Nouailhat, F. (1985). Etat de mal épileptique de l'adulte. Etude épidémiologique et clinique en réanimation. *Revue d'Electroencéphalographie et de Neurophysiologie Clinique*, **15**, 277–285.

Gowers, W.R. (1881). *Epilepsy and other chronic convulsive diseases*. London: Churchill.

Gowers, W.R. (1888). *A manual of diseases of the nervous system*. London: Churchill.

Gowers, W.R. (1901). *Epilepsy and other chronic convulsive disorders*, 2nd edn. London: Churchill.

Graham, J.K. (1978). A comparison of the absorption of phenobarbitone given via the oral and intravenous routes. *Clinical and Experimental Neurology*, **15**, 154–158.

Graves, C.L., McDermott, R.W. & Bidwai, A. (1974). Cardiovascular effects of isoflurane in surgical patients. *Anesthesiology*, **41**, 486–489.

Greenblatt, D.J. & Divoll, M. (1983). Diazepam versus lorazepam: relationship of drug distribution to duration of clinical action. In *Status epilepticus. Mechanisms of brain damage and treatment.* Advances in Neurology, vol. 34, ed. A.V. Delgado-Escueta, C.G. Wasterlain, D.M. Treiman & R.J. Porter, pp. 487–491. New York: Raven Press.

Greenblatt, D.J. & Koch-Weser, J. (1975*a*). Clinical pharmacokinetics. Part I. *New England Journal of Medicine*, **293**, 702–705.

Greenblatt, D.J. & Koch-Weser, J. (1975*b*). Drug therapy: clinical pharmacokinetics second of two parts. *New England Journal of Medicine*, **293**, 964–976.

Greenblatt, D.J., Miller, L.G. & Shader, R.I. (1987). Clonazepam pharmacokinetics, brain uptake, and receptor interactions. *Journal of Clinical Psychiatry*, **48** (suppl.), 4–11.

Greenblatt, D.J., Shader, R.I., Franke, K., MacLaughlin, D.S., Harmatz, J.S., Allen, M.D., Werner, A. & Woo, E. (1979). Pharmacokinetics and bioavailability of intravenous, intramuscular and oral lorazepam in humans. *Pharmacological Science*, **68**, 57–63.

Griffith, P.A. & Karp, H.R. (1980). Lorazepam in therapy for status epilepticus. *Annals of Neurology*, **7**, 493.

Griffiths, T., Evans, M.C. & Meldrum, B.S. (1983). Intracellular calcium accumulation in rat hippocampus during seizures induced by bicuculline or L-allylglycine. *Neuroscience*, **10**, 385–395.

Griffiths, T., Evans, M.C. & Meldrum, B.S. (1984). Status epilepticus: the reversibility of calcium loading and acute neuronal pathological changes in the rat hippocampus. *Neuroscience*, **12**, 557–567.

Grossman, R.A., Hamilton, R.W., Morse, B.M., Penn, A.S. & Goldberg, M. (1974). Nontraumatic rhabdomyolysis and acute renal failure. *New England Journal of Medicine*, **291**, 807–811.

Guberman, A., Cantu-Reyna, G., Stuss, D. & Broughton, R. (1986). Nonconvulsive generalised status epilepticus: clinical features, neuropsychological testing, and long-term follow-up. *Neurology*, **36**, 1284–1291.

Gugler, P., Manion, C.V. & Azaroff, D.L. (1976). Phenytoin: pharmacokinetics and bioavailability. *Clinical Pharmacology and Therapeutics*, **19**, 135–142.

Gupta, S.R., Naheedy, M.H., Elias, D. & Rubino, F.A. (1988). Postinfarction seizures: a clinical study. *Stroke*, **19**, 1477–1481.

Hajnšek, F. & Dürrigl, V. (1970). Some aspects of so-called petit mal status. *Electroencephalography and Clinical Neurophysiology*, **28**, 322.

Halliday, A.M. (1967). The electrophysiology study of myoclonus in man. *Brain*, **90**, 241–284.

Hamilton, N.G. & Matthews, T. (1979). Aphasia: the sole manifestation of focal status epilepticus. *Neurology*, **29**, 745–748.

Handforth, A. & Ackermann, R.F. (1992). Hierarchy of seizure states in the electrogenic limbic status epilepticus model: behavioral and electrographic observations of initial states and temporal progression. *Epilepsia*, **33**, 589–600.

Hardiman, O., Burke, T., Phillips, J., Murphy, S., O'Moore, B., Staunton, H. & Farrell, M.A. (1988). Microdysgenesis in resected temporal neocortex: incidence and clinical significance in focal epilepsy. *Neurology*, **38**, 1041–1047.

Harding, B.N., Egger, J., Portmann, B. & Erdohazi, M. (1986). Progressive neuronal degeneration of childhood with liver disease: a pathological study. *Brain*, **109**, 181–206.

Hariga, M. & Ectors, L. (1974). De la lidocaíne comme agent anticomitial. *Acta Paediatrica Belgica*, **28**, 315–327.

333

Harris, R. & Tizard, J.P.M. (1960). The electroencephalogram in neonatal convulsions. *Journal of Pediatrics*, **57**, 501–520.

Harvey, P.K.P., Higenbottam, T.W. & Loh, L. (1975). Chlormethiazole in treatment of status epilepticus. *British Medical Journal*, **2**, 603–605.

Harvey, S.C. (1985). Hypnotics and sedatives. In *The pharmacological basis of therapeutics*, 7th edn, ed. A. Goodman Gilman, L. Goodman & A. Gilman, pp. 339–371. New York: Macmillan Publishing Co.

Hauser, W.A. (1981). The natural history of febrile seizures. In *Febrile seizures*, ed. R.B. Nelson & J.H. Ellenberg, pp. 5–17. New York: Raven Press.

Hauser, W.A. (1983). Status epilepticus: frequency, etiology and neurological sequelae. In *Status epilepticus. Mechanisms of brain damage and treatment* Advances in Neurology, vol. 34, ed. A.V. Delgado-Escueta, C.G. Wasterlain, D.M. Treiman & R.J. Porter, pp. 3–14. New York: Raven Press.

Hauser, W.A. (1990). Status epilepticus: epidemiologic considerations. *Neurology*, **40** (suppl. 2), 9–13.

Hayashi, T. (1954). Effects of sodium glutamate on the nervous system. *Keio Journal of Medicine*, **3**, 183–192

Heath, R.G. (1986). Studies with deep electrodes in patients intractably ill with epilepsy and other disorders. In *What is epilepsy? The clinical and scientific basis of epilepsy*, ed. M.R. Trimble & E.H. Reynolds, pp. 126–138. Edinburgh: Churchill Livingstone.

Heathfield, K.W.G. (1972). Isolated petit-mal status presenting de novo in middle age. *Lancet*, **i**, 492.

Heberden, W. (1802). Commentarii de morborum historia et curatione. London: Payne.

Heinemann, U. (1987). Basic mechanisms of the epilepsies. In *Textbook of clinical neurophysiology*, ed. A.M. Halliday, S.R. Butler & R. Paul, pp. 497–534. New York: John Wiley.

Heinemann, U. & Jones, R.S.G. (1990). Neurophysiology. In *Comprehensive epileptology*, ed. M. Dam & L. Gram, pp. 17–42. New York: Raven Press.

Heintel, H. (1969). Status von tonischen Dämmerattacken. *Archiv für Psychiatrie und Nervenkrankheiten*, **212**, 117–125.

Heintel, H. (1972). *Status epilepticus: etiology, clinical aspects and lethality – a clinical-statistical analysis*. Stuttgart: Gustav Fischer Verlag.

Hellström-Westas, L., Rosén, I. & Svenningsen, N.W. (1985). Silent seizures in sick infants in early life: diagnosis by continuous cerebral function monitoring. *Acta Paediatrica Scandinavica*, **74**, 741–748.

Hellström-Westas, L., Svenningsen, N.W., Westgren, U., Rosén, I. & Lagerström, P.-O. (1992). Lidocaine for treatment of severe seizures in newborn infants. II. Blood concentrations of lidocaine and metabolites during intravenous infusion. *Acta Paediatrica Scandinavica*, **81**, 35–39.

Hellström-Westas, L., Westgren, U., Rosén, I. & Svenningsen, N.W. (1988). Lidocaine for treatment of severe seizures in newborn infants. I. Clinical effects and cerebral electrical activity monitoring. *Acta Paediatrica Scandinavica*, **77**, 79–84.

Hempel, F.G., Kariman, K. & Saltzman, H.A. (1980). Redox transitions in mitochondria of cat cerebral cortex with seizures and hemorrhagic hypotension. *American Journal of Physiology*, **238**, H249–H256.

Henriksen, G.F. (1973). Status epilepticus partialis with fear as clinical expression. *Epilepsia*, **14**, 39–46.

Henriksen, O. (1985). Discussion of myoclonic epilepsies and Lennox-Gastaut syndromes. In *Epileptic syndromes in infancy, childhood and adolescence*, ed. J. Roger, C. Dravet, M. Bureau, F.E. Dreifuss & P. Wolf, pp. 100–105. London: John Libbey.

Hersch, E.L. & Billings, R.F. (1988). Acute confusional state with status petit mal as a withdrawal syndrome – and five year follow-up. *Canadian Journal of Psychiatry*, 33, 157–159.

Hess, R., Scollo-Lavizzari, G. & Wyss, F.E. (1971). Borderline cases of petit mal status. *European Neurology*, 5, 137–154.

Hillestad, L., Hansen, T., Melsom, H. & Drivenes, A. (1974). Diazepam metabolism in normal man. 1. Serum concentrations and clinical effects after intravenous, intramuscular, and oral administration. *Clinical Pharmacology and Therapeutics*, 16, 479–484.

Hilz, M.J., Bauer, J., Claus, D., Stefan, H. & Neundörfer, B. (1992). Isoflurane anaesthesia in the treatment of convulsive status epilepticus. *Journal of Neurology*, 239, 135–137.

Hirsch, E., Marescaux, C., Maquet, P., Metz-Lutz, M.N., Kiesman, M., Salmon, E., Franck, G. & Kurtz, D. (1990). Landau–Kleffner syndrome: a clinical and EEG study of five cases. *Epilepsia*, 31, 756–767.

Hitt, B.A., Mazze, R.I., Cousins, M.J., Edmunds, H.N., Barr, G.A. & Trudell, J.R. (1974). Metabolism of isoflurane in Fischer 344 rats and man. *Anaesthesiology*, 40, 62–67.

Holaday, D.A., Fiserova-Bergerova, V., Latto, I.P. & Zumbiel, M.D. (1975). Resistance of isoflurane to biotransformation in man. *Anesthesiology*, 43, 325–332.

Holmes, G.L. (1991). Do seizures cause brain damage? *Epilepsia*, 32 (suppl. 5), S14-S28.

Holmes, G.L., McKeever, M. & Saunders, Z. (1981). Epileptiform activity in aphasia of childhood: an epiphenomenon? *Epilepsia*, 22, 631–639.

Holmes, G.L. & Thompson, J.L. (1988). Effects of kainic acid on seizure susceptibility in the developing brain. *Developmental Brain Research*, 39, 51–59.

Holtzman, D.M., Kaku, D.A. & So, Y.T. (1989). New-onset seizures associated with human immunodeficiency virus infection: causation and clinical features in 100 cases. *American Journal of Medicine*, 87, 173–177.

Homan, R.W. & Unwin, D.H. (1989). Benzodiazepines: lorazepam. In *Antiepileptic drugs*, 3rd edn, ed. R. Levy, K. Mattson, B. Meldrum, J.K. Penry & F.E. Dreifuss, pp. 841–854. New York: Raven Press.

Homan, R.W. & Walker, J.E. (1983). Clinical studies of lorazepam in status epilepticus. In *Status epilepticus. Mechanisms of brain damage and treatment*. Advances in Neurology, vol. 34, ed. A.V. Delgado-Escueta, C.G. Wasterlain, D.M. Treiman & R.J. Porter, pp. 493–498. New York: Raven Press.

Horder, J.M. (1978). Fatal chlormethiazole poisoning in chronic alcoholics. *British Medical Journal*, 1, 693–694.

Horton, R.W., Meldrum, B.S., Pedley, T.A. & McWilliam, J.R. (1980). Regional cerebral blood flow in the rat during prolonged seizure activity. *Brain Research*, 192, 399–412.

Houdart, R. & Laborit, G. (1965). L'hémineurine. Thérapeutique de l'état de mal épileptique. Encéphale, 54, 440–445.

Houdart, R. & Laborit, G. (1966). L'hémineurine thérapeutique de l'état de mal épileptique. *Agressologie*, 7, 109–114.

Houghton, G.W., Richens, A., Toseland, P.A., Davidson, S. & Falconer, M.A. (1975). Brain concentrations of phenytoin, phenobarbitone and primidone in epileptic patients. *European Journal of Clinical Pharmacology*, 9, 73–78.

Howard, F.M., Seybold, M.E. & Reiher, J. (1968). The treatment of recurrent convulsions with intravenous injection of diazepam. *Medical Clinics of North America*, 52, 977–987.

Howell, S.J.L., Owen, L. & Chadwick, D.W. (1989). Pseudostatus epilepticus. *Quarterly Journal of Medicine*, 71, 507–519.

Hrachovy, R.A. & Frost, J.D. (1989). Infantile spasms: a disorder of the developing nervous system. In *Problems and concepts in developmental neurophysiology*, ed. P. Kellaway & J.L. Noebels, pp. 131–147. Baltimore, MD: Johns Hopkins University Press.

Hrachovy, R.A. & Frost, J.D. (1990). Infantile spasms. In *Comprehensive epileptology*, ed. M. Dam & L. Gram. pp. 113–121. New York: Raven Press

Hrachovy, R.A., Frost J.D. & Kellaway, P. (1984). Hypsarrhythmia: variations on a theme. *Epilepsia*, **25**, 317–325.

Hrachovy, R.A., Frost J.D., Pollack, M. & Glaze, D.G. (1987). Serological HLA typing in infantile spasms. *Epilepsia*, **28**, 613–617.

Hrachovy, R.A., Frost, J.D., Shearer, W.T., Schlactus, J.L., Mizrahi, E.M. & Glaze, D.E. (1985). Immunological evaluations of patients with infantile spasms. *Annals of Neurology*, **18**, 414.

Hughes, D.R., Sharpe, M.D. & McLachlan, R.S. (1992). Control of epilepsia partialis continua and secondarily generalized status epilepticus with isoflurane. *Journal of Neurology, Neurosurgery and Psychiatry*, **55**, 739–740.

Hunter, R.A. (1959/60). Status epilepticus: history, incidence and problems. *Epilepsia*, **1**, 162–188.

Hutchison, R. (1930). A danger from paraldehyde. *British Medical Journal*, **1**, 718.

Hwang, P.A., Gilday, D.L., Spire, J.-P., Hosny, H., Chugani, H.T., Garnett, S., Theodore, W. & Laxer, K.D. (1991). Chronic focal encephalitis of Rasmussen: functional neuroimaging studies with positron emission tomography and single-photon emission computed tomography scanning. In *Chronic encephalitis and epilepsy: Rasmussen's syndrome*, ed. F. Andermann, pp. 61–72. London: Butterworth-Heinemann.

Hymes, J.A. (1985). Seizure activity during isoflurane anesthesia. *Anesthesia and Analgesia*, **64**, 367–368.

Hyser, C.L. & Drake, M.E. (1984). Status epilepticus after baclofen withdrawal. *Journal of the National Medical Association*, **76**, 537–538.

Iivanainen, M., Bergström, L., Nuutila, A. & Viukari, M. (1984). Psychosis-like absence status of elderly patients: successful treatment with sodium-valproate. *Journal of Neurology, Neurosurgery and Psychiatry*, **47**, 965–969.

Ingvar, M. & Siesjö, B.K. (1983). Local blood flow and glucose consumption in the rat brain during sustained bicuculline induced seizures. *Acta Neurologica Scandinavica*, **69**, 128–144.

Jaffe, R. & Christoff, N.J. (1967). Intravenous diazepam in seizure disorders. *Electroencephalography and Clinical Neurophysiology*, **23**, 77–96.

Jalling, B. (1974). Plasma and cerebrospinal fluid concentrations of phenobarbital in infants given single doses. *Developmental Medicine and Child Neurology*, **16**, 781–793.

Jalling, B., Boreus, L.O., Kallberg, N. & Agurell, S. (1973). Disappearance from the newborn of circulating prenatally administered phenobarbital. *European Journal of Clinical Pharmacology*, **6**, 234–238.

Janovich, D.G., Shabino, C.L., Noorani, A., Bittle, B.K. & Osborne, J.S. (1990). Intravenous midazolam suppression of pentylenetetrazol-induced epileptogenic activity in a porcine model. *Critical Care Medicine*, **18**, 313–316.

Janz, D. (1960). Status epilepticus und Stirnhirn. *Deutsche Zeitschrift für Nervenheilkunde*, **180**, 562–594.

Janz, D. (1961). Conditions and causes of status epilepticus. *Epilepsia*, **2**, 170–177.

Janz, D. (1964). Status epilepticus and frontal lobe lesions. *Journal of the Neurological Sciences*, **1**, 446–457.

Janz, D. (1983). Etiology of convulsive status epilepticus. In *Status epilepticus. Mechanisms of brain damage and treatment*. Advances in Neurology, vol. 34, ed. A.V. Delgado-

Escueta, C.G. Wasterlain, D.M. Treiman & R.J. Porter, pp. 47–54. New York: Raven Press.

Janz, D. & Kautz, G. (1963). Ätiologie und Therapie des status epilepticus. *Deutsche Medizinische Wochenschrift*, **88**, 2189–2195.

Jasper, H.H. & van Gelder, N.M. (eds.) (1983). *Basic mechanisms of neuronal hyperexcitability.* New York: Alan R. Liss.

Jawad, S., Oxley, J., Wilson, J. & Richens, A. (1986). A pharmacodynamic evaluation of midazolam as an antiepileptic compound. *Journal of Neurology, Neurosurgery and Psychiatry*, **49**, 1050–1054.

Jawad, S., Richens, A. & Oxley, J. (1984). Pharmacodynamic and clinical evaluation of midazolam in epilepsy. *Acta Neurologica Scandinavica*, **70**, 219.

Jayakar, P.B. & Seshia, S.S. (1991). Electrical status epilepticus during slow-wave sleep: a review. *Journal of Clinical Neurophysiology*, **8**, 299–311.

Jeavons, P.M., Bower, B.D. & Dimitrakoudi, M. (1973). Long-term prognosis of 150 cases of 'West Syndrome'. *Epilepsia*, **14**, 153–164.

Jefferys, J.G.R. (1990). Basic mechanisms of focal epilepsies. *Experimental Physiology*, **75**, 127–162.

Jefferys, J.G.R. (1993). The pathophysiology of epilepsies. In *A textbook of epilepsy*, ed. J. Laidlaw A. Richens & D. Chadwick, pp. 241–276. Edinburgh: Churchill Livingstone.

Jeffreys, J.G.R. & Roberts, R. (1987). The biology of epilepsy. In *Epilepsy*, ed. A. Hopkins, pp. 19–81. London: Chapman & Hall.

Johnson, M.H. & Jones, S.N. (1985). Status epilepticus, hypothermia and metabolic chaos in a man with agenesis of the corpus callosum. *Journal of Neurology, Neurosurgery and Psychiatry*, **48**, 480–483.

Jostell, K.-G. (1987). *Pharmacokinetics of chlormethiazole in man and influence of altered physiological conditions.* Uppsala: Acta Universitatis Upsaliensis: comprehensive summaries of Uppsala dissertations from the Faculty of Pharmacy, 31.

Jostell K.-G. Agurell, S , Allgen, L.-G., Kuylenstierna, B., Lindgren, J.E., Aberg, G. & Osterlof, G. (1978). Pharmacokinetics of chloromethiazole in healthy adults. *Acta Pharmacologica et Toxicologica*, **43**, 180–189.

Jumao-as, A. & Brenner, R.P. (1990). Myoclonic status epilepticus: a clinical and electroencephalographic study. *Eurology*, **40**, 1199–1202.

Jusko, W.J., Gretsch, M. & Gassett, R. (1973). Precipitation of diazepam from intravenous preparations. *Journal of the American Medical Association*, **225**, 176.

Juul-Jensen, P. & Denny-Brown, D. (1966). Epilepsia partialis continua. *Archives of Neurology*, **15**, 563–578.

Kanazawa, O., Sengoku, A. & Kawai, I. (1989). Oculoclonic status epilepticus. *Epilepsia*, **30**, 121–123.

Kaneko, S., Kurahashi, K., Fujita, S., Fukushima, Y., Sato, T. & Hill, R.G. (1983). Potentiation of GABA by midazolam and its therapeutic effect against status epilepticus. *Folia Psychiatrica et Neurologica Japonica*, **37**, 307–309.

Kanto, J.H., Pihlajamaki, K.K. & Tisalo, E.U.M. (1974). Concentrations of diazepam in adipose tissue of children. *British Journal of Anaesthesia*, **46**, 168.

Kaplan, S.A., Alexander, K., Jack, M.L., Puglisi, C.V., De Silva, J.A.A., Lee, T.L. & Weinfeld, R.E. (1973) Pharmacokinetic profiles of diazepam in dog and humans and of flunitrazepam in dog. *Journal of Pharmaceutical Science*, **63**, 527–532.

Karbowski, K. (1980). Status psychomotoricus. Berne: Hans Huber.

Kellaway, P. & Chao, D. (1955). Prolonged status epilepticus in petit mal. *Electroencephalography and Clinical Neurophysiology*, **7**, 145.

Kellaway, P. & Hrachovy, R.A. (1983). Status epilepticus in newborns: a perspective on neonatal seizures. In *Status epilepticus. Mechanisms of brain damage and treatment*. Advances in Neurology, vol. 34, ed. A.V. Delgado-Escueta, C.G. Wasterlain, D.M. Treiman & R.J. Porter, pp 93–99. New York: Raven Press.

Kellaway, P., Hrachovy, R.A., Frost, J.D. & Zion, T. (1979). Precise characterization and quantification of infantile spasms. *Annals of Neurology*, 6, 214–218.

Kellaway, P. & Mizrahi, E.M. (1987). Neonatal seizures. In: *Epilepsy: electroclinical syndromes*, ed. H. Lüders & R.J. Lesser, pp. 13–47. London: Springer-Verlag.

Kellermann, K. (1978). Recurrent aphasia with subclinical bioelectric status epilepticus during sleep. *European Journal of Pediatrics*, 128, 207–212.

Ketz, E., Bernoulli, C. & Siegfried, J. (1973). Clinical and EEG study of clonazepam (Ro 5-4023) with particular reference to status epilepticus. *Acta Neurologica Scandinavica*, 49, 47–53.

Kinnier Wilson, J.V. & Reynolds, E.H. (1990). Translation and analysis of a cuneiform text forming part of a Babylonian treatise on epilepsy. *Medical History*, 34, 185–198.

Kinnier Wilson, S.A. (1940). *Neurology*, vol. 3. London: Arnold and Co.

Kitagawa, T., Takahashi, K., Matsushima, K. & Kawahara, R. (1979). A case of prolonged confusion after temporal lobe psychomotor status. *Folia Psychiatrica et Neurologica Japonica*, 33, 279–284.

Kivity, S. & Lerman, P. (1992). Stormy onset with prolonged loss of consciousness in benign childhood epilepsy with occipital paroxysms. *Journal of Neurology, Neurosurgery and Psychiatry*, 55, 45–48.

Klotz, U., Antonin, K.H., Brugel, H. & Bieck, P.R. (1977). Disposition of diazepam and its major metabolite desmethyldiazepam in patients with liver disease. *Clinical Pharmacology and Therapeutics*, 21, 430–436.

Knight, R.T. & Cooper, J. (1986). Status epilepticus manifesting as reversible Wernicke's aphasia. *Epilepsia*, 27, 301–304.

Knudsen, F.U. (1977). Plasma-diazepam in infants after rectal administration in solution and by suppository. *Acta Paediatrica Scandinavica*, 66, 563–567.

Knudsen, F.U. (1979). Rectal administration of diazepam in solution in the acute treatment of convulsions in infants and children. *Archives of Disease in Childhood*, 54, 855–857.

Kobayashi, K., Murakami, N., Yoshinaga, H., Enoki, H., Ohtsuka, Y. & Ohtahara, S. (1988). Nonconvulsive status epilepticus with continuous diffuse spike and wave discharges during sleep in childhood. *Japanese Journal of Psychiatry and Neurology*, 42, 509–514.

Koepp, P. & Lagenstein, I. (1978). Acquired epileptic aphasia. *Journal of Pediatrics*, 92, 164–166.

Kofke, W.A., Young, R.S.K., Davis, P., Woelfel, S.K., Gray, L., Johnson, D., Gelb, A., Meeke, R., Warner, D.S., Pearson, K.S., Gibson, J.R., Koncelik, J. & Wessel, H.B. (1989). Isoflurane for refractory status epilepticus: a clinical series. *Anesthesiology*, 71, 653–659.

Kojewnikoff, A.Y. (1895*a*). Eine besondere Form von corticaler Epilepsie. *Neurologie Zentralblatt*, 14, 47–48.

Kojewnikoff, A.Y. (1895*b*). [A particular type of cortical epilepsy] transl. D.M. Asher, 1991. In *Chronic encephalitis and epilepsy: Rasmussen's syndrome*, ed. F. Andermann, pp. 245–262. London: Butterworth-Heinemann.

Koren, G., Butt, W., Rajchgot, P., Mayer, J., Whyte, H., Pape, K. & MacLeod, S.M. (1986). Intravenous paraldehyde for seizure control in newborn infants. *Neurology*, 36, 108–111.

Korttila, K., Sothman, A. & Andersson, P. (1976). Polyethylene glycol as a solvent for diazepam: bioavailability and clinical effects after intramuscular administration, comparison of oral, intramuscular and rectal administration, and precipitation from intravenous solutions. *Acta Pharmacologica et Toxicologica*, **39**, 104–117.

Kramer, R.E., Lüders, H., Lesser, R.P., Weinstein, M.R., Dinner, D.S., Morris, H.H. & Wyllie, E. (1987). Transient focal abnormalities of neuroimaging studies during focal status epilepticus. *Epilepsia*, **28**, 528–532.

Kreisman, N.R., LaManna, J.C., Rosenthal, M. & Sick, T.J. (1981). Oxidative metabolic responses with recurrent seizures in rat cerebral cortex: role of systemic factors. *Brain Research*, **218**, 175–188.

Kreisman, N.R., Magee, J.C. & Brizzee, B.L. (1991). Relative hypoperfusion in rat cerebral cortex during recurrent seizures. *Journal of Cerebral Blood Flow and Metabolism*, **11**, 77–87.

Kroth, N. (1967). Status with psychomotor attacks. *Electroencephalography and Clinical Neurophysiology*, **23**, 183–184.

Krumholz, A., Stern, B.J. & Weiss, H.D. (1988). Outcome from coma after cardiopulmonary resuscitation: relation to seizures and myoclonus. *Neurology*, **38**, 401–405.

Kruse, R. & Blankenhorn, V. (1973). Zusammenfassender Erfahrungsbericht über die klinische Anwendung und Wirksamkeit von Ro 5–4023 (Clonazepam) auf verschiedene Formen epileptischer Anfälle. *Acta Neurologica Scandinavica*, **49** (suppl. 53), 60–71.

Kubová, H. & Mareš, P. (1992). The effect of ontogenetic development on the anticonvulsant activity of midazolam. *Life Sciences*, **50**, 1665–1672.

Kugoh, T. & Hosokawa, K. (1977). Mental dullness associated with left frontal continuous focal discharge. *Folia Psychiatrica et Neurologica Japonica*, **31**, 473–480.

Kumar, A. & Bleck, T.P. (1992). Intravenous midazolam for the treatment of refractory status epilepticus. *Critical Care Medicine*, **20**, 483–488.

Kuzniecky, R., Berkovic, S., Andermann, F., Melanson, D., Olivier, A. & Robitaille, Y. (1988). Focal cortical myoclonus and rolandic cortical dysplasia: clarification by magnetic resonance imaging. *Annals of Neurology*, **23**, 317–325.

Kuzniecky, R. & Rosenblatt, B. (1987). Benign occipital epilepsy: a family study. *Epilepsia*, **28**, 346–350.

Labate, C., Magaudda, A., Fava, C., Meduri, M. & Di Perri, R. (1991). Hemispheric brain atrophy following unilateral status epilepticus. *Bollettino di Lega Italiana Contro L'Epilessia*, **74**, 103–104.

Lacey, D.J. (1988). Status epilepticus in children and adults. *Journal of Clinical Psychiatry*, **49**, 12 (suppl.), 33–35.

Lacey, D.J., Singer, W.D., Horwitz, S.J. & Gilmore, H. (1986). Clinical and laboratory observations: lorazepam therapy in status epilepticus in children and adolescents. *Journal of Pediatrics*, **108**, 771–774.

Lacey, J.R. & Penry, J.K. (1976). *Infantile spasms*. New York: Raven Press.

Lalji, D., Hosking, C.S. & Sutherland, J.M. (1967). Diazepam ('Valium') in the control of status epilepticus. *Medical Journal of Australia*, **1**, 542–545.

Lampl, Y., Eshel, Y., Gilad, R. & Sarova-Pinchas, I. (1990). Chloral hydrate in intractable status epilepticus. *Annals of Emergency Medicine*, **19**, 674–676.

Landau, W.M. (1992). Landau–Kleffner syndrome: an eponymic badge of ignorance. *Archives of Neurology*, **49**, 353–359.

Landau, W.M. & Kleffner, F. (1957). Syndrome of acquired aphasia with convulsive disorder in children. *Neurology*, **7**, 523–530.

Langdon, D.E., Harlan, J.R. & Bailey, R.L. (1973). Thrombophlebitis with diazepam used intravenously. *Journal of the American Medical Association*, **223**, 184–185.

Langmoen, I.A., Hegstad, E. & Berg-Johnsen, J. (1992). An experimental study of the effect of isoflurane on epileptiform bursts. *Epilepsy Research*, **11**, 153–157.

Langslet, A., Meberg, A., Bredesen, J.E. & Lunde, P.K.M. (1978). Plasma concentrations of diazepam and *N*-desmethyldiazepam in newborn infants after intravenous, intramuscular, rectal and oral administration. *Acta Paediatrica Scandinavica*, **67**, 699–704.

Lanzi, G. & Bojardi, A. (1978). Illustrazione di un caso di afasia acquisita. *Neuropsichiatria Infantile*, **206**, 135–156.

Lason, W., Simpson, J.N. & McGinty, J.F. (1988). Effects of D-aminophosphonovalerate on behavioural and histological changes induced by systemic kainic acid. *Neuroscience Letters*, **87**, 23–28.

Laxenaire, M., Tridon, P. & Poiré, P. (1966). Effect of chlormethiazole in treatment of delirium tremens and status epilepticus. *Acta Psychiatrica Scandinavica*, **42** (suppl. 192), 87–102.

Lee, S.H. & Goldberg, H.I. (1977). Hypervascular pattern associated with idiopathic focal status epilepticus. *Radiology*, **125**, 159–163.

Lee, S.I. (1985). Nonconvulsive status epilepticus: ictal confusion in later life. *Archives of Neurology*, **42**, 778–781.

Lehmann, A. (1987). Alterations in hippocampal extracellular amino acids and purine catabolites during limbic seizures induced by folate injections into the rabbit amygdala. *Neuroscience*, **22**, 573–578.

Lehmann, A., Hagberg, H., Jacobson, I. & Hamberger, A. (1985). Effects of status epilepticus on extracellular amino acids in the hippocampus. *Brain Research*, **359**, 147–151

Lehmann, J., Etienne, P., Cheney, D.L. & Wood, P.L. (1991). NMDA receptors and their ion channels. In *Neurotransmitters and epilepsy*. Frontiers of clinical neuroscience, vol. 11, ed. R.S. Fisher & J.T. Coyle, pp. 147–166. New York: Wiley-Liss.

Lemmen, L.J., Klassen, M. & Duiser, B. (1978). Intravenous lidocaine in the treatment of convulsions. *Journal of the American Medical Association*, **239**, 2025.

Lennox, W. (1945). The petit mal epilepsies: their treatment with tridione. *Journal of the American Medical Association*, **129**, 1069–1073.

Lennox, W. (1960). *Epilepsy and related disorders*. Boston, MA: Little Brown.

Lennox, W.G. & Davis, J.P. (1950). Clinical correlates of the fast and slow spike wave electroencephalogram. *Pediatrics*, **5**, 626–644.

Lennox-Buchthal, M.A. (1974). Febrile convulsions. In *Handbook of clinical neurology*, vol. 15 *The Epilepsies*, ed. O. Magnus & A.M. Lorentz de Haas, pp. 246–263. Amsterdam: North Holland Publishing Co.

Leppik, I.E. (1986). Status epilepticus. *Neurologic Clinics*, **4**, 633–643.

Leppik, I.E. (1990). Status epilepticus: the next decade. *Neurology*, **40** (suppl. 2), 4–9.

Leppik, I.E., Derivan, A.T., Homan, R.W., Walker, J., Ramsay, R.E. & Patrick, B. (1983*a*). Double-blind study of lorazepam and diazepam in status epilepticus. *Journal of the American Medical Association*, **249**, 1452–1454.

Leppik, I.E., Patrick, B.K. & Cranford, R.E. (1983*b*). Treatment of acute seizures and status epilepticus with intravenous phenytoin. In *Status epilepticus. Mechanisms of brain damage and treatment*. Advances in Neurology, vol. 34, ed. A.V. Delgado-Escueta, C.G. Wasterlain, D.M. Treiman & R.J. Porter, pp. 447–452. New York: Raven Press.

Lerique-Koechlin, A., Mises, J., Lossky, D., Daveau, M. & De Grammont (1967). Etiologie de l'état de mal chez l'enfant. In *Les états de mal épileptiques*, ed. H. Gastaut, J. Roger & H. Lob, pp. 239–245. Paris: Masson.

340

Lerman, P., Lerman-Sagie, T. & Kivity, S. (1991). Effect of early corticosteroid therapy for Landau–Kleffner syndrome. *Developmental Medicine and Child Neurology*, **33**, 257–266.

Lerner-Natoli, M., Rondouin, G., Belaidi, M., Baldy-Moulinier, M. & Kamenka, J.M. (1991). *N*-[1-(2-Thienyl)cyclohexyl]-piperidine (TCP) does not block kainic acid-induced status epilepticus but reduces secondary hippocampal damage. *Neuroscience Letters*, **122**, 174–178.

Levin, S. (1952). Epileptic clouded states: a review of 52 cases. *Journal of Nervous and Mental diseases*, **116**, 215–225.

Levy, R., Dreifuss, F.E., Mattson, R., Meldrum, B. & Penry, J.K. (eds.) (1989). *Antiepileptic drugs*, 3rd edn. New York: Raven Press.

Levy, R.J. & Krall, R.L. (1984). Treatment of status epilepticus with lorazepam. *Archives of Neurology*, **41**, 605–611.

Levy, S.R., Abroms, I.F., Marshall, P.C. & Rosquete, E.E. (1985). Seizures and cerebral infarction in the full-term newborn. *Annals of Neurology*, **17**, 366–370.

Lévy-Alcover, M.A. & Goulon, M. (1967). Etude E.E.G. d'états de mal comitiaux révélateurs de porphyrie. In *Les états de mal épileptiques*, ed. H. Gastaut, J. Roger & H. Lob, pp. 229–237. Paris: Masson.

Lim, J., Yagnik, P., Schraeder, P. & Wheeler, S. (1986). Ictal catatonia as a manifestation of nonconvulsive status epilepticus. *Journal of Neurology, Neurosurgery and Psychiatry*, **49**, 833–836.

Lingam, S., Bertwistle, H., Elliston, H. & Wilson, J. (1980). Problems with intravenous chlormethiazole (Heminevrin) in status epilepticus. *British Medical Journal*, **1**, 155–156.

Link, M.J., Anderson, R.E. & Meyer, F.B. (1991). Effects of magnesium sulfate on pentylenetetrazol-induced status epilepticus. *Epilepsia*, **32**, 543–549.

Linter, C.M. & Linter, S.P.K. (1986). Severe lactic acidosis following paraldehyde administration. *British Journal of Psychiatry*, **149**, 650–651.

Lion, P. (1967). A case of post-traumatic petit mal status. *Electroencephalography and Clinical Neurophysiology*, **22**, 96–97.

Lipman, I., Isaacs, E. & Suter, C. (1971). Petit mal status: a variety of non-convulsive status epilepticus. *Diseases of the Nervous System*, **32**, 342–345.

Livingston, J.H. & Brown, J.K. (1987). Non-convulsive status epilepticus resistant to benzodiazepines. *Archives of Disease in Childhood*, **62**, 41–44.

Livingston, S., Torres, I., Pauli, L. & Rider, R.V. (1965). Petit mal epilepsy: results of a prolonged follow up study of 117 patients. *Journal of the American Medical Association*, **194**, 227–232.

Lloyd, K.G., Bossi, L., Morselli, P.L., Munari, C., Rougier, M. & Loiseau, H. (1986). Alterations of GABA-mediated synaptic transmission in human epilepsy. In *Basic mechanisms of the epilepsies: molecular and cellular approaches*. Advances in Neurology, vol. 44, ed. A.V. Delgado-Escueta, A.A. Ward Jr, D.M. Woodbury & R.J. Porter, pp. 1033–1044. New York: Raven Press.

Lob, H., Roger, J., Soulayrol, R., Regis, H. & Gastaut, H. (1967). Les états de mal généralisés à l'expression confusionelle. In *Les états de mal épileptiques*, ed. H. Gastaut, J. Roger & H. Lob, pp. 91–109. Paris: Masson.

Lockman, L.A. (1983). Phenobarbital dosage for neonatal seizures. In *Status epilepticus. Mechanisms of brain damage and treatment*. Advances in Neurology, vol. 34, ed. A.V. Delgado-Escueta, C.G. Wasterlain, D.M. Treiman & R.J. Porter, pp. 505–508. New York: Raven Press.

Lockman, L.A. (1989). Paraldehyde. In *Antiepileptic drugs*, 3rd edn, ed. R.H. Levym, F.E. Dreifuss, R.A. Mattson, B.S. Meldrum & J.K. Penry, pp. 881–886. New York: Raven Press.

Lockman, L.A. (1990). Treatment of status epilepticus in children. *Neurology*, **40** (suppl. 2), 43–46.

Lockman, L.A., Kriel, R., Zaske, D., Thompson, T. & Virnig, N. (1979). Phenobarbital dosage for control of neonatal seizures. *Neurology*, **29**, 1445–1449.

Löhler, J. & Peters, U.H. (1974). Epilepsia partialis continua (Kozevnikov-Epilepsie). *Fortschritte der Neurologie-Psychiatrie*, **42**, 185–212.

Loiseau, P. & Cohadon, F. (1970). *Le petit mal et ses frontières*. Paris: Masson.

Lombroso, C.T. (1966). Treatment of status epilepticus with diazepam. *Neurology*, **16**, 629–634.

Lombroso, C.T. (1983). Prognosis in neonatal seizures. In *Status epilepticus. Mechanisms of brain damage and treatment*. Advances in Neurology, vol. 34, ed. A.V. Delgado-Escueta, C.G. Wasterlain, D.M. Treiman & R.J. Porter, pp. 101–113. New York: Raven Press.

Loonen, M.G.B. & van Dongen, H.R. (1990). Acquired childhood aphasia. Outcome one year after onset. *Archives of Neurology*, **47**, 1324–1328.

Lothman, E.W. (1990). The biochemical basis and pathophysiology of status epilepticus. *Neurology*, **40** (suppl. 2), 13–23.

Lothman, E.W. & Bertram, E.H. (1993). Epileptogenic effects of status epilepticus. *Epilepsia*, **34** (suppl. 1), S59–S70.

Lothman, E.W., Bertram, E.H., Beckenstein, J.W. & Perlin, J.B. (1989). Self-sustaining limbic status epilepticus induced by 'continuous' hippocampal stimulation: electrographic and behavioural characteristics. *Epilepsy Research*, **3**, 107–119.

Lothman, E.W., Bertram, E.H., Kapur, J. & Stringer, J.L. (1990). Recurrent spontaneous hippocampal seizures in the rat, as a chronic seqeula to limbic status epilepticus. *Epilepsy Research*, **6**, 110–118.

Lothman, E.W. & Collins, R.C. (1981). Kainic acid induced limbic seizures: metabolic, behavioural, electroencephalographic and neuropathologic correlates. *Brain Research*, **218**, 299–318.

Lothman, E.W., Collins, R.C. & Ferrendelli, J.A. (1981). Kainic acid induced limbic seizures: electrophysiologic studies. *Neurology*, **31**, 806–812.

Lou, H.C., Brandt, S. & Bruhn. P. (1977). Progressive aphasic epilepsy with a self-limited course. In *Epilepsy: the eighth international symposium*, ed. J.K. Penry, pp. 295–303. New York: Raven Press.

Low, L., Stephenson, J.B.P. & Goel, K.M. (1980). Prolonged intravenous use of chlormethiazole (Heminevrin). *British Medical Journal*, **1**, 484.

Lowenstein, D.H. & Alldredge, B.K. (1993). Status epilepticus in an urban public hospital in the 1980s. *Neurology*, **43**, 483–488.

Lowenstein, D.H. & Aminoff, M.J. (1992). Clinical and EEG features of status epilepticus in comatose patients. *Neurology*, **42**, 100–104.

Lowenstein, D.H., Aminoff, M.J. & Simon, R.P. (1988). Barbiturate anesthesia in the treatment of status epilepticus: clinical experience of 14 patients. *Neurology*, **38**, 395–400.

Lüders, H. (ed.) (1992). *Epilepsy surgery*. New York: Raven Press.

Lugaresi, E., Pazzaglia, P. & Tassinari, C.A. (1971). Differentiation of absence status and 'temporal lobe status'. *Epilepsia*, **12**, 77–87.

Lyon, G. & Gastaut, H. (1985). Considerations of the significance attributed to unusual cerebral histological findings recently described in eight patients with primary generalised epilepsy. *Epilepsia*, **26**, 365–367.

Lysons, D. (1772). *Practical essays upon intermitting fevers, dropsies, diseases of the liver, the epilepsy etc.* Bath: Hazard.

McBride, M.C., Dooling, E.C. & Oppenheimer, E.Y. (1981). Complex partial status epilepticus in young children. *Annals of Neurology*, **9**, 526–530.

McGreal, D.A. (1958). The emergency treatment of convulsions in childhood. *Practitioner*, **181**, 719–723.

MacKenzie, S.J., Kapadia, F. & Grant, I.S. (1990). Propofol infusion for control of status epilepticus. *Anaesthesia*, **45**, 1043–1045.

MacKichan, J., Duffner, P.K. & Cohen, M.E. (1979). Adsorption of diazepam to plastic tubing. *New England Journal of Medicine*, **301**, 332–333.

McKinney, W. & McGreal, D.A. (1974). An aphasic syndrome in children. *Journal of the Canadian Medical Association*, **110**, 637–639.

McMorris, S. & McWilliam, P. (1969). Status epilepticus in infants and young children treated with parenteral diazepam. *Archives of Disease in Childhood*, **44**, 604–611.

McWilliam, P.K.A. (1958). Intravenous phenytoin sodium in continuous convulsions in children. *Lancet*, **2**, 1147–1149.

Magnussen, I., Oxlund, H.R.W., Alsbirk, K.E. & Arnold, E. (1979). Absorption of diazepam in man following rectal and parenteral administration. *Acta Pharmacologica et Toxicologica*, **45**, 87–90.

Mäkelä, J.P. & Iivanainen, M., Pieninkeroinen, I.P., Waltimo, O. & Lahdensuu, M. (1993). Seizures associated with propofol anesthesia. *Epilepsia*, **34**, 832–835.

Manford, M. & Shorvon, S.D. (1992). Prolonged sensory or visceral symptoms: an under-diagnosed form of focal, non-convulsive (simple partial) status epilepticus. *Journal of Neurology, Neurosurgery and Psychiatry*, **55**, 714–716.

Manhire, A.R. & Espir, M. (1974). Treatment of status epilepticus with sodium valproate. *British Medical Journal*, **3**, 808.

Mann, L.B. (1954). Status epilepticus occurring in petit mal. *Bulletin of the Los Angeles Neurological Society*, **19**, 96–109.

Manning, D.J. & Rosenbloom, L. (1987). Non-convulsive status epilepticus. *Archives of Disease in Childhood*, **62**, 37–40.

Mantovani, J.F. & Landau, W.M. (1980). Acquired aphasia with convulsive disorder: course and prognosis. *Neurology*, **30**, 524–529.

Maquet, P., Hirsch, E., Dive, D., Salmon, E., Marescaux, C. & Franck, C. (1990). Cerebral glucose utilization during sleep in Landau–Kleffner: a PET study. *Epilepsia*, **31**, 778–783.

Marescaux, C., Hirsch, E., Finck, S., Maquet, P., Schlumberger, E., Sellal, F., Metz-Lutz, M.N., Alembik, Y., Salmon, E., Franck, E. & Kurtz, D. (1990). Landau–Kleffner syndrome: a pharmacologic study of five cases. *Epilepsia*, **31**, 768–777.

Margerison, J.H. & Corsellis, J.A.N. (1966). Epilepsy and the temporal lobes: a clinical electroencephalographic and neuropathological study of the brain with particular reference to the temporal lobes. *Brain*, **89**, 499–530.

Mark, L.C., Burns, J.J., Campomanes, C.I., Ngai, S.H., Trousof, N., Papper, E.M. & Brodie, B.B. (1958). The passage of thiopental into brain. *Journal of Pharmacology and Experimental Therapeutics*, **123**, 35–38.

Markand, O.N. (1977). Slow spike–wave activity in EEG and associated clinical features: often called 'Lennox' or 'Lennox–Gastaut' syndrome. *Neurology*, **27**, 746–757.

Markand, O.N., Wheeler, G.L. & Pollack, S.L. (1978). Complex partial status epilepticus (psychomotor status). *Neurology*, **28**, 189–196.

Markowitsch, H.J. (1992). The neuropsychology of hanging: an historical perspective. *Journal of Neurology, Neurosurgery and Psychiatry*, **55**, 507–512.

Marsden, C.D., Hallett, M. & Fahn, S. (1982). The nosology and pathophysiology of myoclonus. In *Movement disorders*, ed. C.D. Marsden & S. Fahn, pp. 196–248. London: Butterworths.

Martin, D. & Hirt, H.R. (1973). Clinical experience with clonazepam (Rivotril) in the treatment of epilepsies in infancy and childhood. *Neuropädiatrie*, **4**, 245–266.

Massa, T. & Niedermeyer, E. (1968). Convulsive disorders during the first three months of life. *Epilepsia*, **9**, 1–9.

Matthews, P.M., Andermann, F. & Arnold, D.L. (1991). Proton magnetic resonance spectroscopy study of chronic encephalitis and epilepsy. In *Chronic encephalitis and epilepsy: Rasmussen's syndrome*, ed. F. Andermann, pp. 73–77. London: Butterworth-Heinemann.

Mattson, R.H. (1972). Other antiepileptic drugs: the benzodiazepines. In *Antiepileptic drugs*, ed. D.M. Woodbury, J.K. Penry & R.P. Schmidt, pp. 497–516. New York: Raven Press.

Mayeux, R., Alexander, M.P., Benson, D.F., Brandt, J. & Rosen, J. (1979). Poriomania. *Neurology*, **29**, 1616–1619.

Mayeux, R. & Lüders, H. (1978). Complex partial status epilepticus: case report and proposal for diagnostic criteria. *Neurology*, **28**, 957–961.

Mayhue, F.E. (1988). IM midazolam for status epilepticus in the emergency department. *Annals of Emergency Medicine*, **17**, 643–645.

Maytal, J., Novak, G.P. & King, K.C. (1991). Lorazepam in the treatment of refractory neonatal seizures. *Journal of Child Neurology*, **6**, 319–323.

Maytal, J., Shinnar, S., Moshé, S.L. & Alvarez, L.A. (1989). Low morbidity and mortality of status epilepticus in children. *Pediatrics*, **83**, 323–331.

Meberg, A., Langslet, A., Bredesen, J.E. & Lunde, P.K.M. (1978). Plasma concentration of diazepam and *N*-desmethyldiazepam in children after a single rectal or intramuscular dose of diazepam. *European Journal of Clinical Pharmacology*, **14**, 273–276.

Meencke, H.-J. (1985). Neuronal density in the molecular layer of the frontal cortex in primary generalised epilepsy. *Epilepsia*, **26**, 450–454.

Meencke, H.-J. (1991). Pathology of childhood epilepsies. *Cleveland Clinic Journal of Medicine*, **56** (suppl. 1), S111-S120.

Meencke, H.J. (1994). Minimal developmental disturbances in epilepsy and MRI. In *Magnetic resonance scanning and epilepsy*, ed. S.D. Shorvon, D.R. Fish, F. Andermann, G. Bydder & H. Stefan. London: Plenum Press, in press.

Meencke, H.-J. & Janz, D. (1984). Neuropathological findings in primary generalised epilepsy: a study of eight cases. *Epilepsia*, **25**, 8–21.

Meencke, H.-J. & Janz, D. (1985). The significance of microdysgenesis in primary generalised epilepsy: and answer to the considerations of Lyon and Gastaut. *Epilepsia*, **26**, 368–371.

Meierkord, H. & Shorvon, S.D. (1990). Epilepsie bei Neuroakanthozytose. *Nervenarzt*, **61**, 692–694.

Meierkord, H., Will, B., Fish, D. & Shorvon, S. (1991). The clinical features and prognosis of pseudoseizures diagnosed using video-EEG telemetry. *Neurology*, **41**, 1643–1646.

Meiners, L.C., Valk, J., Jansen, G.H. & Luyten, P.R. (1994). MR of epilepsy: three observations. In *Magnetic resonance scanning and epilepsy*, ed. S.D. Shorvon, D.R. Fish, F. Andermann, G. Bydder & H. Stefan. London: Plenum Press, in press.

Melamed, E. (1976). Reactive hyperglycaemia in patients with acute stroke. *Journal of the Neurological Sciences*, **29**, 267–275.

Meldrum, B.S. (1983). Metabolic factors during prolonged seizures and their relation to cell death. In *Status epilepticus. Mechanisms of brain damage and treatment*. Advances in Neurology, vol. 34, ed. A.V. Delgado-Escueta, C.G. Wasterlain, D.M. Treiman & R.J. Porter, pp. 261–275. New York: Raven Press.

Meldrum, B.S. (1986). Cell damage in epilepsy and the role of calcium cytotoxicity. In *Basic mechanisms of the epilepsies: molecular and cellular approaches*. Advances in Neurology, vol. 44, ed. A.V. Delgado-Escueta, A.A. Ward, D.M. Woodbury, R.J. Porter, pp. 849–855. New York: Raven Press.

Meldrum, B.S. & Brierley, J.B. (1973). Prolonged epileptic seizures in primates: ischemic cell change and its relation to ictal physiological events. *Archives of Neurology*, **28**, 10–17.

Meldrum, B.S. & Corsellis J.A.N. (1984). Epilepsy. In *Greenfield's neuropathology*, 4th edn, ed. J. Hume Adams, J.A.N. Corsellis & L.W. Duchen, pp. 921–950. New York: Raven Press.

Meldrum, B.S., Ferendelli, J.A. & Wieser, H.G. (eds.) (1988). *Anatomy of epileptogenesis*. London: John Libbey.

Meldrum, B.S., Horton, R.W., Bloom, S.R., Butler, J. & Keenan, J. (1979). Endocrine factors and glucose metabolism during seizures in baboons. *Epilepsia*, **20**, 527–534.

Meldrum, B.S. & Horton, R.W. (1973). Physiology of status epilepticus in primates. *Archives of Neurology*, **28**, 1–9.

Meldrum, B.S. & Horton, R.W. (1980). Effects of the bicyclic GABA agonist, THIP, on myoclonic and seizure responses in mice and baboons with reflex epilepsy. *European Journal of Pharmacology*, **61**, 231–237.

Meldrum, B.S., Horton, R.W. & Brierley, J.B. (1974). Epileptic brain damage in adolescent baboons following seizures induced by allylglycine. *Brain*, **97**, 407–418.

Meldrum, B.S. & Nilsson, B. (1976). Cerebral blood flow and metabolic rate early and late in prolonged epileptic seizures induced in rats by bicuculline. *Brain*, **99**, 523–542.

Meldrum, B.S., Vigouroux, R.A. & Brierley, J.B. (1973). Systemic factors and epileptic brain damage. *Archives of Neurology*, **29**, 82–87.

Menini, C., Meldrum, B.S., Riche, D., Silva-Comte, C. & Stutzmann, J.M. (1980). Sustained limbic seizures induced by intra-amygdaloid kainic acid in the baboon: symptomatology and neuropathological consequences. *Annals of Neurology*, **8**, 501–509

Menini, C. & Naquet, R. (1986). Les myoclonies: des myoclonies du *Papio papio* à certaines myoclonies humaines. *Revue Neurologique*, **142**, 3–28.

Merlis, S. (1960). Status epilepticus in petit mal: a case report. *Pediatrics*, **26**, 654–656.

Messing, R.O., Closson, R.G. & Simon, R.P. (1984). Drug-induced seizures: a 10-year experience. *Neurology*, **34**, 1582–1586.

Meyer, A., Beck, E. & Shepherd, M. (1955). Unusually severe lesions in the brain following status epilepticus. *Journal of Neurology, Neurosurgery and Psychiatry*, **18**, 24–33.

Michaels, R.L. & Rothman, S.M. (1990). Glutamate neurotoxicity in vitro: antagonist pharmacology and intracellular calcium concentrations. *Journal of Neuroscience*, **10**, 283–292.

Mikati, M.A., Lee, W.L. & DeLong, G.R. (1985). Protracted epileptiform encephalopathy: an unusual form of partial complex partial epilepticus. *Epilepsia*, **26**, 563–571.

Milde, L.N. & Milde, J.H. (1986). Preservation of cerebral metabolites by etomidate during incomplete cerebral ischemia in dogs. *Anesthesiology*, **65**, 272–277.

Miller, P. & Kovar, I. (1983). Chlormethiazole in the treatment of neonatal status epilepticus. *Postgraduate Medical Journal*, **59**, 801–802.

Milligan, N., Dhillon, S., Oxley, J. & Richens, A. (1982). Absorption of diazepam from the rectum and its effects on interictal spikes in the EEG. *Epilepsia*, **23**, 323–331.

Mitchell, W.G. & Crawford, T.O. (1990). Lorazepam is the treatment of choice for status epilepticus. *Journal of Epilepsy*, **3**, 7–10.

Mizrahi, E.M. & Kellaway, P. (1987). Characterisation and classification of neonatal seizures. *Neurology*, **37**, 1837–1844.

Moe, P.G. (1971). Spike–wave stupor. *American Journal of Diseases of Children*, **121**, 307–313.

Monod, N. & Dreyfus-Brisac, C. (1972). Neonatal status epilepticus. In *Handbook of EEG and clinical neurophysiology*, vol. 15B, ed. A. Rémond, pp. 38–52. Amsterdam: Elsevier Publishing Co.

Moore, R.G., Triggs, E.J., Shanks, C.A. & Thomas, J. (1975). Pharmacokinetics of chlormethiazole in humans. *European Journal of Clinical Pharmacology*, **8**, 353–357.

Mori, T., Kato, H., Ikeda, S. & Morizaki, I. (1977). Antiepileptic activity of clonazepam: a benzodiazepine antiepileptic. II. Effects of intravenous injection of clonazepam. *Brain and Nerve*, **29**, 171–180.

Morikawa, T., Seino, M., Osawa, R. & Yagi, K. (1985). Five children with continuous spike–wave discharges during sleep. In *Epileptic syndromes in infancy, childhood and adolescence*, ed. J. Roger, C. Dravet, M. Bureau, F.E. Dreifuss & P. Wolf, pp. 205–215. London: John Libbey.

Morikawa, T., Seino, M., Watanabe, Y., Watanabe, M. & Yagi, K. (1989). Clinical relevance of continuous spike–waves during slow wave sleep. In *The Eighth epilepsy international symposium*, ed. J. Manelis, E. Bental, J.N. Loeber & F.E. Dreifuss, pp. 359–363. New York: Raven Press.

Morin, A.M. & Wasterlain, C.G. (1983). Role of receptors for neurotransmitters in status epilepticus. In *Status epilepticus. Mechanisms of brain damage and treatment*. Advances in Neurology, vol. 34, ed. A.V. Delgado-Escueta, C.G. Wasterlain, D.M. Treiman & R.J. Porter, pp. 369–374. New York: Raven Press.

Morrison, G., Chiang, S.T., Koepke, H.H. & Walker, B.R. (1984). Effect of renal impairment and hemodialysis on lorazepam kinetics. *Clinical Pharmacology and Therapeutics*, **35**, 646–652.

Msall, M., Shapiro, B., Balfour, P.B., Niedermeyer, E. & Capute, A.J. (1986). Acquired epileptic aphasia: diagnostic aspects of progressive language loss in preschool children. *Clinical Pediatrics*, **25**, 248–251.

Munari, C., Casaroli, D., Matteuzzi, G. & Pacifico, L. (1979). The use of althesin in drug-resistant status epilepticus. *Epilepsia*, **20**, 475–483.

Munari, C., Soncini, M., Brunet, P., Musolino, A., Chodkiewicz, J.P., Talairach, J. & Bancaud, J. (1985). Sémiologie électroclinique des crises temporales subintrantes. *Revue d'Electroencéphalographie et de Neurophysiologie Clinique*, **15**, 289–298.

Murasaki, M. & Takahashi, A. (1988). Complex partial status epilepticus. *Japanese Journal of Psychiatry*, **42**, 515–519.

Muskens, L.J.J. (1928). *Epilepsy: comparative pathogenesis, symptoms and treatment*, pp. 356–358. London: Balliere, Tindall and Cox.

Nadler, J.V. (1981). Kainic acid as a tool for the study of temporal lobe epilepsy. *Life Sciences*, **29**, 2031–2042

Nadler, J.V., Okazaki, M.M., Gruenthal, M., Ault, B. & Armstrong, D.R. (1986). Kainic acid seizures and neuronal cell death: insights from studies of selective lesions and drugs.

In *Excitatory amino acids and epilepsy*. Advances in Experimental Medicine and Biology, vol. 203, ed. R. Schwartz & Y. Ben-Ari, pp. 673–686. New York: Plenum Press.

Naquet, R., Soulayrol, R., Dolce, G., Tassinari, C.A., Broughton, R. & Loeb, H. (1965). First attempt at treatment of experimental status epilepticus in animals and spontaneous status epilepticus in man with diazepam. *Electroencephalography and Clinical Neurophysiology*, **18**, 424–427.

Nation, R.L., Learoyd, B., Barber, J. & Triggs, E.J. (1976). The pharmacokinetics of chlormethiazole following intravenous administration in the aged. *European Journal of Clinical Pharmacology*, **10**, 407–415.

Nelson, K.B. & Ellenberg, J.H. (eds.) (1981). *Febrile seizures*. New York: Raven Press.

Nevander, G., Ingvar, M., Auer, R.N. & Siesjo B.K. (1985). Status epilepticus in well oxygenated rats causes neuronal necrosis. *Annals of Neurology*, **18**, 281–290.

Niedermeyer, E. (1968). The Lennox–Gastaut syndrome: a severe type of childhood epilepsy. *Electroencephalography and Clinical Neurophysiology*, **24**, 283.

Niedermeyer, E. & Degen, R. (eds.) (1988). *The Lennox Gastaut syndrome*. Neurology and Neurobiology, vol. 45. New York: Alan R. Liss.

Niedermeyer, E., Fineyre, F., Riley, T. & Uematsu. S. (1979). Absence status (petit mal status) with focal characteristics. *Archives of Neurology*, **36**, 417–421.

Niedermeyer, E. & Khalifeh, R. (1965). Petit mal status ('spike–wave stupor'): an electroclinical appraisal. *Epilepsia*, **6**, 250–262.

Nicol, C.F., Tutton, J.C. & Smith, B.H. (1969). Parenteral diazepam in status epilepticus. *Neurology*, **19**, 332–343.

Nicoll, J.M.V. (1986). Status epilepticus following enflurane anaesthesia. *Anaesthesia*, **41**, 927–930.

Nightingale, S. & Welch, J. (1982). Psychometric assessment in absence status. *Archives of Neurology*, **39**, 516–519.

Noach, E.L. & van Rees, H. (1964). Intestinal distribution of intravenously administered diphenylhydantoin in the rat. *Archives of International Pharmacodynamics and Therapeutics*, **150**, 52–61.

Noach, E.L., Woodbury, D.M. & Goodman, L.S. (1958). Studies on the absorption, distribution, fate and excretion of 4-^{14}C-labelled diphenylhydantoin. *Journal of Pharmacology and Experimental Therapeutics*, **122**, 301–314.

Noel, P., Cornil, A., Chailly, P. & Flament-Durand, J. (1977). Mesial temporal haemorrhage consequent on status epilepticus. *Journal of Neurology, Neurosurgery and Psychiatry*, **40**, 932–935.

Norman, R.M. (1964). The neuropathology of status epilepticus. *Medicine, Science and the Law*, **4**, 46–51.

Novak, J., Corke, P. & Fairley, N. (1971). 'Petit mal status' in adults. *Diseases of the Nervous System*, **32**, 245–248.

Obeso, J.A., Rothwell, J.C. & Marsden, C.D. (1985). The spectrum of cortical myoclonus. *Brain*, **108**, 193–224.

Ochs, H.R., Busse, J., Greenblatt, D.J. & Allen, M.D. (1980). Entry of lorazepam into cerebrospinal fluid. *British Journal of Clinical Pharmacology*, **10**, 405–406.

O'Donohoe, N.V. (1979). *Epilepsies of childhood*. London: Butterworths.

Oguni, H., Andermann, F. & Rasmussen, T.B. (1991). The natural history of chronic encephalitis and epilepsy: a study of the MNI series of forty-eight cases. In *Chronic encephalitis and epilepsy: Rasmussen's syndrome*, ed. F. Andermann, pp. 7–36. Boston, MA: Butterworth-Heinemann.

Ohtahara, S., Ohtsuka, Y., Yamatogi, Y. & Oka, E. (1987). The early-infantile epileptic encephalopathy with suppression-burst: developmental aspects. *Brain and Development*, 9, 371–376.

Ohtahara, S., Ohtsuka, Y., Yamatogi, Y., Oka, E. & Inoue, H. (1992). The early-infantile epileptic encephalopathy with suppression-bursts. In *Epileptic syndromes in infancy, childhood and adolescence*, 2nd edn. ed. J. Roger, M. Bureau, C. Dravet, F.E. Dreifuss, A. Perret & P. Wolf, pp. 25–35. London: John Libbey.

Ohtahara, S., Ohtsuka, Y., Yoshinaga, H., Iyoda, K., Amano, R., Yamatogi, Y. & Oka, E. (1988). Lennox–Gastaut syndrome: etiological considerations. In *The Lennox–Gastaut syndrome*. Neurology and Neurobiology, vol. 45, ed. E. Niedermeyer & R. Degen, pp. 47–64. New York: Alan R. Liss.

Ohtahara, S., Oka, E., Bau, T., Yamatogi, Y. & Inoue, H. (1970). The Lennox syndrome. Electroencephalographic study. *Clinical Neurology*, 10, 617–625.

Ohtahara, S., Oka, E., Yamatogi, Y., Ohtsuka, Y., Ishida, T., Ichiba, N., Ishida, S. & Miyake, S. (1979). Non-convulsive status epilepticus in childhood. *Folia Psychiatrica et Neurologica Japonica*, 33, 345–351.

Olivier, A. (1991). Corticectomy for the treatment of seizures due to chronic encephalitis. In *Chronic encephalitis and epilepsy: Rasmussen's syndrome*, ed. F. Andermann, pp. 205–212. Boston, MA: Butterworth-Heinemann.

Oller-Daurella, L. (1973). Evolution et pronostic du syndrome de Lennox-Gastaut. In *Evolution and prognosis of epilepsies*, ed. E. Lugaresi, P. Pazzaglia & C.A. Tassinari, pp. 155–164. Bologna: Aulo Gaggi.

Oller-Daurella, L. & Oller, L. (1988). The Lennox–Gastaut syndrome: synopsis. In *The Lennox Gastaut syndrome*. Neurology and Neurobiology, vol. 45, ed. E. Niedermeyer & R. Degen, pp. 387–398. New York: Alan R. Liss.

Olney, J.W. (1985). Excitatory transmitters and epilepsy-related brain damage. *International Review of Neurobiology*, 27, 337–362.

Olney J.W. (1986). Inciting excitotoxic cytocide among central neurons. In *Excitatory amino acids and epilepsy*. Advances in Experimental Medicine and Biology, vol. 203, ed. R. Schwarcz & Y. Ben-Ari, pp. 631–646. New York: Plenum Press.

Olney, J.W., Collins, R.C. & Sloviter, R.S. (1986). Excitotoxic mechanisms of epileptic brain damage. In *Basic mechanisms of the epilepsies: molecular and cellular approaches*. Advances in Neurology, vol. 44, ed. A.V. Delgado-Escueta, A.A. Ward Jr, D.M. Woodbury & R.J. Porter, pp. 857–878. New York: Raven Press.

Olney, J.W., de Gubareff, T. & Labruyère, J. (1983a). Seizure related brain damage induced by cholinergic agents. *Nature*, 301, 520–522.

Olney, J.W., de Gubareff, T. & Sloviter, R.S. (1983b). 'Epileptic' brain damage in rats induced by sustained electrical stimulation of the perforant path. 11. Ultrastructural analysis of acute hippocampal pathology. *Brain Research Bulletin*, 10, 699–712.

Olney, J.W., Fuller, T.A., Collins, R.C. & de Gubareff, T. (1980). Systemic dipiperidinoethane mimics the convulsant and neurotoxic action of kainic acid. *Brain Research*, 200, 231–235.

Olney, J.W., Fuller, T. & de Gubareff T. (1979). Acute dendrotoxic changes in the hippocampus of kainate treated rats. *Brain Research*, 176, 91–100.

Olney, J.W., Rhee, V. & Ho, O.L. (1974). Kainic acid: a powerful neurotoxic analogue of glutamate. *Brain Research*, 77, 507–512.

Omorokov, L.I. (1927). [Kozhevnikov's epilepsy in Siberia] transl. by D.M. Asher, 1991. In *Chronic encephalitis and epilepsy: Rasmussen's syndrome*, ed. F. Andermann, pp. 263–269. Boston, MA: Butterworth-Heinemann.

Orlowski, J.P., Erenberg, G., Lüders, H., & Cruse, R.P. (1984). Hypothermia and barbiturate coma for refractory status epilepticus. *Critical Care Medicine*, **12**, 367–372.

Ormandy, G.C., Jope, R.S. & Snead, O.C. (1989). Anticonvulsant actions of MK-801 on the lithium-pilocarpine model of status epilepticus in rats. *Experimental Neurology*, **106**, 172–180.

Osawa, T., Seino, M., Miyokashi, M., Yamamoto, K., Kakagawa, N., Yagi, K., Hirata, T., Morikawa, T. & Wada, T. (1977). Therapy-resistant epilepsy with long-term history. Slow spike and wave syndrome. In *Epilepsy. The eighth international symposium*, ed. J.K. Penry, pp. 63–68. New York: Raven Press.

Osorio, I. & Reed, R.C. (1988). Phenobarbital for status epilepticus. *Neurology*, **38**, 1504–1505.

Osorio, I. & Reed, R.C. (1989). Treatment of refractory generalised tonic-clonic status epilepticus with pentobarbital anaesthesia after high-dose phenytoin. *Epilepsia*, **30**, 464–471.

Ounsted, C., Lindsay, J. & Norman, R. (1966). Biological factors in temporal lobe epilepsy. *Clinics in Developmental Medicine*, **22**, 1–135.

Oxbury, J.M. & Whitty, C.W.M. (1971a). Causes and consequences of status epilepticus in adults: a study of 86 cases. *Brain*, **94**, 733–744.

Oxbury, J.M. & Whitty, C.W.M. (1971b). The syndrome of isolated epileptic status. *Journal of Neurology, Neurosurgery and Psychiatry*, **34**, 182–184.

Painter, M.J., Minnigh, B., Mollica, L. & Alvin, J. (1987). Binding profiles of anticonvulsants in neonates with seizures. *Annals of Neurology*, **22**, 413.

Painter, M.J., Pippenger, C., Wasterlain, C., Barmada, M., Pitlick, W., Carter, G. & Abern, S. (1981). Phenobarbital and phenytoin in neonatal seizures: metabolism and tissue distribution. *Neurology*, **31**, 1107–1112.

Pakalnis, A., Drake, M.E. & Phillips, B. (1991). Neuropsychiatric aspects of psychogenic status epilepticus. *Neurology*, **41**, 1104–1106.

Panayiotopoulos, C.P. (1989). Benign childhood epilepsy with occipital paroxysms: a 15-year prospective study. *Annals of Neurology*, **26**, 51–56.

Paquier, P.F., van Dongen, H.R. & Loonen, C.B. (1992). The Landau–Kleffner syndrome or 'acquired aphasia with convulsive disorder': long term follow up of six children and a review of the recent literature. *Archives of Neurology*, **49**, 354–359.

Parke, T.J., Stevens, J.E., Rice, A.S.C., Greenway, C.L., Bray, R.J., Smith, P.J., Waldmann, C.S. & Verghese, C. (1992). Metabolic acidosis and fatal myocardial failure after propofol infusions in children: five case reports. *British Medical Journal*, **305**, 613–616.

Parsonage, M.J. & Norris, J.W. (1967). Use of diazepam in treatment of severe convulsive status epilepticus. *British Medical Journal*, **3**, 85–88.

Partinen, M., Kovanen, J. & Nilsson, E. (1981). Status epilepticus treated with barbiturate anaesthesia with continuous monitoring of cerebral function. *British Medical Journal*, **282**, 520–521.

Pascual, J., Ciudad, J. & Berciano, J. (1992). Role of lidocaine (lignocaine) in managing status epilepticus. *Journal of Neurology, Neurosurgery and Psychiatry*, **55**, 49–51.

Pascual, J., Sedano, M.J., Polo, J.M. & Berciano, J. (1988). Intravenous lidocaine for status epilepticus. *Epilepsia*, **29**, 584–589.

Pascual-Castroviejo, I., Martin, V.L., Bermejo, A.M. & Higueras, A.P. (1992). Is cerebral arteritis the cause of the Landau-Kleffner syndrome? Four cases in childhood with angiographic study. *Canadian Journal of Neurological Sciences*, **19**, 46–52.

Passouant, P., Cadilhac, J., Ribstein, M., Delange, M. & Castan, P. (1967). Les états de mal partiels. In *Les états de mal épileptique: compte rendu de la réunion européenne d'information électroencéphalographique*, Xth Colloque de Marseille 1962, ed. H. Gastaut, J. Roger & H. Lob, pp. 152–181. Paris: Masson.

Passouant, P., Duc, N. & Cadilhac, J. & Minvielle, J. (1957). Accès confusionnel de longue durée et décharge épileptique temporale au cours de l'évolution d'une paralysie générale. *Revue Neurologique*, **96**, 329–332.

Patry, G., Lyagoubi, S. & Tassinari, C.A. (1971). Subclinical 'electrical status epilepticus' induced by sleep in children. *Archives of Neurology*, **24**, 242–252.

Patsalos, P.N., Bell, D.M., Richards, G., Sander, J.W.A.S., Oxley, J.R., Dhillon, S. & Cromarty, J. (1991). Pharmacokinetic evaluation of intravenous and intramuscular midazolam in patients with epilepsy. *Epilepsia*, **32** (suppl. 1), 29.

Pauca, A.L. & Dripps, R.D. (1973). Clinical experience with isoflurane (Forane). *British Journal of Anaesthesia*, **45**, 697–703.

Penfield, W.P. (1927). The mechanisms of cicatricial contraction in brain. *Brain*, **50**, 499–517.

Penfield, W.P. & Humphries, S. (1940). Epileptogenic lesions of the brain: a histological study. *Archives of Neurology and Psychiatry*, **43**, 240–261.

Penfield, W.P. & Jasper, H.H. (1954). *Epilepsy and the functional anatomy of the human brain.* Boston, MA: Little Brown.

Pentikäinen, P.J., Neuvonen, P.J. & Jostell, K.-G. (1980). Pharmacokinetics of chlormethiazole in healthy volunteers and patients with cirrhosis of the liver. *European Journal of Clinical Pharmacology*, **17**, 275–284.

Pentikäinen, P.J., Valtonen, V.V. & Miettinen, T.A. (1976). Deaths in connection with chlormethiazole (Heminevrin) therapy. *International Journal of Clinical Pharmacology*, **14**, 225–230.

Perlin, J.B., Churn, S.B., Lothman, E.W. & DeLorenzo, R.J. (1992). Loss of type 11 calcium/calmodulin-dependent kinase activity correlates with stages of development of electrographic seizures in status epilepticus in rat. *Epilepsy Research*, **11**, 111–118.

Perry, T.L. & Hansen, S. (1981). Amino acid abnormalities in epileptogenic foci. *Neurology*, **31**, 872–876.

Petersen, U., Koepp, P., Solmsen, M. & von Villiez, T. (1978). Aphasie im Kindesalter mit EEG Verndärungen. *Neuropädiatrie*, **9**, 84–96.

Petroff, O.A.C., Prichard, J.W., Behar, K.L., Alger, J.R. & Shulman, R.G. (1984). In vivo phosphorus nuclear magnetic resonance spectroscopy in status epilepticus. *Annals of Neurology*, **16**, 169–177.

Pfleger, L. (1880). Beobachtungen uber schrumpfung und Sclerose des Ammonshornes bei Epilepsie. *Allgemeine Zeitschrift für Psychiatrie*, **36**, 359–365.

Phillips, R.E. & Solomon, T. (1990). Cerebral malaria in children. *Lancet*, **336**, 1355–1359.

Phillips, S.A. & Shanahan, R.J. (1989). Etiology and mortality of status epilepticus in children. *Archives of Neurology*, **46**, 74–76.

Piatt, J.H. & Schiff, S.J. (1984). High dose barbiturate therapy in neurosurgery and intensive care. *Neurosurgery*, **15**, 427–444.

Pilke, A., Partinen, M. & Kovanen, J. (1984). Status epilepticus and alcohol abuse: an analysis of 82 status epilepticus admissions. *Acta Neurologica Scandinavica*, **70**, 443–450.

Pinder, R.M., Brogden, R.N., Speight, T.M. & Avery, G.S. (1976). Clonazepam: a review of its pharmacological properties and therapeutic efficacy in epilepsy. *Drugs*, **12**, 321–361.

Pisani, F., Gallitto, G. & Di Perri, R. (1991). Could lamotrigine be useful in status epilepticus? A case report. *Journal of Neurology, Neurosurgery and Psychiatry*, **54**, 845–846.

Plouin, P. (1985). Benign neonatal convulsions (familiar and nonfamilial). In *Epileptic syndromes in infancy, childhood and adolescence*, ed. J. Roger, C. Dravet, M. Bureau, F.E. Dreifuss & P. Wolf, pp. 2–11. London: John Libbey.

Plouin, P. (1992). Benign idiopathic neonatal convulsions (familial and non-familial). In *Epileptic syndromes in infancy, childhood and adolescence*, 2nd edn, ed. J. Roger, M. Bureau, C. Dravet, F.E. Dreifuss, A. Perret & P. Wolf, pp. 3–11. London: John Libbey.

Plouin, P., Sternberg, B., Bour, F. & Lerique, A. (1981). Etats de mal néonataux d'étiologie indéterminée. *Revue d'Electroencéphalographie et de Neurophysiologie Clinique*, **11**, 385–389.

Poiré, R., Royer, P., Degraeve, M. & Rustin, C. (1963). Traitement des états de mal épileptiques par le 'CTZ base' (dérivé de la fraction thiazolique de la vitamine B1). Etude électroclinique. *Revue Neurologique*, **108**, 112–126.

Porter, R.J. & Layzer, R.B. (1975). Plasma albumin concentration and diphenylhydantoin in man. *Archives of Neurology*, **32**, 298–303.

Porter, R.J. & Penry, J.K. (1983). Petit mal status. In *Status epilepticus. Mechanisms of brain damage and treatment*. Advances in Neurology, vol. 34, ed. A.V. Delgado-Escueta, C.G. Wasterlain, D.M. Treiman & R.J. Porter, pp. 61–67. New York: Raven Press.

Poulton, T.J. & Ellington R.J. (1984). Seizure associated with induction of anesthesia with isoflurane. *Anesthesiology*, **61**, 471–476.

Power, C., Poland, S.D., Blume, W.T., Girvin, J.P. & Rice, G.P.A. (1990). Cytomegalovirus and Rasmussen's encephalitis. *Lancet*, **336**, 1282–1284.

Prensky, A.L., Raff, M.C., Moore, M.J. & Schwab, R.S. (1967). Intravenous diazepam in the treatment of prolonged seizure activity. *New England Journal of Medicine*, **276**, 779–784.

Prichard, J.C. (1822). *A treatise on diseases of the nervous system*. London: Underwood.

Primavera, A., Bo, G.P. & Venturi, S. (1988). Aphasic status epilepticus. *European Neurology*, **28**, 255–257.

Prince, D.A. (1985). Physiological mechanisms of focal epileptogenesis. *Epilepsia*, **26** (suppl. 1), S3–S14.

Pritchard, P.B., Holmstrom, V.L., Roitzsch, J.C. & Giacinto, J. (1985). Epileptic amnesic attacks: benefit from antiepileptic drugs. *Neurology*, **35**, 1188–1189.

Pritchard, P.B. & O'Neal, D.B. (1984). Nonconvulsive status epilepticus following metrizamide myelography. *Annals of Neurology*, **16**, 252–254.

Privitera, M.D., Morris, G.L. & Gilliam F. (1991). Postictal language assessment and lateralisation of complex partial seizures. *Annals of Neurology*, **30**, 391–396.

Pulsinelli, W.A., Levy, D.E., Sigabee, B., Scherer, P. & Plum, F. (1983). Increased damage after ischemic stroke in patients with hyperglycemia with or without established diabetes. *American Journal of Medicine*, **74**, 540–544.

Putnam, T.J. & Merritt, H.H. (1941). Dullness as an epileptic equivalent. *Archives of Neurology*, **45**, 797–813.

Racy, A., Osborn, M.A., Vern, B.A. & Molinari, G.F. (1980). Epileptic aphasia: first onset of prolonged monosymptomatic status epilepticus in adults. *Archives of Neurology*, **37**, 419–422.

Radvanyi-Bouvet, M.F., Vallecalle, M.H., Morel-Kahn, F., Relier, J.P. & Dreyfus-Brisac, C. (1985). Seizures and electrical discharges in premature infants. *Neuropediatrics*, **16**, 143–148.

Raines, A., Blake, G.J., Richardson, B. & Gilbert, M.B. (1979). Differential selectivity of several barbiturates on experimental seizures and neurotoxicity in the mouse. *Epilepsia*, **20**, 105–113.

Raines, A., Henderson, T.R., Swinyard, E.A. & Dretchen, K.L. (1990). Comparison of midazolam and diazepam by the intramuscular route for the control of seizures in a mouse model of status epilepticus. *Epilepsia*, **31**, 313–317.

Ramsey, R.E. (1989). Pharmacokinetics and clinical use of parenteral phenytoin, phenobarbital, and paraldehyde. *Epilepsia*, **30** (suppl. 2), S1–S3.

Ramsey, R.E. (1993). Treatment of status epilepticus. *Epilepsia*, **34** (suppl. 1), S71–S81.

Ramsey, R.E., Hammond, E.J., Perchalski, R.J. & Wilder, B.J. (1979). Brain uptake of phenytoin, phenobarbital, and diazepam. *Archives of Neurology*, **36**, 535–539.

Rapin, I., Mattis, S., Rowan, A.J. & Golden, G.G. (1977). Verbal auditory agnosia in children. *Developmental Medicine and Child Neurology*, **19**, 192–207.

Rapport R.L. II, Harris, A.B., Friel, P.N. & Ojemann, G.A. (1975). Human epileptic brain: Na, K ATPase activity and phenytoin concentrations. *Archives of Neurology*, **32**, 549–554.

Rashkin, M.C., Youngs, C. & Penovich, P. (1987). Pentobarbital treatment of refractory status epilepticus. *Neurology*, **37**, 500–503.

Rasmussen, T., Olszweski, J. & Lloyd-Smith, D.L. (1958). Focal seizures due to chronic localized encephalitis. *Neurology*, **8**, 435–445.

Ravnik, I. (1985). A case of Landau–Kleffner syndrome: effect of intravenous diazepam. In *Epileptic syndromes in infancy, childhood and adolescence*, ed. J. Roger, C. Dravet, M. Bureau, F.E. Dreifuss & P. Wolf, pp. 192–193. London: John Libbey.

Raymond, A.A., Cook, M., Fish, D.R. & Shorvon, S.D. (1993). Cortical dysgenesis in adults with epilepsy. In *Magnetic resonance scanning and epilepsy*, ed. S.D. Shorvon, D.R. Fish, F. Andermann, G. Bydder & H. Stefan. London: Plenum Press, in press.

Rémy, C., Jourdil, N., Villemain, D., Favel, P. & Genton, P. (1992). Intrarectal diazepam in epileptic adults. *Epilepsia*, **33**, 353–358.

Rennick, M., Perez-Borja, C. & Rodin, E.A. (1969). Transient mental deficits associated with recurrent prolonged epileptic clouded state. *Epilepsia*, **10**, 397–405.

Ribak, C.E. (1986). Contemporary methods in neurocytology and their application to the study of epilepsy. In *Basic mechanisms of the epilepsies: molecular and cellular approaches*. Advances in Neurology, vol. 44, ed. A.V. Delgado-Escueta, A.A. Ward Jr, D.M. Woodbury & R.J. Porter, pp. 739–764. New York: Raven Press.

Ribak, C.E., Hunt, C.A., Barkay, R.A.E. & Oertel, W.H. (1986). A decrease in the number of GABAergic somata is associated with the preferential loss of GABAergic terminals at epleptic foci. *Brain Research*, **363**, 78–90.

Ribak, C.E. & Reiffenstein, R.J. (1982). Selective inhibitory synapse loss in chronic cortical slabs: a morphological basis for epileptic susceptibility. *Canadian Journal of Physiology and Pharmacology*, **60**, 864–870.

Richard, P. & Brenner, R.P. (1980). Absence status: case reports and a review of the literature. *L'Encéphale*, **6**, 385–392.

Richard, M.O., Chiron, C., d'Athis, P., Aubourg, P., Dulac, O. & Olive, G. (1993). Phenytoin monitoring in status epilepticus in infants and children. *Epilepsia*, **34**, 144–150.

Riela, A.R., Sires, B.P. & Penry, J.K. (1991). Transient magnetic resonance imaging abnormalities during partial status epilepticus. *Journal of Child Neurology*, **6**, 143–145.

Ripamonti, L., Cerullo, A., Provini, F., Plazzi, G., Avoni, P. & Tinuper, P. (1991). Stato di male alla chisusura degli occhi. *Bollettino di Lega Italiana Contro L'Epilessia*, **74**, 105–106.

Roberts, E. (1986). Failure of GABAergic inhibition: a key to local and global seizures. In *Basic mechanisms of the epilepsies: molecular and cellular approaches*. Advances in Neurology, vol. 44, ed. A.V. Delgado-Escueta, A.A. Ward Jr, D.M. Woodbury & R.J. Porter, pp. 319–342. New York: Raven Press.

Roberts, M.A. & Humphreys, P.R.D. (1988). Prolonged complex partial status epilepticus: a case report. *Journal of Neurology, Neurosurgery and Psychiatry*, **51**, 586–592.

Robinson, L.J. (1938). Intravenous paraldehyde narcosis for pneumoencephalography. *New England Journal of Medicine*, **219**, 114–117.

Robitaille, Y. (1991). Neuropathologic aspects of chronic encephalitis. In *Chronic encephalitis and epilepsy: Rasmussen's syndrome*, ed. F. Andermann, pp. 79–110. Boston, MA: Butterworth-Heinemann.

Robson, D.J., Blow, C., Gaines, P., Flanagan, R.J. & Henry, J.A. (1984). Accumulation of heminevrin during intravenous infusion. *Intensive Care Medicine*, **10**, 315–316.

Rodriguez, I. & Niedermeyer, E. (1982). The aphasia-epilepsy syndrome in children: electroencephalographic aspects. *Clinical Electroencephalography*, **13**, 23–35.

Roger, J., Bureau, M., Dravet, C., Dalla Bernardina, B., Tassinari, C.A., Revol, J., Challamel, J. & Taillandier, P.I. (1972). Les hémiplégies cérébrales infantiles. Les données EEG et les manifestations épileptiques en relation avec l'hémiplégie cérébrale infantile. *Revue d'Electroencéphalographie et de Neurophysiologie Clinique*, **2**, 5–28.

Roger, J., Bureau, M., Dravet, C., Dreifuss, F.E., Perret, A. & Wolf, P. (eds.) (1992). *Epileptic syndromes in infancy, childhood and adolescence*, 2nd edn. London: John Libbey.

Roger, J., Dravet, C., Bureau, M., Dreifuss, F.E. & Wolf, P. (eds.) (1985). *Epileptic syndromes in infancy, childhood and adolescence*. London: John Libbey.

Roger, J., Lob, H. & Tassinari, C.A. (1974). Status epilepticus. In *Handbook of clinical neurology*, vol. 15. The epilepsies, ed. O. Magnus & A.M. Lorentz de Haas, pp. 145–188. Amsterdam: North Holland Publishing Company.

Roger, J., Rémy, C., Bureau, M., Oller Daurella, L., Beaumanoir, A., Favel, P. & Dravet, C. (1987). Le syndrome de Lennox–Gastaut de l'adulte. *Revue Neurologique*, **143**, 401–405.

Rohr-Le Floch, J., Gauthier, G. & Beaumanoir, A. (1988). Etats confusionnels d'origine épileptique intérêt de l'EEG fait en urgence. *Revue Neurologique*, **144**, 6–7, 425–436.

Ropper, A.H., Kofke, W.A., Bromfield, E.B. & Kennedy, S.K. (1986). Comparison of isoflurane, halothane, and nitrous oxide in status epilepticus. *Annals of Neurology*, **19**, 98–99.

Rose, A.L. & Lombroso, C.T. (1970). Neonatal seizure states: a study of clinical, pathological and electroencephalographic features in 137 full-term babies with a long-term follow-up. *Pediatrics*, **45**, 404–405.

Rosenbaum, D.H., Siegel, M., Barr, W.B. & Rowan, A.J. (1986). Epileptic aphasia. *Neurology*, **36**, 822–825.

Rossier, A., Caldera, R. & Le-Oc-Mach, A. (1973). Les convulsions néonatales. Etude de 53 cas. *Annales de Pédiatrie*, **20**, 869–876.

Rowan, A.J. & Scott, D.F. (1970). Major status epilepticus: a series of 42 patients. *Acta Neurologica Scandinavica*, **46**, 573–584.

Rubinstein, B.K., Walton, N.Y. & Treiman, D.M. (1992). Cardiac hypertrophy secondary to status epilepticus. *Epilepsia*, **33** (suppl. 3), 4.

Rumpl, E. & Hinterhuber, H. (1981). Unusual 'spike–wave stupor' in a patient with manic-depressive psychosis treated with amitriptyline. *Journal of Neurology*, **226**, 131–135.

Rust, R.S. & Dodson, W.E. (1989). Phenobarbital: absorption, distribution and excretion.

In *Antiepileptic drugs*, 3rd edn, ed. R.H. Levy, F.E. Dreifuss, R.A. Mattson, B.S. Meldrum & J.K. Penry, pp. 293–304. New York: Raven Press.

Sacquegna, T., Pazzaglia, P., Baldrati, A., De Carolis, P., Gallassi, R. & Maccheroni, M. (1981). Status epilepticus with cognitive symptomatology in a patient with partial complex epilepsy. *European Neurology*, **20**, 319–325.

Sakaki, T., Abe, K., Hoshida, T., Morimoto, T., Tsunoda, S., Okuchi, K., Miyamoto, A. & Furuya, H. (1992). Isoflurane in the management of status epilepticus after surgery for lesion around the motor area. *Acta Neurochirurgica*, **116**, 38–43.

Sallman, A., Goldberg, M. & Wombolt, D. (1981). Secondary hyperparathyroidism manifesting as acute pancreatitis and status epilepticus. *Archives of Internal Medicine*, **141**, 1549–1550.

Sammaritano, M., Andermann, F., Melanson, D., Pappius, H.M., Camfield, P., Aicardi, J. & Sherwin, A. (1985). Prolonged focal cerebral edema associated with partial status epilepticus. *Epilepsia*, **26**, 334–339.

Sander, J.W.A.S., Hart, Y.M., Johnson, A.L. & Shorvon, S.D. (1990). National general practice study of epilepsy: newly diagnosed epileptic seizures in a general population. *Lancet*, **336**, 1267–1271.

Sano, K. & Malamud, N. (1953). The clinical significance of sclerosis of the cornu ammonis. *Archives of Neurology and Psychiatry*, **70**, 40–53.

Sato, S. (1989). Benzodiazepines: clonazepam. In *Antiepileptic drugs*, 3rd edn, ed. R. Levy, R. Mattson, B. Meldrum, J.K. Penry & F.E. Dreifuss, pp. 765–774. Raven Press: New York.

Sato, S. & Dreifuss, F.E. (1973). Electroencephalographic findings in a patient with developmental expressive aphasia. *Neurology*, **23**, 181–185.

Sawhney, I.M.S., Suresh, N., Dhand, U.K. & Chopra, J.S. (1988). Acquired aphasia with epilepsy – Landau–Kleffner syndrome. *Epilepsia*, **29**, 283–287.

Sawyer, G.T., Webster, D.D. & Schut, L.J. (1968). Treatment of uncontrolled seizure activity with diazepam. *Journal of the American Medical Association*, **203**, 913–918.

Scheibel, M.E., Paul, L. & Fried, I. (1983). Some structural substrates of the epileptic state. In *Basic mechanisms of neuronal hyperexcitability*, ed. H.H. Jasper & N.M. van Gelder, pp. 109–130. New York: Alan R. Liss.

Scheibel, M.E. & Scheibel, A.B. (1973). Hippocampal pathology in temporal lobe epilepsy. A golgi survey. In *Epilepsy. Its phenomena in man*, ed. M.A.B. Brazier, pp. 311–337. New York: Raven Press.

Schmidt, D. (1985). Benzodiazepines – an update. In *Recent advances in epilepsy*, vol. 2, ed. T.A. Pedley & B.S. Meldrum, pp. 125–135. Edinburgh: Churchill Livingstone.

Schmidt, D. (1989). Diazepam. In *Antiepileptic drugs*, 3rd edn, ed. R. Levy, R. Mattson, B. Meldrum, J.K. Penry & F.E. Dreifuss, pp. 735–764. New York: Raven Press.

Scholtz, W. (1933). Uber die entstehung des hirnbefundes bei der Epilepsie. *Zeitschrift für die Gesamte Neurologie und Psychiatrie*, **145**, 471–515.

Schwab, R.S. (1953). A case of status epilepticus in petit mal. *Electroencephalography and Clinical Neurophysiology*, **5**, 441–442.

Schwartz, M.S. & Scott, D.F. (1971). Isolated petit mal status presenting de novo in middle age. *Lancet*, **2**, 1399–1401.

Schwartzkroin, P.A. (1986). Hippocampal slice in experimental and human epilepsy. In *Basic mechanisms of the epilepsies: molecular and cellular approaches*. Advances in Neurology, vol. 44, ed. A.V. Delgado-Escueta, A.A. Ward Jr, D.M. Woodbury & R.J. Porter, pp. 991–1010. New York: Raven Press.

354

Schwartzkroin, P.A. & Wheal, H.V. (eds.) (1984). *Electrophysiology of epilepsy*. London: Academic Press.

Scott, D.B., Beamish, D., Hudson, I.N. & Jostell, K.-G. (1980). Prolonged infusion of chlormethiazole in intensive care. *British Journal of Anaesthesia*, **52**, 541–545.

Scott, J.S. & Masland, R.L. (1952). Occurrence of 'continuous symptoms' in epilepsy patients. *Neurology*, **2**, 297–301.

Seow, L.T., Mather, L.E. & Roberts, J.E. (1981). An integrated study of pharmacokinetics and pharmacodynamics of chlormethiazole in healthy young volunteers. *European Journal of Clinical Pharmacology*, **19**, 263–269.

Shaner, D.M., McCurdy, S.A., Herring, M.O. & Gabor, A.J. (1988). Treatment of status epilepticus: a prospective comparison of diazepam and phenytoin versus phenobarbital and optional phenytoin. *Neurology*, **38**, 202–207.

Sherwin, A.L. (1988). Guide to neurochemical analysis of surgical specimens of human brain. *Epilepsy Research*, **2**, 281–288.

Sherwin, A.L., Eisen, A.A. & Sokolowski, C.D. (1973). Anticonvulsant drugs in human epileptogenic brain: correlation of phenobarbital and diphenylhydantoin levels with plasma. *Archives of Neurology*, **29**, 73–77.

Sherwin, A.L., Quesney, F., Gauthier, S., Olivier, A., Robitaille, Y., McQuaid, P., Harvey, C. & van Gelder, N. (1984). Enzyme changes in actively spiking areas of human epileptic cerebral cortex. *Neurology*, **34**, 927–933.

Sherwin, A.L., Robitaille, Y., Quesney, F., Olivier, A., Villemure, J., LeBlanc, R., Feindel, W., Andermann, E., Gotman, J., Andermann, F., Ethier, R. & Kish, S. (1988). Excitatory amino acids are elevated in human epileptic cerebral cortex. *Neurology*, **38**, 920–923.

Sherwin, A.L. & van Gelder, N.M. (1986). Amino acid and catecholamine markers of metabolic abnormalities in human focal epilepsy. In *Basic mechanisms of the epilepsies: molecular and cellular approaches*. Advances in Neurology, vol. 44. ed. A.V. Delgado-Escueta, A.A. Ward Jr, D. M. Woodbury & R.J. Porter, pp. 1011–1032. New York: Raven Press.

Shields, W.D. (1989). Status epilepticus. *Pediatric Clinics of North America*, **36**, 383–393.

Shinnar, S., Maytal, J., Krasnoff, L. & Moshé, S.L. (1992). Recurrent status epilepticus in children. *Annals of Neurology*, **31**, 598–604.

Shorvon, S.D. (1987). Non-convulsive status epilepticus. *Lancet*, **i**, 958–959.

Shorvon, S.D. (1989). Pseudostatus epilepticus. *Lancet*, **ii**, 485.

Shorvon, S.D. (1992). Classification and clinical characteristics of epilepsy. In *Diseases of the nervous system: clinical neurobiology*, vol. 2, 2nd edn, ed. A.K. Asbury, G.M. McKhann & W.I. McDonald, pp. 906–915. Philadelphia: WB Saunders.

Shorvon, S.D. (1993). Tonic–clonic status epilepticus. *Journal of Neurology, Neurosurgery and Psychiatry*, **56**, 125–134.

Shoumaker, R.D., Bennett, D.R., Bray, P.F. & Curless, R.G. (1974). Clinical and EEG manifestations of an unusual aphasic syndrome in children. *Neurology*, **24**, 10–16.

Siesjö, B.K. & Wieloch, T. (1986). Epileptic brain damage: pathophysiology and neuro-chemical pathology. In *Basic mechanisms of the epilepsies: molecular and cellular approaches*. Advances in Neurology, vol. 44, ed. A.V. Delgado-Escueta, A.A. Ward Jr, D.M. Woodbury & R.J. Porter, pp. 813–847. New York: Raven Press.

Sieveking, E.H. (1857). *On epilepsy and epileptiform seizures*. London.

Silverberg Shalev, R.S. & Amir, N. (1983). Complex partial status epilepticus. *Archives of Neurology*, **40**, 90–92.

355

Simon, R.P. (1985). Physiologic consequences of status epilepticus. *Epilepsia*, 26 (suppl. 1), S58-S66.

Simon, R.P. & Aminoff, M.J. (1980). Clinical aspects of status epilepticus in an unselected urban population. *Transactions of the American Neurological Association*, 105, 46–49.

Simon, R.P. & Aminoff, M.J. (1986). Electrographic status epilepticus in fatal anoxic coma. *Annals of Neurology*, 20, 351–355.

Simon, R.P., Bayne, L.L., Tranbaugh, R.F. & Lewis, F.R. (1982). Elevated pulmonary lymph flow and protein content during status epilepticus in sheep. *Journal of Applied Physiology*, 52, 91–95.

Simon, R.P., Copeland, J.R., Benowitz, N.L., Jacob P. III, & Bronstein, J. (1987). Brain phenobarbital uptake during prolonged status epilepticus. *Journal of Cerebral Blood Flow and Metabolism*, 7, 783–788.

Simpson, H., Habel, A.H. & George, E.L. (1977). Cerebrospinal fluid acid-base status and lactate and pyruvate concentrations after convulsions of varied duration and aetiology in children. *Archives of Disease in Childhood*, 52, 844–849.

Singhal, P.C., Chugh, K.S. & Gulati, D.R. (1978). Myoglobinuria and renal failure after status epilepticus. *Neurology*, 28, 200–201.

Sironi, V.A., Cabrini, G., Porro, M.G., Ravagnati, L. & Marossero, F. (1980). Antiepileptic drug distribution in cerebral cortex, Ammon's horn, and amygdala in man. *Journal of Neurosurgery*, 523, 686–692.

Sloper, J.J., Johnson, P. & Powell, T.P.S. (1980). Selective degeneration of interneurons in the motor cortex of infant monkeys following controlled hypoxia: a possible cause of epilepsy. *Brain Research*, 198, 204–209.

Sloviter, R.S. (1983). Epileptic brain damage in rats induced by sustained electrical stimulation of the perforant path. 1. Acute electrophysiological and light microscopic studies. *Brain Research Bulletin*, 10, 675–697.

Sloviter, R.S. (1986). On the role of seizure activity and endogenous excitatory amino acids in mediating seizure associated hippocampal damage. In *Excitatory amino acids and epilepsy*. Advances in Experimental Medicine and Biology, vol. 203, ed. R. Schwarcz & Y. Ben-Ari, pp. 659–672. New York: Plenum Press.

Sloviter, R.S. (1987). Decreased hippocampal inhibition and a selective loss of interneurons in experimental epilepsy. *Science*, 235, 73–76.

Smith, R.D., Brown, B.S., Maher, R.W. & Matier, W.L. (1989). Pharmacology of ACC-9653 (phenytoin prodrug). *Epilepsia*, 30 (suppl. 2), S15–S21.

Snead, O.C. & Hosey, L.C. (1985). Exacerbation of seizures in children by carbamazepine. *New England Journal of Medicine*, 313, 916–921.

Snead, O.C. & Miles, M.V. (1985). Treatment of status epilepticus in children with rectal sodium valproate. *Journal of Pediatrics*, 106, 323–325.

Snodgrass, S.M., Tsuburaya, K. & Ajmone-Marsan, C. (1989). Clinical significance of periodic lateralised epileptiform discharges: relationship with status epilepticus. *Journal of Clinical Neurophysiology*, 6, 159–172.

So, N., Berkovic, S., Andermann, F., Kuzniecky, R., Gendron, D. & Quesney, L.F. (1989). Myoclonus epilepsy and ragged-red fibres (MERRF). 2. Electrophysiological studies and comparison with other progressive myoclonus epilepsies. *Brain*, 112, 1261–1276.

Soderfeldt, B., Kalimo, H., Losson, Y. & Siesjo, B. (1983). Histopathological changes in rat brain during bicuculline-induced status epilepticus. In *Status epilepticus: mechanisms of brain damage and treatment*, Advances in Neurology, vol. 34, ed. A.V. Delgado-Escueta, C.G. Wasterlain, D.M. Treiman & R.J. Porter, pp. 169–175. New York: Raven Press.

356

Somerville, E.R. & Bruni, J. (1983). Tonic status epilepticus presenting as confusional state. *Annals of Neurology*, **13**, 549–551.

Sommer, W. (1880). Erkrankung des Ammonshorns als ätiologisches Moment der Epilepsie. *Archiv für Psychiatrie Nervenkrankheiten*, **10**, 631–675.

Sorel, L. & Dusaucy-Bauloye, A. (1958). A propos de 21 cas d'hypsarhythmia de Gibbs. Son traitement spectaculaire par l'A.C.T.H. *Acta Neurologica et Psychiatrica Belgica*, **58**, 130–141.

Sorel, L., Mechler, L. & Harmant, J. (1981). Comparative trial of intravenous lorazepam and clonazepam in status epilepticus. *Clinical Therapeutics*, **4**, 326–336.

Sowa, M.V. & Pituck, S. (1989). Prolonged spontaneous complex visual hallucinations and illusions as ictal phenomena. *Epilepsia*, **30**, 524–526.

Sparenborg, S., Brennecke, L.H., Jaax, N.K. & Braitman, D.J. (1992). Dizocilpine (MK-801) arrests status epilepticus and prevents brain damage induced by soman. *Neuropharmacology*, **31**, 357–368.

Sperber, E.F., Wong, B.Y., Wurpel, J.N. & Moshé, S.L. (1987). Nigral infusion of muscimol or bicuculline facilitates seizures in developing rats. *Brain Research*, **465**, 243–250.

Spielmeyer, W. (1927). Die Pathogenese des Epilepetischen Krampfes. *Zeitschrift für die Gesamte Neurologie und Psychiatrie*, **109**, 501–515.

Stanley, J.H. (1980). Rectal disease in a patient with delirium tremens. *Journal of the American Medical Association*, **243**, 1749–1750.

Stanley, T.V. (1982). Oral chlormethiazole in childhood epilepsy. *Archives of Disease in Childhood*, **57**, 242–243.

Stanski, D.R., Mihm, F.G., Rosenthal, M.H. & Kalman, S.M. (1980). Pharmacokinetics of high-dose thiopental used in cerebral resuscitation. *Anesthesiology*, **53**, 169–171.

Steriade, M. & Llinas, R.R. (1988). The functional states of the thalamus and associated neuronal interplay. *Physiological Reviews*, **68**, 649–742.

Sternbach, L.H. (1980). The benzodiazepine story. In *Benzodiazepines today and tomorrow*, ed. R.G. Priest, U. Vianna Filho, R. Amrein & M. Skreta, pp. 5–19. London: MTP Press.

Stone, W.E. & Javid, M.J. (1983). Effects of anticonvulsants and other agents on seizures induced by intracerebral L-glutamate. *Brain Research*, **264**, 165–167.

Storchheim, F. (1933). Status epilepticus treated by magnesium sulphate, injected intravenously. *Journal of American Medical Association*, **101**, 1313–1314.

Sung, C.-Y. & Chu, N.-S. (1989a). Status epilepticus in the elderly: etiology, seizure type and outcome. *Acta Neurologica Scandinavica*, **80**, 51–56.

Sung, C.-Y. & Chu, N.-S. (1989b). Epileptic seizures in intracerebral haemorrhage. *Journal of Neurology, Neurosurgery and Psychiatry*, **52**, 1273–1276.

Sung, C.-Y. & Chu, N.-S. (1990). Epileptic seizures in thrombotic stroke. *Journal of Neurology*, **237**, 166–170.

Sutherland, J.M. & Tait, H. (1969). *The epilepsies. Modern diagnosis and treatment*. Edinburgh: Livingstone.

Svedin, C.-O. (1966). Tissue distribution of chlormethiazole and compatability with ethanol and certain drugs. *Acta Psychiatrica Scandinavica*, **42** (suppl. 192), 23–25.

Takeda, A. (1988). Complex partial status epilepticus of frontal lobe origin. *Japanese Journal of Psychiatry and Neurology*, **42**, 525–530.

Tanaka, S., Sako, K., Tanaka, T. & Yonemasu, Y. (1989). Regional calcium accumulation and kainic acid (KA)-induced limbic seizure status in rats. *Brain Research*, **478**, 385–390

357

Tanganelli, P. & Regesta, G. (1991). Refractory tonic generalised status epilepticus. *European Neurology*, **31**, 413–418.

Tarnow, J., Eberlein, H.J., Oser, G., Patchke, D., Schneider, E., Schweichel, E. & Wilde, J. (1977). Hämodynamik, myokardkontraktilität, ventrikelmolumina und sauerstoffversorgung des herzens unter verschiedenen inhalationsanaethetika. *Anaesthetist*, **26**, 220–230.

Tassinari, C.A., Bureau, M., Dalla Bernardina, B. & Roger, J. (1992). Epilepsy with continuous spikes and waves during slow sleep – otherwise described as ESES (epilepsy with electrical status epilepticus during slow sleep). In *Epileptic syndromes in infancy, childhood and adolescence*, 2nd edn, ed. J. Roger, M. Bureau, C. Dravet, F.E. Dreifuss, A. Perret & P. Wolf, pp. 245–256. London: John Libbey.

Tassinari, C.A., Bureau, M., Dravet, C., Dalla Bernardina, B. & Roger, J. (1985). Epilepsy with continuous spikes and waves during slow sleep. In *Epileptic syndromes in infancy, childhood and adolescence*, ed. J. Roger, C. Dravet, M. Bureau, F.E. Dreifuss & P. Wolf, pp. 194–204. London: John Libbey,

Tassinari, C.A., Bureau, M. & Thomas, P. (1992). Epilepsy with myoclonic absences. In *Epileptic syndromes in infancy, childhood and adolescence*, 2nd edn, ed. J. Roger, M. Bureau, C. Dravet, F.E. Dreifuss, A. Perret & P. Wolf, pp. 151–160. London: John Libbey.

Tassinari, C.A., Daniele, O., Michelucci, R., Bureau, M., Dravet, C. & Roger, J. (1983). Benzodiazepines: efficacy in status epilepticus. In *Status epilepticus: mechanisms of brain damage and treatment*. Advances in Neurology, vol. 34, ed. A.V. Delgado-Escueta, C.G. Wasterlain, D.M. Treiman & R.J. Porter, pp. 465–475. New York: Raven Press.

Tassinari, C.A., Dravet, C. & Roger, J. (1977a). Encephalopathy related to electrical status epilepticus during slow sleep. *Electroencephalography and Clinical Neurophysiology*, **43**, 529.

Tassinari, C.A., Dravet, C., Roger, J., Cano, J.P. & Gastaut. H. (1972). Tonic status epilepticus precipitated by intravenous benzodiazepine in five patients with Lennox–Gastaut syndrome. *Epilepsia*, **13**, 421–435.

Tassinari, C.A., Terzano, G. & Capocchi, G., Dalla Bernardina, B., Vigevano, F., Daniele, O., Valladier, C., Dravet, C. & Roger, J. (1977b). Epileptic seizures during sleep in children. In *Epilepsy. The eighth international symposium*, ed. J.K. Penry, pp. 345–354. New York: Raven Press.

Taverner, D. & Bain, W.A. (1958). Intravenous lidocaine as an anticonvulsant in status epilepticus and serial epilepsy. *Lancet*, **ii**, 1145–1157.

Taylor, J. (1931). *Selected writings of John Hughlings Jackson*, vol. 1. *On epilepsy and epileptiform convulsions*. London: Hodder & Stoughton.

Taylor, R.L. (1981). Magnesium sulfate for AIP seizures. *Neurology*, **31**, 1371–1372.

Temkin, O. (1971). *The falling sickness: a history of epilepsy from the Greeks to the beginnings of modern neurology*, 2nd edn. London and Baltimore: Johns Hopkins Press.

Terzano, M.G., Gemignani, F. & Mancia, D. (1978). Petit mal status with myoclonus: case report. *Epilepsia*, **19**, 385–392.

Thomas, J.E., Reagan, T.J. & Klass, D.W. (1977). Epilepsia partialis continua: a review of 32 cases. *Archives of Neurology*, **34**, 266–275.

Thomas, P., Beaumanoir, A., Genton, P., Dolisi, C. & Chatel, M. (1992). 'De novo' absence status of late onset: report of 11 cases. *Neurology*, **42**, 104–110.

Thompson, S.M. & Gähwiler, B.H. (1989). Activity-dependent disinhibition. 1. Repetitive stimulation reduces IPSP driving force and conductance in the hippocampus in vitro. *Journal of Neurophysiology*, **61**, 501–511.

Thompson, S.W. & Greenhouse, A.H. (1968). Petit mal status in adults. *Annals of Internal Medicine*, **68**, 1271–1279.

Thurston, J.H., Liang, H.S., Smith, J.S. & Valentini, E.J. (1968). New enzymatic method

358

for measurement of paraldehyde: correlation of effects with serum and CSF levels. *Journal of Laboratory and Clinical Medicine*, **72**, 699–704.

Tinuper, P., Aguglia, U., Laudadio, S. & Gastaut, H. (1987). Prolonged ictal paralysis: electroencephalographic confirmation of its epileptic nature. *Clinical Electroencephalography*, **18**, 12–14.

Todt, H. & Eysold, R. (1988). Long-term observations. In *The Lennox Gastaut syndrome*. Neurology and Neurobiology, vol. 45, ed. E. Niedermeyer & R. Degen, pp. 377–386. New York: Alan R. Liss

Tomson, T., Svanborg, E. & Wedlund, J.-E. (1986). Nonconvulsive status epilepticus: high incidence of complex partial status. *Epilepsia*, **27**, 276–285.

Toner, W., Howard, P.J., Dundee, J.W. & McIlroy, P.D.A. (1979). Estimation of plasma thiopentone. *Anaesthesia*, **34**, 657–660.

Toner, W., Howard, P.J., McGowan, W.A.W. & Dundee, J.W. (1980). Another look at acute tolerance to thiopentone. *British Journal of Anaesthesia*, **52**, 1005–1008.

Toone, B.K. & Roberts, J. (1979). Status epilepticus: an uncommon hysterical conversion syndrome. *Journal of Nervous and Mental Diseases*, **167**, 548–552.

Tortella, F.C., Long, J.B. & Holaday, J.W. (1985). Endogenous opioid systems: physiological role in the self-limitation of seizures. *Brain Research*, **332**, 174–178.

Toso, V., Moschini, M., Gagnin, G. & Antoni, D. (1981). Aphasie acquise de l'enfant avec épilepsie. Trois observations et revue de la littérature. *Revue Neurologique*, **137**, 425–434.

Treiman, D.M. (1993). Generalised convulsive status epilepticus in the adult. *Epilepsia*, **34** (suppl. 1) S2–S11.

Treiman, D.M., De Giorgio, C.M., Ben-Menachem, E., Gehret, D., Nelson, L., Salisbury, S. M., Barber, K.O. & Wickboldt, C.L. (1985). Lorazepam versus phenytoin in the treatment of generalised convulsive status epilepticus: report of an ongoing study. *Neurology*, **35** (suppl. 1), 284.

Treiman, D.M. & Delgado-Escueta, A.V. (1980). Status epilepticus. In *Critical care of neurologic and neurosurgical emergencies*, ed. R.A. Thompson & J.R. Green, pp. 53–99. New York: Raven Press.

Treiman, D.M. & Delgado-Escueta, A.V. (1983). Complex partial status epilepticus. In *Status epilepticus: mechanisms of brain damage and treatment*. Advances in Neurology, vol. 34, ed. A.V. Delgado-Escueta, C.G. Wasterlain, D.M. Treiman & R.J. Porter, pp. 69–81. New York: Raven Press.

Treiman, D.M., Delgado-Escueta, A.V. & Clark, M.A. (1981). Impairment of memory following prolonged complex partial status epilepticus. *Neurology*, **31** (suppl. 4(ii)), 109.

Treiman, D.M., Gunawan, S., Walton, N.Y., Meyers, P.D. & the DVA Status Epilepticus Cooperative Study Group (1992). Serum concentrations of antiepileptic drugs following intravenous administration for the treatment of status epilepticus. *Epilepsia*, **33**, 3.

Treiman, D.M., Walton, N.Y. & Kendrick, C. (1990). A progressive sequence of electroencephalographic changes during generalised convulsive status epilepticus. *Epilepsy Research*, **5**, 49–60.

Tridon, P. & Weber, M. (1973). Conduite du traitement des états de mal épileptiques par le Ro 05–4023 (clonazepam). *Semaine des Hôpitaux de Paris*, **49** (suppl.), 29.

Trimble, M.R. (1991). *The psychoses of epilepsy*. New York: Raven Press.

Trimble, M.R. & Reynolds, E.H. (1986). *What is epilepsy? The clinical and scientific basis of epilepsy*. London: Churchill Livingstone.

Troupin, A.S., Mendius, J.R., Cheng, F. & Risinger, M.W. (1986). MK-801. In *New anticonvulsant drugs*, ed. B.S. Meldrum & R.J. Porter, pp. 191–201. London: John Libbey.

Trousseau, A. (1868a). *Lectures on clinical medicine delivered at the Hôtel Dieu, Paris*, vol. 1, transl. P.V. Bazire. London: New Sydenham Society.

Trousseau, A. (1868b). *Clinique médicale de L'Hôtel-Dieu de Paris*, tome premier. Paris: Baillière et fils.

Tsao, C.Y. (1992). Generalised tonic-clonic status epilepticus in a child with cat-scratch disease and encephalopathy. *Clinical Electroencephalography*, **23**, 65–67.

Tsukamoto, S., Horiike, N., Hisanaga, M. & Utsumi, S. (1980). The efficacy of lidocaine in status epilepticus. *Brain and Nerve*, **32**, 363–368.

Tucker, W.M. & Forster, F.M. (1950). Petit mal epilepsy occurring in status. *Archives of Neurology and Psychiatry*, **64**, 823–827.

Turcant, A., Delhumeau, A., Premel-Cabic, A., Granry, J.-C., Cottineau, C., Six, P. & Allain, P. (1985). Thiopental pharmacokinetics under conditions of long-term infusion. *Anesthesiology*, **63**, 50–54.

Turner, W.A. (1907). *Epilepsy: a study of idiopathic condition*. London: Macmillan.

Vadja, F.J.F., Symington, G.R. & Bladin, P.F. (1977). Rectal valproate in intractable status epilepticus. *Lancet*, **i**, 359–360.

Vajda, F., Williams, F.M., Davidson, S., Falconer, M.A. & Breckenridge, A. (1974). Human brain, cerebrospinal fluid, and plasma concentration of diphenylhydantoin and phenobarbital. *Clinical Pharmacology and Therapeutics*, **15**, 597–603.

Valin, A., Cepeda, C., Rey, E. & Naquet, R. (1981). Opposite effects of lorazepam on two kinds of myoclonus in the photosensitive Papio papio. *Electroencephalography and Clinical Neurophysiology*, **52**, 647–651.

Van den Berg, B.J. & Yerushalmy, J. (1969). Studies on convulsive disorders in young children. I. Incidence of febrile and nonfebrile convulsions by age and other factors. *Pediatric Research*, **3**, 298–304.

Van der Kleijn, E., Baars, A.M., Vree, T.B. & Van der Dries, A. (1983). Clinical pharmacokinetics of drugs used in the treatment of status epilepticus. In *Status epilepticus: mechanisms of brain damage and treatment*. Advances in Neurology, vol. 34, ed. A.V. Delgado-Escueta, C.G. Wasterlain, D.M. Treiman & R.J. Porter, pp. 421–440. New York: Raven Press.

van Gelder, N.M. (1986) The hyperexcited brain: glutamic acid release and failure of inhibition. In *Excitatory amino acids and epilepsy*. Advances in Experimental Medicine and Biology, vol. 203, ed. R. Schwarcz & Y. Ben-Ari, pp. 331–347. New York: Plenum Press.

van Gelder, N.M., Sherwin, A.L. & Rasmussen, T. (1972). Amino acid content of epileptogenic human brain: focal versus surrounding regions. *Brain Research*, **40**, 385–393.

van Harskamp, F., van Dongen, H.R. & Loonen, M.C.B. (1978). Acquired aphasia with convulsive disorder in children: a case study with seven years follow up. *Brain and Language*, **6**, 405–409.

Van Huffelen, A.C. & Magnus, O. (1976). The treatment of status epilepticus with clonazepam. *Nederlands Tijdschrift voor Geneeskunde*, **120**, 1734–1738.

VanLandingham, K.E. & Lothman, E.W. (1991a). Self-sustaining limbic status epilepticus. 11. Role of hippocampal commissures in metabolic responses. *Neurology*, **41**, 1950–1957.

VanLandingham, K.E. & Lothman, E.W. (1991b). Self sustaining limbic status epilepticus. 1. Acute and chronic cerebral metabolic studies, Limbic hypermetabolism and neocortical hypometabolism. *Neurology*, **41**, 1942–1949.

Van Ness, P.C. (1990). Pentobarbital and EEG burst suppression in treatment of status epilepticus refractory to benzodiazepines and phenytoin. *Epilepsia*, **31**, 61–67.

Van Orman, C.B. & Darwish, H.-Z. (1985). Efficacy of phenobarbital in neonatal seizures. *Canadian Journal of Neurological Sciences*, **12**, 95–99.

Van Rossum, J., Groeneveld-Ockhuysen, A.A.W. & Arts, R.J.H.M. (1985). Psychomotor status. *Archives of Neurology*, **42**, 989–993.

Van Sweden, B. (1985). Toxic 'ictal' confusion in middle age: treatment with benzodiazepines. *Journal of Neurology, Neurosurgery and Psychiatry*, **48**, 472–476.

Van Sweden, B. & Mellerio, F. (1988). Toxic ictal confusion. *Journal of Epilepsy*, **1**, 157–163.

Varma, N.K. & Lee, S.I. (1992). Nonconvulsive status epilepticus following electroconvulsive therapy. *Neurology*, **42**, 263–264.

Vercelletto, M. & Gastaut, J.L. (1981). Les épilepsies débutant après soixante ans. *Revue d'Electroencéphalographie et de Neurophysiologie Clinique*, **11**, 537–544.

Verhagen, W.I.M., Renier, W.O., ter Laak, H., Jaspar, H.H.J. & Gabreels, F.J.M. (1988). Anomalies of the cerebral cortex in a case of epilepsia partialis continua. *Epilepsia*, **29**, 57–62.

Verity, C.M. & Golding, J. (1991). Risk of epilepsy after febrile convulsions: a national cohort study. *British Medical Journal*, **303**, 1373–1376.

Victor, M. & Brausch, C. (1967). The role of abstinence in the genesis of alcoholic epilepsy. *Epilepsia*, **8**, 1–20.

Vignaendra, V., Loh, T.G. & Lim, C.L. (1976). Petit mal status in a patient with chronic renal failure. *Medical Journal of Australia*, **2**, 258–259.

Viswanathan, C.T., Booker, H.E. & Welling, P.G. (1978). Bioavailability of oral and intramuscular phenobarbital. *Journal of Clinical Pharmacology*, **18**, 100–105.

Vizioli, R. & Magliocco, E.B. (1953). Clinical and laboratory notes: a case of prolonged petit mal seizures. *Electroencephalography and Clinical Neurophysiology*, **5**, 439–440.

Vollmer, M.E., Weiss, H., Beanland, C. & Krumholz, A. (1985). Prolonged confusion due to absence status following metrizamide myelography. *Archives of Neurology*, **42**, 1005–1008.

Volpe, J.J. (1977). Neonatal seizures. *Clinics in Perinatology*, **4**, 43–63.

Volpe, J.J. (1981). *Neurology and the newborn*. Philadelphia: W.B. Saunders.

Volpe, J.J. (1987). *Neurology of the newborn. Major problems in clinical pediatrics*, 2nd edn, vol. 22. Philadelphia: W.B. Saunders.

Völzke, E. & Doose, H. (1979). Petit mal status and dementia. *Epilepsia*, **20**, 183.

von Albert, H.-H. (1983). A new phenytoin infusion concentrate for status epilepticus. In *Status epilepticus: mechanisms of brain damage and treatment*. Advances in Neurology, vol. 34, ed. A.V. Delgado-Escueta, C.G. Wasterlain, D.M. Treiman & R.J. Porter, pp. 453–456. New York: Raven Press.

Walker, J.E., Homan, R.W., Vasko, M.R., Crawford, I.L., Bell, R.D. & Tasker, W.G. (1979). Lorazepam in status epilepticus. *Annals of Neurology*, **6**, 207–213.

Wallace, S.J. (1988). *The child with febrile seizures*. London: Butterworth.

Wallin, A., Nergardh, A. & Hynning, P.-A. (1989). Lidocaine treatment of neonatal convulsions, a therapeutic dilemma. *European Journal of Clinical Pharmacology*, **36**, 583–586.

Wallis, W., Kutt, H. & McDowell, F. (1968). Intravenous diphenyl hydantoin treatment of acute repetitive seizures. *Neurology*, **18**, 513–525.

Walton, N.Y. (1993). Systemic effects of generalised convulsive status epilepticus. *Epilepsia* **34**, (suppl. 1).

Walton, N.Y. & Treiman, D.M. (1989). Phenobarbital treatment of status epilepticus in a rodent model. *Epilepsy Research*, **4**, 216–221.

Walton, N.Y. & Treiman, D.M. (1990). Lorazepam treatment of experimental status epilepticus in the rat: relevance to clinical practice. *Neurology*, **40**, 990–994.

Walton, N.Y. & Treiman, D.M. (1992). Treatment of experimental status epilepticus with a potent new GABA uptake inhibitor. *Epilepsia*, **33** (suppl. 3), 3.

Waltregny, A. & Dargent, J. (1975). Preliminary study of parenteral lorazepam in status epilepticus. *Acta Neurologica Belgica*, **75**, 219–229.

Wasterlain C.G. (1974). Mortality and morbidity from serial seizures: an experimental study. *Epilepsia*, **15**, 155–174.

Wasterlain, C.G. (1978). Neonatal seizures and brain growth. *Neuropadiatrie*, **9**, 213–228.

Wasterlain, C.G. & Dwyer, B.E. (1983). Brain metabolism during prolonged seizures in neonates. In *Status epilepticus: mechanisms of brain damage and treatment*. Advances in Neurology, vol. 34, ed. A.V. Delgado-Escueta, C.G. Wasterlain, D.M. Treiman & R.J. Porter, pp. 241–260. New York: Raven Press.

Wasterlain, C.G., Fujikawa, D.G., Penix, L. & Sankar, R. (1993). Pathophysiological mechanisms of brain damage from status epilepticus. *Epilepsia*, **34** (suppl. 1), S37–S53.

Watson, W.A., Godley, P.J., Garriott, J.C., Bradberry, J.C. & Puckett, J.D. (1986). Blood pentobarbital concentrations during thiopental therapy. *Drug Intelligence and Clinical Pharmology*, **20**, 283–287.

Wauquier, A. (1983). A profile of etomidate: a hypnotic, anticonvulsant and brain protective compound. *Anaesthesia*, **38** (suppl.), 26–33.

Wechsler, I.S. (1940). Intravenous injection of paraldehyde for the control of convulsions. *Journal of the American Medical Association*, **114**, 2198.

Weiermann, G. & Jacobi, G. (1988). An analysis of clinical and electrographic data in 120 patients with Lennox–Gastaut syndrome. In *The Lennox–Gastaut syndrome*. Neurology and Neurobiology, vol. 45, ed. E. Niedermeyer & R. Degen, pp. 399–408. New York: Alan R. Liss.

Weiner, R.D., Volow, M.R., Gianturco, D.T. & Cavenar, J.O. (1980*a*). Seizures terminable and interminable with ECT. *Neuroscience Letters*, **87**, 23–28.

Weiner, R.D., Whanger, A.D., Erwin, C.W. & Wilson, W.P. (1980*b*). Prolonged confusional state and EEG seizure activity following concurrent ECT and lithium use. *American Journal of Psychiatry*, **137**, 1452–1453.

Weiss, J.H., Hartley, D.M., Koh, J. & Choi, D.W. (1990). The calcium channel blocker nifedipine attenuates slow excitatory amino acid neurotoxicity. *Science*, **247**, 1474–1477.

Wells, C.E. (1975). Transient ictal psychosis. *Archives of General Psychiatry*, **32**, 1201–1203.

Wells, C.R., Labar, D.R. & Solomon, G.E. (1992). Aphasia as the sole manifestation of simple partial status epilepticus. *Epilepsia*, **33**, 84–87.

West, W.J. (1841). On a peculiar form of infantile convulsions. *Lancet*, pp. 724–725.

Westmoreland, B.F. & Gomez, M.R. (1987). Infantile spasms (West syndrome). In *Epilepsy: electroclinical syndromes*, ed. H. Lüders & R.P. Lesser, pp. 49–72. London: Springer-Verlag.

Westreich, G. & Kneller, A.W. (1972). Intravenous lidocaine for status epilepticus. *Minneapolis Medicine*, **55**, 807–808.

Whitty, C.W.M. & Taylor, M. (1949). Treatment of status epilepticus. *Lancet*, **ii**, 591–594.

Wieser, H.G. (1980). Temporal lobe or psychomotor status epilepticus: a case report. *Electroencephalography and Clinical Neurophysiology*, **48**, 558–572.

Wieser, H.G., Graf, H.P., Bernoulli, C. & Siegfried, J. (1977). Quantitative analysis of intracerebral recordings in epilepsia partialis continua. *Electroencephalography and Clinical Neurophysiology*, **44**, 14–22.

Wieser, H.G., Hailemariam, S., Regard, M. & Landis, T. (1985). Unilateral limbic epileptic status activity: stereo EEG, behavioral, and cognitive data. *Epilepsia*, **26**, 19–29.

Wieser, H.G., Swartz, B.E., Delgado-Escueta, A.V., Bancaud, J., Walsh, G.O., Maldonado, H. & Saint-Hilaire, J.M. (1992). Differentiating frontal lobe seizures from temporal lobe seizures. In *Frontal lobe seizures and epilepsies*. Advances in Neurology, vol. 57, ed. P. Chauvel, A.V. Delgado-Escueta, E. Halgren, & J. Bancaud, pp. 267–285. New York: Raven Press.

Wilder, B.J. (1983). Efficacy of phenytoin in the treatment of status epilepticus. In *Status epilepticus. Mechanisms of brain damage and treatment*. Advances in Neurology, vol. 34, ed. A.V. Delgado-Escueta, C.G. Wasterlain, D.M. Treiman & R.J. Porter, pp. 441–446. New York: Raven Press.

Wilder, B.J., Ramsay, R.E., Willmore, L.J., Feussner, G.F., Perchalski, R.J. & Shumate, J.B. (1977). Efficacy of intravenous phenytoin in the treatment of status epilepticus: kinetics of central nervous system penetration. *Annals of Neurology*, **1**, 511–518.

Wilensky, A.J., Friel, P.N., Levy, R.H., Comfort, C.P. & Kaluzny, S.P. (1982). Kinetics of phenobarbital in normal subjects and epileptic patients. *European Journal of Clinical Pharmacology*, **23**, 87–92.

Wilks, S. (1878). *Lectures on diseases of the nervous system*. London: Churchill.

Williams, D. (1956). The structure of emotions reflected in epileptic experiences. *Brain*, **79**, 29–67.

Williams, P.L., Warwick, R., Dyson, M. & Bannister, L.H. (eds.) (1989). *Gray's Anatomy*, 37th edn. Edinburgh: Churchill Livingstone.

Williamson, P.D., Spencer, D.D., Spencer, S.S., Novelly, R.A. & Mattson, R.H. (1985). Complex partial status epilepticus: a depth-electrode study. *Annals of Neurology*, **18**, 647–654.

Willis, T. (1667). *Pathologiae cerebri et nervosi generis specimen. In quo agitur de morbis convulsivis et de scorbuto*, transl. S. Pordage, 1681. London: Dring.

Wilson, P.J.E. (1968). Treatment of status epilepticus in neurosurgical patients with diazepam ('Valium'). *British Journal of Clinical Practice*, **22**, 21–24.

Winocour, P.H., Waise, A., Young, G. & Moriarty, K.J. (1989). Severe, self-limiting lactic acidosis and rhabdomyolysis accompanying convulsions. *Postgraduate Medical Journal*, **65**, 321–322.

Wolf, P. (1970). Zur Klinik und Psychopathologie des status psychomotoricus. *Nervenarzt*, **41**, 603–610.

Wong, R.K.S., Traub, R.D. & Miles, R. (1986). Cellular basis of neuronal synchrony in epilepsy. In *Basic mechanisms of the epilepsies: molecular and cellular approaches*. Advances in Neurology, vol. 44. ed. A.V. Delgado-Escueta, A.A. Ward Jr, D. M. Woodbury & R.J. Porter, pp. 583–592. New York: Raven Press.

Wood, P.R., Browne, G.P.R. & Pugh, S. (1988). Propofol infusion for the treatment of status epilepticus. *Lancet*, **i**, 480–481.

Woodbury, D.M. (1989). Phenytoin: absorption, distribution, and excretion. In *Antiepileptic drugs*, 3rd edn, ed. R. Levy, R. Mattson, B. Meldrum, J.K. Penry & F.E. Dreifuss, pp. 177–195. New York: Raven Press.

Woodbury, D.M. & Swinyard, E.A. (1972). Diphenylhydantoin: absorption, distribution, and excretion. In *Antiepileptic drugs*, ed. D.M. Woodbury, J.K. Penry & R.P. Schmidt, pp. 113–126. New York: Raven Press.

Woodson, F.G. (1943). Sciatic nerve injury due to the intramuscular injection of paraldehyde. *Journal of the American Medical Association*, **121**, 1343–1344.

Worster-Drought, C. (1971). An unusual form of acquired aphasia in children. *Developmental Medicine and Child Neurology*, **13**, 563–71.

Wroblewski, B.A. & Joseph, A.B. (1992). The use of intramuscular midazolam for acute seizure cessation or behavioral emergencies in patients with traumatic brain injury. *Clinical Neuropharmacology*, **15**, 44–49.

Wroe, S.J., Ellershaw, J.E., Whittaker, J.A. & Richens, A. (1987). Focal motor status epilepticus following treatment with azlocillin and cefotaxamine. *Medical Toxicology*, **2**, 233–234.

Yaffe, K. & Lowenstein, D.H. (1992). Pentobarbital coma for refractory status epilepticus: prognostic factors in the outcome of 17 patients. *Neurology*, **42** (suppl. 3), 263.

Yager, J.Y., Cheang, M. & Seshia, S.S. (1988). Status epilepticus in children. *Canadian Journal of Neurological Sciences*, **15**, 402–405.

Yanny, H.F. & Christmas, D. (1988). Propofol infusions for status epilepticus. *Anaesthesia*, **43**, 514.

Yasuhara, A., Yoshida, H., Hatanaka, T., Sugimoto, T., Kobayashi, Y. & Dyken, E. (1991). Epilepsy with continuous spike–waves during slow sleep and its treatment. *Epilepsia*, **32**, 59–62.

Yeoman, P., Hutchinson, A., Byrne, A., Smith, J. & Durham, S. (1989). Etomidate infusions for the control of refractory status epilepticus. *Intensive Care Medicine*, **15**, 255–259.

Young, G.B., Blume, W.T., Bolton, C.F. & Warren, K.G. (1980). Anesthetic barbiturates in refractory status epilepticus. *Canadian Journal of Neurological Sciences*, **7**, 291–292.

Young, R.S.K., Fripp, R.R., Yagel, S.K., Werner, J.C., McGrath, G. & Schuler, H.G. (1985). Cardiac dysfunction during status epilepticus in the neonatal pig. *Annals of Neurology*, **18**, 291–297.

Young, R.S.K., Osbakken, M.D., Briggs, R.W., Yagel, S.K., Rice, D.W. & Goldberg, S. (1985). *Annals of Neurology*, **18**, 14–20.

Young, R.S.K., Ropper, A.H., Hawkes, D., Woods, M. & Yohn, P. (1983). Pentobarbital in refractory status epilepticus. *Pediatric Pharmacology*, **3**, 63–67.

Zappoli, R. (1955). Two cases of prolonged epileptic twilight state with almost continuous 'wave–spikes'. *Electroencephalography and Clinical Neurophysiology*, **7**, 421–423.

Zappoli, R., Zaccara, G., Rossi, L., Arnetoli, G. & Amantini, A. (1983). Combined partial temporal and secondary generalised status epilepticus: report of a case with fear bouts followed by prolonged confusion. *European Neurology*, **22**, 192–204.

Index

Abscess, cerebral
  infantile spasm *(table) 45*
  neonatal SE *table) 38*
  tonic–clonic SE 69
  see also Cerebral infection
Absence continuing, *see* Absence SE
Absence SE
  adult onset, *see De novo* absence SE of
      late onset
  atypical absence SE
    clinical and EEG forms 103, 104,
        105, *(fig.) 106*
    emergency treatment 308, 309–10
    prognosis and outcome 309
    see also Lennox–Gastaut syndrome;
        Mental retardation
  causes 83–4
  comparison of petit mal, psychomotor
      and frontal SE *(table) 82*
  EEG 82
  early descriptions iii, 7–8, 13–14, 76
  frequency 31, 79–82, *(table) 32*
  myoclonic–astatic epilepsy 47–8
  nosological problems and
      differentiation of typical and
      atypical absence epilepsy 76–8
  synonyms *(table) 77*
  typical absence SE (petit mal SE)
    clinical and EEG form, 79–83
    emergency treatment 290
    frequency 79
    prognosis and outcome 308
Absorption of drugs *see* Pharmacokinetics
    of antiepileptic drugs; *and specific
    drugs*
Acetazolamide, myoclonic–astatic
    epilepsy 289
Acetylcholine, neurotransmitter in
    SE 167, 174, *(table) 172*

Acidosis
  experimental SE 151, 160, 163–5
  tonic–clonic SE *(table) 55*, 58, 178
  see also Lactate; Lactic acidosis
Acquired epileptic aphasia
        (Landau–Kleffner syndrome)
    and aphasia in adult nonconvulsive
        status 111
  causes 51
  clinical and EEG features 51–2
  emergency treatment 289–90
  and ESES 50–1
  and Lennox–Gastaut syndrome 103
  pathophysiology 52
  prognosis and outcome 307–8
Active metabolites, antiepileptic drugs
        193, *(table) 193*
Acute tubular necrosis, tonic–clonic SE
        61
Administration of drugs, *see*
        Pharmacokinetics of antiepileptic
        drugs; *and specific drugs*
Adrenaline
  neurotransmitter in SE *(table) 172*
  release in tonic–clonic SE 54, 57
Adrenocorticoid steroids
  in epilepsia partialis continua 287
  in infantile spasm 287, 303
  in neonatal SE, 288, 303
  in refractory SE 287, 303
  in slow wave sleep and aphasia 289–90
Adrenoleucodystrophy, tonic–clonic SE
        46
Adult-onset absence SE, *see De novo*
        absence SE of late onset
Alcohol
  complex partial SE, 129
  de novo absence SE of late onset 136
  tonic–clonic SE 67, 71

Allylglycine-induced experimental SE 160–1, 171

Alper's disease
epilepsia partialis continua 97
Lennox–Gastaut syndrome *(table) 102*
neuropathological features 154
tonic–clonic SE 61

Althesin 286

Alzheimer's disease, myoclonic SE in coma *(table) 99*

Ammon's horn sclerosis 139, 153–5; *see also* Hippocampus and amygdala; Neuropathology of SE

Amino acids, epileptogenesis 172

Aminoaciduria, neonatal SE *(table) 38*

Anaerobic glycosis, ATP levels in SE 151

Anaesthetic drugs
neonatal SE *(table) 38*
treatment of SE 201–2, 262
see also Etomidate; Isoflurane; Pentobarbitone; Propofol; Thiopentone

Angelman syndrome, myoclonic SE 47

Anterior operculum syndrome 48

Antiepileptic drug treatment, failure 202–3

Antiepileptic drugs
causing SE 71
early and established tonic–clonic SE 198, 201, 223–62
ideal drug 195–8
maintenance, long-term 202
pharmacokinetics 183–94
premonitory tonic–clonic SE 198, 203–23
refractory tonic–clonic SE: anaesthesia 201–2, 262–87
withdrawal, toxic causes of tonic–clonic SE 70–1
see also Drugs, antiepileptic *and specific drugs*

Aphasia, nonconvulsive simple partial status 111–12, 113; *see also* Acquired epileptic aphasia

Apparent volume of distribution *(table) 191*, 190–2; *see also specific drugs (absorption and distribution)*

Aspartate, neurotransmitter in SE 169, 173, *(table) 173*

ATP
cerebral levels in human and experimental SE 58, 151
levels in cardiac muscle 60

Atypical absence SE, *see* Absence SE

Aura, prolonged (simple partial SE) 114

Autism, and SE in mental retardation *(table) 73*

Autonomic changes, tonic–clonic SE 54

Azlocillin, epilepsia partialis continua 97

Behavioural disturbances, *see* Psychosis and behavioural disturbance

Benign childhood epilepsy syndromes
benign occipital epilepsy 48–9
benign rolandic epilepsy 48
emergency treatment 289
prognosis and outcome 306–7

Benign familial neonatal convulsions 41, 303, *(table) 38*

Benign myoclonic epilepsy in infants, 46, 289, 303; *see also* Myoclonic epilepsies

Benign neonatal convulsions 41, 303, *(table) 38*

Benign neonatal sleep myoclonus *(table) 38*

Benzodiazepines
emergency treatment 287–92
withdrawal, adult-onset absence SE 136–7
see also Clonazepam; Diazepam; Lorazepam; Midazolam

Berger, Hans 2, 13, 18

Bicêtre, Paris 2, 4, 5

Bicuculline-induced experimental SE 145–51, 158–60, 166, 171

Bilirubin encephalopathy, neonatal SE *(table) 38*

Biotin-responsive progressive myoclonic epilepsy 110

Bismuth poisoning, myoclonic SE in coma *(table) 99*

Blood pressure, tonic–clonic SE 57–8

Blood sugar, changes, tonic–clonic SE 57–8

Blood vessel blowouts, cause of SE 157

Blood–brain barrier 185–6

Borderline petit mal SE, *see* Absence SE

Boston Collaborative Drug Surveillance Program, drug-induced convulsions 70–1

Boundary conditions
definition and classification 25–6
electrographic SE with subtle clinical signs 130
emergency treatment 291–2
epileptic behavioural disturbance and psychosis 131–5
prolonged postictal confusional states 131, *(figs.) 132, 133*

Bourneville, Desiré Magloir 5–6, 19

Bright, Richard 8

Bromides
historical notes 285–6
in tonic–clonic SE 289

Bronchodilators, causing SE 71

Burst suppression
monitoring SE 181–2
myoclonic status in coma 100

Caelius Aurelianus 1

Calcium, intracellular
cell damage 171–3
cerebral energy 150
termination of seizure activity 150

Calcium receptor blockers, in adjunctive therapy 287

Calmeil, Louis Florentin 2, 18

Calmodulin kinase, genetic susceptibility 174

Canadian descriptions of EPC 85–6

Carbamazepine, oral therapy of complex partial SE 291

Carbon dioxide narcosis, myoclonic SE in coma *(table) 99*

Carbon monoxide poisoning, myoclonic SE in coma *(table) 99*

Cardiac arrhythmia, in tonic–clonic SE 54, 60, 179, *(tables) 55, 180*

Cardiac failure, in tonic–clonic SE 60, *(table) 180*

Cardiac hypertrophy, in SE 60

Cardiac output, in SE *(table) 55*

Cardiopulmonary surgery, myoclonic SE in coma *(table) 99*

Cardiorespiratory function
depression, and sedatives 195–6
and resuscitation, tonic–clonic SE 176

Cardiovascular disease, *see* Cerebrovascular disease

Cat scratch fever, and SE 72

Catecholamine release, in tonic–clonic SE 54, 58, *(table) 55*

Cefotaxime, epilepsia partialis continua 97

Cell damage in SE, *see* Cerebral damage

Central venous pressure, in tonic–clonic SE *(table) 55*

Centroencephalographic condition of prolonged disturbance of consciousness (CCC), *see* Absence SE

Cerebellum, pathological changes in SE 152–64, *(tables) 159, 164*

Cerebral arteritis, acquired epileptic aphasia 51

Cerebral cortex, damage in SE 152–64, *(tables) 159, 164*

Cerebral autoregulation, in SE *(table) 55*

Cerebral blood flow, evolution of change in SE *(table) 55*

Cerebral damage
allylglycine-induced seizures in baboons 160–1
cause of tonic–clonic SE 67–9
neuropathology 151–65, *(tables) 159, 164*
role of excitatory transmission 170–3
seizure-caused vs hypoglycaemia, hypoxia 163–5
status-induced 152–65, *(table) 180*
see also Gliosis and neuronal loss

Cerebral development, *see* Fetal cerebral development

Cerebral energy metabolism, neurophysiology of SE 150–1

Cerebral function monitor, electroencephalography 181–2, *(fig.) 181*

Cerebral hypoxia, in tonic–clonic SE 54–7, *(table) 55*, 69–70, *(table) 180*

Cerebral infection
  complex partial SE, 129
  electric SE during slow wave sleep
    (ESES) 49
  epilepsia partialis continua *(table) 97*
  infantile spasm 40, *(table) 45*
  myoclonic SE in coma *(table) 99*
  neonatal SE *(table) 38*
  outcome of neonatal SE *(table) 302*
  presenting as SE *(table) 69*
  SE in mental retardation *(table) 73*
  tonic–clonic SE 67, 69, *(table) 68*
Cerebral haemorrhage, infarction
    (table) 180; see also Cerebrovascular
    disease
Cerebral ischaemia, cerebral damage in
    158–60, 153–8, 163–5, *(table) 164*
Cerebral malformation
  cause of neonatal SE *(table) 38*
  neonatal myoclonic encephalopathy
    40
  outcome of neonatal SE *(table) 302*
Cerebral metabolism, evolution of change
    in SE *(table) 55*
Cerebral oedema, in SE *(table) 55*, 59,
    (table) 180, 182
Cerebral palsy
  early infantile epileptic encephalopathy
    40
  Lennox–Gastaut syndrome *(table) 102*
Cerebral side-effects of drugs 195
Cerebral venous thrombosis *(table) 180*
Cerebral trauma
  complex partial SE 129
  epilepsia partialis continua *(table) 97*
  infantile spasm *(table) 45*
  myoclonic SE in coma 98, *(table) 99*
  SE in mental retardation *(table) 73*
  tonic–clonic SE 67–8, 76, *(table) 68*
Cerebral tumour
  acquired epileptic aphasia 51
  complex partial SE *(fig.) 126*, 129
  epilepsia partialis continua *(table) 97*
  infantile spasm *(table) 45*
  presenting as SE *(table) 69*
  SE in mental retardation *(table) 73*
  tonic–clonic SE 67, *(table) 68*, 69, 76
Cerebrovascular disease
  complex partial SE 129

epilepsia partialis continua *(table) 97*
infantile spasm 44, *(table) 45*
neonatal SE *(table) 38*, 40
presenting as SE *(table) 69*
myoclonic SE in coma *(table) 99*
outcome of SE *(table) 302*
SE in mental retardation *(table) 73*
tonic–clonic SE 67–9, *(table) 68*
Ceroid lipofuscinoses
  childhood myoclonic SE 46
  progressive myoclonic epilepsy 110
Charcot, Jean-Martin iii, 4, 8, 19, 21
Childhood myoclonic epilepsies, *see*
    Myoclonic epilepsies
Childhood SE
  clinical forms 41–52
  emergency treatment 288–9
  influence of age on cause *(table) 42*
  prognosis and outcome 297–307
  see also specific conditions
Chloral, in SE 286
Chlormethiazole 224–30
  absorption and distribution 224,
    *(tables) 185, 191, 193, (figs.) 225,
    227*
  administration and dosage *(tables) 199,
    229*, 229–30
  biotransformation and excretion
    (table) 193, 225–6
  clinical effects 226–8
  in established SE *(table) 199*, 201
  pharmacokinetic properties *(table) 191*,
    193
  structure 224
  summary 229–30, *(table) 230*
  toxic effects 228–9
Chromosomal anomalies
  neonatal SE *(table) 38*
  SE in mental retardation *(table) 73*
Clark, L. Pierce (& Prout) 9–12, 20
Classification of SE 14–17, 23–7
  Commission on Classification and
    Terminology, International
    League against Epilepsy (1985)
    16, 110
  criteria 25, 27
  *International Classification of Seizure Type
    (1970)* 15–16; revision (1982)
    16

Les Colloques de Marseille (Xth 1962) 14–17
new classification 25–7, *(table) 26*
seizure type classification 23–4, 110–11, *(table) 24*
Clearance, defined 192
antiepileptic drug 192, *(table) 191*
Clinical forms of SE
confined largely to infancy and childhood 41–52
confined to adult life 135–7
in late childhood and adult life 53–135
in the neonatal period 34–41
pseudostatus epilepticus 137–8
Clonazepam 230–5
absorption and distribution 183, *(tables) 185, 191, 193,* 231–2
administration and dosage *(table) 199,* 234, *(table) 234*
biotransformation and excretion *(table) 193,* 232
clinical effects 232–3
in early SE 199–200, *(table) 199*
pharmacokinetic properties *(table) 191,* 193
structure 231
summary 234–5, *(table) 234*
toxic effects 233
Clorazepate, antiepileptic action and use in SE 286–7
Colman, Walter Stacy 4, 19
Coma, *see* myoclonic SE in coma
Complex partial SE 116–30
anatomical site 128–9
causes 129–30
clinical features 118–27, *(figs.) 120, 122, 124, 125*
behavioural and psychological features 122–3
comparison with absence status 81, *(table) 82*
confusion 119
fluctuation and cycling of clinical and EEG features 116–18, 126–7, 128
motor features 120–1
other features 123–7
patterns 119
speech and language disturbance 123

definition and subclassification 116–18
electroencephalography 116–18, 127–8
emergency treatment 291–2
frequency 31, *(table) 32*
historical notes 11, 14, 116–17
prognosis and outcome 311
Confusional states
absence SE 79–80
confined to adult life (late-onset) 135–7
complex partial SE 119, 129
prolonged postictal 131
Congenital causes of tonic–clonic SE 72–5
prognosis and outcome *(table) 302*
Consumptive coagulopathy, in SE *(table) 55*
Contrast media, causing SE 71, 97
Convulsant drugs, *see* Allylglycine; Bicuculline; Flurothyl; Kainic acid; Penicillin
Coronary resuscitation, myoclonic SE in coma *(table) 99*
Corticosubcortical reverberating circuits 149
Corticosteroids, *see* Adrenocorticoid steroids
CT (computed X-ray tomography)
emergency investigation in tonic–clonic SE 178
in complex partial SE 129
Cytochrome *c* deficiency, epilepsia partialis continua and Alper's disease 97

De novo absence SE of late onset
clinical features and causes 136–7
emergency treatment 290
prognosis and outcome 311–12
Decompression injury, myoclonic SE in coma *(table) 99*
Definition of SE 21–3
Les Colloques de Marseille (Xth 1962) 14–17
WHO dictionary 21
Dentato-rubro-pallido-luysian atrophy, myoclonic SE 110
Dexamethasone 287

D-Glyceric acidaemia, childhood
myoclonic SE 46
Dialysis syndrome, myoclonic SE in
coma *(table) 99*
Diazepam 203–13
absorption 183, 184, *(table) 185*, 204–5
active metabolites 193
administration and dosage 211, 212,
(tables) 199, 200, 212
biotransformation and excretion
(table) 193, 207
clinical effects *(table) 193*, 207–9
distribution *(tables) 191, 193*, 205–7,
(fig.) 206
drug concentrations in blood and brain,
experimental model *(fig.) 246*
effects on EEG *(figs.) 106, 124*, 208,
(fig.) 210
in early SE 199–200
in febrile SE 288–9
pharmacokinetic properties *(table) 191*,
193
in premonitory stage of SE 198
structure 203
summary *(table) 212*
toxic effects 209–11
Disseminated intravascular coagulation
complication of SE 60
emergency treatment 179, *(table) 180*
Disseminated postinfectious
encephalomyelitis, myoclonic SE
in coma *(table) 99*
Distribution, antiepileptic drug 186–90,
(table) 191
Dopamine, neurotransmitter in SE
(table) 172
Drug intoxication, cause of tonic–clonic
SE 67, 70–1; *see also specific drugs*
Drug overdose, as a cause of myoclonic
SE in coma *(table) 99*
Drug withdrawal
de novo absence SE of late onset 136
neonatal SE *(table) 38*
tonic–clonic SE 67, 70–1, 178
Drug-induced seizures
animal models, hypertension in 60
Boston Collaborative Drug Surveillance
Program 70–1
toxic causes 70–1

Drugs, antiepileptic
absorption and route of administration,
see Pharmacokinetics of
antiepileptic drugs
blood levels and interactions 194
in emergency treatment
failure 202–3
'ideal drug' 195–8
historical notes 285–6
oral therapy
SE other than tonic–clonic 287–92
see also specific substances and conditions
pharmacokinetics 183–94
apparent volume of distribution
190–2
distribution and half-lives 186–90
see also specific drugs and conditions

Echocardiography, in SE 60
Early infantile epileptic encephalopathy
(table) 38, 40, 288, 303
Early myoclonic encephalopathy 44
Electroencephalography, historical notes
13–14
Electrographic SE 52, 79, 100, 103, 104,
105, 130, 131–5, 138
Electroencephalography, *see*
Neurophysiology of SE,
experimental; *and specific conditions*
Electrical SE during slow wave sleep
(ESES)
causes 49
clinical and EEG features 49–51
emergency treatment 289–90
in Lennox–Gastaut syndrome 103
prognosis and outcome 307
Electrocution, cause of myoclonic SE in
coma *(table) 99*
Encephalitis, neonatal SE *(table) 38*
acquired epileptic aphasia 51
epilepsia partialis continua 85–6, 95,
(table) 97
infantile spasm *(table) 45*
Lennox–Gastaut syndrome *(table) 102*
myoclonic SE in coma *(table) 99*
tonic–clonic SE 69
see also Cerebral infection; Rasmussen's
chronic encephalitis
Energy metabolism in SE, cerebral 150–1

Emergency treatment of SE 175–292; *see also specific drugs and conditions*
EPC, *see* Epilepsia partialis continua
Epilepsia minoris continua, *see* Absence SE; Complex parial SE
Epilepsia partialis continua (EPC)
  as focal motor epilepsy 91–4
  causes 95–8, *(table) 97*
  clinical and EEG features *figs.) 86, 88*
  cortical vs subcortical origin and relationship to myoclonus 86–91, *(fig.) 88*
  emergency treatment 290
  frequency *(table) 32*
  historical note 20, 130
  pathological findings 95–8, *(table) 97*
  prognosis and outcome 308–9
  Rasmussen's chronic encephalitis 85–6, 95
  Russian spring–summer tick-borne encephalitis 85
Epilepsy
  acute symptomatic, frequency of SE in 30, *(table) 32*
  established, frequency of SE in 31, *(table) 32*
  newly diagnosed, frequency of SE in 30, *(table) 32*
  see also specific conditions
Epilepsy with myoclonic absences, syndrome of 109
Epileptic twilight state, *see* Absence SE; Complex partial SE
Epileptic twilight state with wave–spikes, *see* Absence SE
Esquirol, Etienne Dominique 4, 19
ESES, *see* Electrical SE during slow wave sleep
Etat confusionnel simple, see Absence SE
Etat de mal généralisé à l'expression confusionelle, see Absence SE
Etat mal frontal polaire 81, *(table) 82; see also* Complex partial SE
Ethosuximide
  absence SE 290
  myoclonic epilepsies of childhood 289
Etomidate 279–82
  administration and dosage *(tables) 199, 281, 281*

clinical effects 279–80
  in refractory status *(table) 199,* 202
  pharmacokinetics *(tables) 185, 191, 193,* 279
  properties *(table) 191,* 193
  structure 279
  summary 281–2, *(table) 281*
  toxic effects 280
Excitatory transmission
  neurochemistry of SE 168–74
  role in cerebral damage 170–3
Excretion, antiepileptic drug 193, *(table) 193*

Febrile convulsions, and ESES 49
Febrile SE in children 45–6, 70
  emergency treatment 288–9
  frequency 28–30, 31, *(table) 32,* 41–2
  HH and HHE syndrome in 304–5
  National Cooperative Perinatal project (NCPP) 304–6
  prognosis and outcome 304–6
Feline penicillin model, generalised epilepsy 149
Ferrier, David 4, 18
Fetal brain development 74–5
  neuronal cell migration 74–5
Flunitrazepam 287
Flurothyl-induced seizures, animal models 163
Focal motor epilepsy, epilepsia partialis continua 91–4
Focal motor SE
  azlocillin 97
  cefotaxime 97
  pathologies 151–8
    animal models 158–65
  see also Epilepsia partialis continua
Foix–Chavany–Marie syndrome 48
Fosphenytoin 286
Frequency of SE 27–32, *(table) 32*
  approximate annual incidence*(table) 32*
  factors influencing 29–30
  population estimates 30–3
  as proportion of all cases 28
  as proportion of hospital admissions 28
  timing of SE 28–9
Frontal lobe, structural lesions, and SE 29–30, 67, 69, 128–9

Frontal polar SE 81*(table) 82; see also*
    Complex partial SE
Fugue, absence SE, Charcot's Parisian
    case 76

Galen 1
Gamma-amino-butyric acid (GABA),
    neurotransmitter in SE 141, 144,
    150, 166, 167–8, *(table) 172*
Gammaglobulins, in infantile spasm 288
Gastaut, H.
    International Classification of Seizure Type
        (1970) 15–16
    Les Colloques de Marseille (Xth 1962)
        15–16
Gaucher's disease
    childhood myoclonic SE 46
    progressive myoclonic epilepsy 110
Gavassetti 1
Generalised epilepsy, *see* Primary
    generalised epilepsy, *and* specific
    conditions
Generalised SE, experimental models
    (*Papio papio*, cortical penicillin and
    other chemical convulsants)
    145–9, 166
    see also specific conditions
Gliosis and neuronal loss
    Chaslin gliosis 156
    extrahippocampal, in SE 155–7,
        Fig.) 156
    hippocampal, in SE 152–5, *(fig.) 154*
    in acquired epileptic aphasia 51
    in experimental animal models 158–9,
        (tables) 159, 164
    see also Cerebral damage in SE
Glucose, intravenous, in tonic–clonic SE
    177–8
Glutamate, neurotransmitter in SE 166,
    168–73, *(table) 172*
D-Glyceric acidaemia, neonates 40
Glycine, neurotransmitter in SE
    (table) 172
GM$_2$ gangliosidosis, progressive
    myoclonic epilepsy 110
Golgi studies of cerebral tissue in SE
    157
Gowers, William Richard 4, 18
Grand mal SE, *see* tonic–clonic SE

Half-life, antiepileptic drug 186–90,
    (table) 191
Hallucinations 113, 123
Head injury, *see* Cerebral trauma
Heat stroke, myoclonic SE in coma
    (table) 99
Heavy metal poisoning, myoclonic SE in
    coma *(table) 99*
Hemiplegia, after febrile SE 304–5
Hepatic failure
    cause of tonic–clonic SE 70
    cause of myoclonic SE in coma
        (table) 99
    result of tonic–clonic SE *(table) 55,*
        60–1, 179, (table) 180
    see also specific drugs
Hepatic metabolism of drugs 192–3
Hexachlorophene, cause of neonatal SE
    (table) 38
HH (HHE) syndrome 304
Hippocrates 1
Hippocampal slice, model of seizure
    propagation and termination 141,
    144, 150
Hippocampus and amygdala
    anatomy and schemes of notation of
        hippocampus 153
    in SE 74, 116, 117–18, 128, 134,
        139–42, 151, 152–5, *(figs.) 153,*
        154, 156–70, (tables) 159, 164,
        305–6, 311
Historical notes iii, 1–20
    classical descriptions of SE 4–13
    early history 1–2
    era of electroencephalography 13–14
    Les Colloques de Marseille and
        definition and classification of SE
        14–17
    origins of SE 2–4
HIV infection, tonic–clonic SE 69
Homocysteic acid, experimental SE 169
Horsley, Victor Alexander 4, 18
Hunter, Richard 2, 18
Hydrocephalus
    Lennox–Gastaut syndrome *(table) 102*
    tonic–clonic SE 71
Hypercapnia, tonic–clonic SE 57
    emergency treatment 179
Hyperglycaemia, in SE *(table) 55, 57–8, 70*

372

Hyperglycinaemia, *see* Nonketotic
  hyperglycinaemia
Hyperkalaemia, tonic–clonic SE 61
Hyperparathyroidism, tonic–clonic SE 70
Hyperpyrexia, in SE 5–6, 10–11,
  (table) 55, 58–9, 179, *(table) 180*
Hypertension, in SE 54, *(table) 55*, 57,
  (table) 180
Hypocalcaemia
  neonatal SE *(table) 38*, 40, 70
  neonatal SE outcome *(table) 302*
Hypoglycaemia
  and cerebral damage 163–5, *(table) 164*
  emergency treatment in tonic–clonic
    SE 177–8
  infantile spasm *(table) 45*
  myoclonic SE in coma *(table) 99*
  neonatal SE 40, *(table) 38*, 70
  outcome of neonatal SE *(table) 302*
  tonic–clonic SE *(table) 55*, 57–8
  tonic–clonic SE in mental retardation
    (table) 73
Hypokalaemia, in SE *(table) 55*
Hypomagnesaemia, neonatal SE
  (table) 38, 40, 70
Hyponatraemia
  myoclonic SE in coma *(table) 99*
  neonatal SE *(table) 38*
  tonic–clonic SE *(table) 55*
Hypotension, in SE *(table) 55*, 57, 178–9,
  (table) 180, 195–6, 203
Hypoxia
  cerebral damage 151, 160, 163–5
  in tonic–clonic SE 54–7, *(table) 55*, 58,
    59, 175–6, *(table) 180*, 203
Hypoxic-ischaemic encephalopathy
  electrical SE during slow wave sleep
    (ESES) 49
  in SE in mental retardation 73
  infantile spasm 44, *(table) 45*
  neonatal SE *(table) 38*, 39–40
  outcome of neonatal SE *(table) 302*
  see also Cerebrovascular disease

Ictal fear 111
Idiopathic generalised epilepsy, *see*
  Primary generalised epilepsy
Inborn errors of metabolism, cause of
  neonatal SE *(table) 38*

Incidence of SE, *see* Frequency of SE
Inclusion body encephalitis 95
Infantile spasm (West syndrome) 8,
  42–5
  causes 44–5, *(table) 45*
  EEG 43–4
  emergency treatment 288
  frequency *(table) 32*, 43
  historical notes 8, 42–3
  Lennox–Gastaut syndrome *(table) 102*,
    103
  prognosis and outcome 303–4
Infection, *see* Cerebral infection
Insulin, causing SE 71
Intensive care unit (ITU), tonic–clonic
  SE 175–82
Intracranial pressure
  in tonic–clonic SE *(table) 55*, 59,
    (table) 180, 182
  monitoring 182
Intravenous lines, tonic–clonic SE 177
International League Against Epilepsy
  (ILAE), *see* Classification of SE
Ionisation, antiepileptic drug 185–6,
  (table) 185
IPSPs, and GABA 141
Iron, extravasated, and epileptogenesis
  157
Isoflurane 274–8
  administration and dosage *(table) 199*,
    277–8, *(table) 278*
  clinical effects 275–6
  in refractory status *(table) 199*, 202
  pharmacokinetics *(tables) 185*, *191*,
    193, 275
  pulmonary excretion 193
  structure 274
  summary 277–8, *(table) 278*
  toxic effects 276–7
Isoniazid, causing SE 71
Iterative tonic–clonic SE 75–6
ITU, *see* Intensive care unit

Jacob–Creutzfeldt disease, myoclonic SE
  in coma 98, *(table) 99*
Jackson, John Hughlings 4, 8, 18, 84

Kainic acid (kainate), in experimental SE
  161–5, 169–73

Ketamine
 anaesthetic treatment of SE 262
 and experimental SE 171
Kojewnikoff, Alexie 8, 13, 20, 85

Lactate
 cerebral concentration in SE *(table) 55*
 CSF concentrations in SE 58
 in cardiac muscle in SE 60
 in epilepsia partialis continua 97
Lactic acidosis
 in experimental status 151, 160
 in tonic–clonic SE *(table) 55*, 178
Lafora body disease
 childhood myoclonic SE 46
 progressive myoclonic epilepsy 110
Lamotrigine
 disseminated intravascular coagulation
  in SE 60
 in tonic-clonic SE 286, 291
Landau–Kleffner syndrome, *see* Acquired
  epileptic aphasia
Language disturbance in SE, *see* Speech
  disturbance in SE
Lennox, William 13–14, 20
Lennox–Gastaut syndrome
 age of onset 103
 and absence SE, comparisons 84
 cause 102, *(table) 102*
 clinical patterns 103–8
  atypical absence SE 104–5, *(fig.) 106*
  minor motor SE (myoclonic
   encephalopathy) 107–8
  subclinical SE 105
  tonic SE 105–7
 differentiation from absence status
  48
 electroencephalography 103, 104, 105,
  (fig.) 106, 107–8, *(fig.) 108*
 emergency treatment 291
 historical notes 101
 mental retardation, specific forms of SE
  in 101–8
 prognosis and outcome 309–10
 underlying pathologies 102
Lethargy, absence SE 80
Leucocytosis, blood and CSF in SE
  (table) 55, 61
Lidocaine, *see* Lignocaine

Lignocaine 235–8
 administration and dosage *(table) 199*,
  237, *(table) 238*
 cause of SE 71
 clinical effects 236–7
 in early SE 199–200, *(table) 199*
 pharmacokinetic properties
  (tables) 185, 191, 193, 235–6
 structure 235
 summary 237–8, *(table) 238*
 toxic effects 237
Limbic SE, experimental *see* Neurophysiology of SE, experimental
Lipid solubility, antiepileptic drug 185–6,
  (table) 185
Lithium, cause of *de novo* absence SE of
  late onset 136
Loading dose, antiepileptic drug 192
Long-term maintenance antiepileptic
  therapy 202
Lorazepam 238–44
 absorption and distribution *(tables) 185,
  191, 193*, 239–41
 administration and dosage *(tables) 199,
  200*, 243, *(table) 244*
 biotransformation and excretion
  (table) 193, 241
 clinical effects 241–3
 drug concentrations in brain and blood,
  experimental models *(Fig.) 240*
 in early SE 199–200, *(tables) 199, 200*
 pharmacokinetic properties *(table) 191*,
  193
 structure 239
 summary 243–4, *(table) 244*
 toxic effects 243
Low birth weight, and SE in mental
  retardation *(table) 73*

Magnesium sulphate
 antiepileptic action 286
 properties 286
Maternal toxaemia, cause of infantile
  spasm *(table) 45*
Magnetic resonance imaging (MRI)
 cerebral oedema in SE 59
 complex partial SE 129
 fractal analysis 72
 neuronal migrational defects 71–5

ventricular enlargement 300
Magnetic resonance spectroscopy (MRS)
    cerebral metabolism in SE 58
    in epilepsia partialis continua 97
    in experimental SE 151
Maintenance antiepileptic therapy,
        long-term 202
Marseilles, Les Colloques de Marseille,
        Xth (1962) 14–17
Meglumine, and SE 71
Membrane phospholipids, breakdown,
        role in SE 174
Meningitis
    electrical SE during slow wave sleep
        (ESES) 49
    infantile spasm *(table) 45*
    neonatal SE *(table) 38*
    tonic–clonic SE 69
    see also Cerebral infection
Mental retardation
    complex partial SE 129
    emergency treatment 292
    frequency 31, 101
    prognosis and outcome 309
    SE in *(table) 73*
    specific forms of SE in 100–8
        atypical absence SE 104–5; *see also*
            Absence SE
        minor motor SE (myoclonic
            encephalopathy) 107–8
        tonic SE 105–7
Mercury, cause of neonatal SE *(table) 38*
Mesial temporal sclerosis, *see*
            Hippocampus and amygdala
Metabolic acidosis, tonic–clonic SE 58
Metabolic disorder
    complex partial SE 129
    de novo absence SE of late onset 136
    emergency treatment 179, *(table) 180*
    infantile spasm 44, *(table) 45*
    myoclonic SE in coma 98, *(table) 98*
    neonatal myoclonic encephalopathy 40
    neonatal SE, *(table) 38*
    presenting as SE *(table) 69*
    SE in mental retardation *(table) 73*
    tonic–clonic SE 67, 70, *(table) 68*
Methylmalonic acidaemia, neonates 40
Methylphenidate, in Lennox–Gastaut
        syndrome 291

Metrizamide, tonic–clonic SE 71, 97
    de novo absence SE of late onset 136
Midazolam 213–18
    absorption and distribution 183,
        (tables) 185, 191, 193, 214,
        (fig.) 216
    administration and dosage *(table) 199,*
        217, *(table) 217*
    biotransformation and excretion
        (table) 193, 214
    clinical effects 214–15
    pharmacokinetic properties
        (tables) 191, 193
    in premonitory stage of SE 198,
        (tables) 199, 200
    structure 213
    summary 217–18, *(table) 217*
    toxic effects 215–16
MK-801, and experimental SE 171
Microdysgenesis 72; *see also* Neuronal
        migrational defects
Minor epileptic SE, *see* Absence SE;
        Complex partial SE
Minor motor SE (myoclonic
        encephalopathy), in
        Lennox–Gastaut syndrome and
        other forms of mental retardation
        107–8
Mitochondrial disease (mitochondrial
        cytopathy)
    childhood myoclonic SE 46
    progressive myoclonic epilepsy 110,
        310
    tonic–clonic SE 71
Mortality and morbidity of SE 293–301
    early mortality and morbidity statistics
        293–4, *(table) 296*
    factors influencing outcome 300–1
    recent studies of morbidity 298–300
    recent studies of mortality 294–8
    in adults *(table) 296*
    see also specific conditions and drugs
Motor activity, tonic–clonic SE 5–6,
        9–11, 53–4
Multiorgan failure, in SE 60, *(table)
        180*
Multiple sclerosis, and SE 71
Myoclonic–astatic epilepsy, *see* Myoclonic
        epilepsies

Myoclonic dystonia 90–1
Myoclonic encephalopathy (minor motor
    SE), in Lennox–Gastaut syndrome
    and other forms of mental
    retardation 107–8
  causes 46
Myoclonic epilepsies
  benign myoclonic epilepsy in infants
    46, 289
  causes 46
  classification 46
  cryptogenic and symptomatic childhood
    myoclonic epilepsies 46, 289,
    306
  mental retardation, myoclonic SE in
    100–8, 290, 309–10
  myoclonic–astatic epilepsy 47–8, 289,
    306
    overlap with Lennox–Gastaut
      syndrome 103
  myoclonic SE in coma 98–100, 290,
    309, *(table) 99*
  myoclonic SE in non-progressive
    encephalopathy 47, 289, 306
  myoclonic SE in primary generalised
    epilepsy 109, 291, 310
  myoclonic SE in progressive
    myoclonicepilepsies 109–10, 290,
    310
  severe myoclonic epilepsy in infants
    46–7, 306
Myoclonic SE in coma, *see* Myoclonic
    epilepsies
Myoclonic SE in nonprogressive
    encephalopathy, *see* Myoclonic
    epilepsies
Myoclonic storm 109
Myoclonus
  absence SE 80
  cortical vs brain stem vs spinal origin
    88–91
  epilepsia artialis continua 86–91
  myoclonic epilepsies of childhood
    46–8
  moyclonic SE in coma 98
  neonatal SE 40–1
  other causes 110
Myoglobinuria, and rhabdomyolysis,
    tonic–clonic SE 60

Na:K-ATPase, termination of seizure
    150
National Cooperative Perinatal Project
    (NCPP), febrile SE 305
National Hospital for the Epileptic and
    Paralysed 4, 18
Neonatal epilepsy syndromes
  benign familial neonatal seizures 41,
    288, 303
  benign neonatal convulsions 41, 288,
    303
  early infantile epileptic encephalopathy
    40, 288, 303
  emergency treatment 288
  frequency 31, *(table) 32*
  neonatal myoclonic encephalopathy 40
  prognosis and outcome 303
  see also Neonatal SE
Neonatal myoclonic encephalopathy
  infantile spasm 44, *(table) 45*
  neonatal SE in *(table) 38*, 40, 288, 303
Neonatal status epilepticus
  causes *(tables) 36, 38*, 38–40, *(table) 39*
  changing trends *(table) 39*
  clinical forms 34–40
  definition 35
  frequency 31, 34–5
  prognosis and outcome 301–3,
    (table) 302
  seizure types 36–7
  see also Neonatal epilepsy syndromes
Neuroacanthocytosis, cause of iterative
    tonic–clonic SE 76
Neuroaxonal dystrophy 110
Neurochemistry of SE 165–74
  excitatory mechanisms 168–74
  inhibitory mechanisms 167–8
Neurocutaneous disorders
  infantile spasm *(table) 45*
  neonatal SE *(table) 38*
  SE in mental retardation *(table) 73*
Neurodevelopmental disorder *(table) 38*,
    41, 44, *(table) 45*, 46, 72–5, *(fig.) 75*,
    (table) 102; *see also specific disorders*
Neuronal migration, fetal brain
    development 74–5
Neuronal migrational defects
  infantile spasm 44, *(table) 45*
  magnetic resonance imaging in 72–5

neonatal SE 40, *(table) 38*
tonic–clonic SE 72–5
Neuronal loss in SE, *see* Gliosis and
    neuronal loss; Cerebral damage
Neuropathology of SE
    comparison with hypoglycaemic and
        ischaemic damage 163–5,
        (table) 164
    experimental pathology and animal
        models 158–65
    historical descriptions 8, 12
    human extrahippocampal pathology
        115–58
    human hippocampal pathology 152–5,
        (fig.) 154
    see also Gliosis and neuronal loss
Neurophysiology of SE, experimental
    animal models 140–1, *(fig.) 145*
    cerebral energy 150–1
    generalised status 145–9
    initiation of seizure activity 140–1
    limbic status 142–5, *(figs.) 142, 143,* 161
    spread and maintenance of seizure
        activity 141–9
    termination of seizure activity 149–50
Neurosarcoidosis *(fig.) 114*
Neurosurgery
    cause of SE 67–8, 76
    emergency treatment of SE 287, 288
Neurotransmitters, in SE 165, 166–74,
    (table) 172; see also specific transmitters
NMDA (*N*-methyl-*D*-aspartate) receptor,
    and epileptogenesis 165, 169, 170–4
NMS, *see* Magnetic resonance
    spectroscopy
Nonconvulsive generalised SE, situational
    related 137
Nonconvulsive simple partial SE 110–16
    classification 110–11
    clinical and EEG forms 111–16,
        (figs.) 112, 114, 115
    emergency treatment 291
    frequency *(table) 32*
    prognosis and outcome 310
    see also Simple partial SE
Nonketotic hyperglycinaemia
    childhood myoclonic SE 46
    epilepsia partialis continua 97
    myoclonic SE in coma *(table) 99*

neonatal myoclonic encephalopathy 40
Noradrenaline
    neurotransmitter in SE *(table) 172*
    release in tonic–clonic SE 47, 54
Nordiazepam, *see* Diazepam,
    biotransformation and excretion
Nystagmoid SE 111

Occipital epilepsy, benign childhood
    epilepsy syndromes 48–9, 307
Oculoclonic SE 111
Ohtahara syndrome (early infantile
    epileptic encephalopathy) *(table)
    38,* 40, 44, *(table) 45,* 288, 303
Opioid neurotransmission in SE 150,
    (table) 172
Opioids, role in SE 150, 173
Oral therapy, SE other than tonic–clonic
    287–92
Organic acidurias, in neonatal SE
    (table) 38
Outcome of SE, *see* Prognosis and
    outcome of SE

Pacemaker cells 141
    synaptic inhibition, termination of
        seizures 149
Paracetamol, in febrile status epilepticus 289
Paraldehyde 218–23
    absorption and distribution 183,
        (tables) 185, 191, 193, 218–19
    intramuscular injection 184,
        (fig.) 184
    administration and dosage *(table) 199,*
        221–2, *(table) 222*
    biotransformation and excretion
        (table) 193, 219
    clinical effects 219–20
    pharmacokinetic properties
        (tables) 191, 193
    in premonitory stage of SE 198,
        (table) 199
    pulmonary excretion 193
    structure 218
    summary 222, *(table) 222*
    toxic effects 220–1
Parenterovite
    acute allergic reactions 195–6
    see also Thiamine

Partial SE, experimental, *see*
Neurochemistry of SE;
Neuropathology of SE;
Neurophysiology of SE
Partial SE, clinical, *see* Complex partial
SE; Epilepsia partialis continua;
Nonconvulsive simple partial SE
Pathology, *see* Neuropathology of SE
Patient monitoring, tonic–clonic SE 177
Pancreatitis, acute *(table) 180*
Penfield, Wilder 13, 20
Penicillin
epilepsia partialis continua 97
feline model of generalised epilepsy 149
neonatal SE *(table) 38*
tonic–clonic SE 71
Pentobarbitone sodium 269–74
administration and dosage *(tables) 199,
273*, 273–4
clinical and toxic effects 270–3
in refractory status *(table) 199*, 202
pharmacokinetics *(tables) 185, 191,
193*, 269–70
structure 269
summary *(table) 273*, 273–4
Periodic lateralised epileptiform
discharges (PLEDS) 37, 61–2,
(figs.) 64, 65
Periodic lateralised spasms 44
Perinatal damage
infantile spasm 44
SE in mental retardation *(table) 73*
tonic–clonic SE 72–5
Petit mal status, *see* Absence SE
Petit mal status like, *see* Absence SE
pH
cerebral in experimental status 151
cerebral in SE 58
effect on drug distribution 185–6
Pharmacokinetics of antiepileptic drugs
blood levels and interactions 194
drug absorption, route of
administration 183–5
drug distribution, metabolism and
excretion *(fig.) 184, (tables) 185,
191, 193*
active metabolites 193
apparent volume of distribution
191–2

blood–brain barrier, lipid solubility
and ionisation 185–6
clearance 192
drug distribution and half-life *(fig.)
185*, 186–9, *(figs.) 187, 188, 190*
excretion 193–4, *(table) 193*
loading dose 192
hepatic metabolism 192–3
ideal antiepileptic drug in
tonic–clonic SE
antiepileptic action 196–7
pharmacokinetics 196–7
physical characteristics, side effects
and selectivity 195
see also specific drugs
Phenobarbitone 254–62
absorption and distribution 183, *(tables)
185, 191, 193*, 255–7, *(fig.) 256*
intramuscular injection *(figs.) 184,
256*
administration and dosage *(tables) 199,
200*, 260, *(table) 261*
biotransformation and excretion
(table) 193, 257–8
clinical effects 258–9
drug concentrations in blood and brain,
experimental model *(fig.) 246*
in established SE *(tables) 199, 200*, 201
pharmacokinetic properties
(tables) 191, 193
structure 254
summary *(table) 261*, 261–2
toxic effects 260
Phenylketonuria, SE in mental
retardation *(table) 73*
Phenytoin 244–54
absorption and distribution 183,
(tables) 185, 191, 193, 245–9
intramuscular injection *(fig.) 184*
administration and dosage *(tables) 199,
200*, 252–3, *(table) 253*
biotransformation and excretion
(table) 193, 249
clinical effects 250–1
drug concentrations in brain and blood,
experimental model *(fig.) 246*
fosphenytoin 286
in established SE *(tables) 199, 200*, 201
loading dose 192

pharmacokinetic properties
(tables) 191, 193
structure 245
summary *(table) 253*, 253–4
toxic effects 251–2
Phosphocreatine, in SE 58
Phospholipids, breakdown, role in SE 174
Pinel, Ph. 4, 19
pK_a *(table) 185*
Poliodystrophy, in progressive myoclonic
epilepsy 110
Porencephaly, in Lennox–Gastaut
syndrome *(table) 102*
Poriomania, iii, 12
Positron emission tomography (PET)
cerebral energy metabolism 150–1
in epilepsia partialis continua 97
Postnatal damage
infantile spasm 44
SE in mental retardation *(table) 73*
Prader-Willi syndrome, myoclonic SE in
47
Prednisone, in infantile spasm 288, 303
Prematurity, and SE in mental
retardation *(table) 73*
Premonitory (prodromal) stage of
tonic–clonic SE 53
emergency treatment 203–23
Prenatal damage
infantile spasm 44
SE in mental retardation *(table) 73*
Pressor therapy, hypotension 178–9
Prevalence of SE, *see* Frequency of SE
Prichard, James Cowles 7, 19
Primary generalised epilepsy
corticosubcortical reverberating
circuits 149
feline penicillin model 149
microdysgenesis in 72, 84
myoclonic status in 109
Prognosis and outcome of SE 293–312
continuing epilepsy 165, 299–300,
305–6
neurological sequelae 297, 298–300,
304–12
ventricular enlargement 300, 305
see also specific conditions; HH (HHE)
syndrome; Mortality and morbidity
of SE

Progressive multifocal
leucoencephalopathy, myoclonic
SE in coma *(table)* 99
Progressive myoclonic epilepsies,
childhood and adult 109–10
emergency treatment 291
prognosis and outcome 310
Prolonged behavioural disturbance as ictal
phenomenon, *see* Absence
SE; Complex partial SE
Prolonged epileptic twilight state, *see*
Absence SE; Complex partial SE
Prolonged epileptic twilight state with
almost continuous wave spikes, *see*
Absence SE; Complex partial SE
Prolonged petit mal automatism, *see*
Absence SE
Propionic acidaemia, neonatal SE 40
Propofol 282–5
administration and dosage *(tables) 199,
200, 284*, 284
clinical effects 283
in refractory status *(tables) 199, 200,*
202
pharmacokinetics *(tables) 185, 191,
193*, 282–5
structure 282
summary *(table) 284*, 285
toxic effects 283–4
Prout, Thomas P., (& Clark), quoted
9–12
Pseudoataxia 107
Pseudodementia 107
Pseudostatus epilepticus 137–8
Psychomotor status epilepticus, clinical
features 82
Psychosis and behavioural disturbance
in absence SE 81–2
in boundary syndromes 131–5, *(fig.) 133*
in complex partial SE 123, *(figs.) 124, 125*
in electrical status during slow wave
sleep 50
in *de novo* absence SE of late onset 136
Psychotropic drugs, causing SE 71
Pulmonary excretion of drugs 193
Pulmonary oedema and pulmonary
arterial hypertension
emergency treatment 179, *(table) 180*
in tonic–clonic SE 59–60

Pulmonary embolus *(table) 180*
Pyridoxine deficiency
    infantile spasm *(table) 45*, 288
    neonatal SE *(table) 38*, 40

Quisqualate-induced seizures,
    experimental SE 169

Rasmussen's chronic encephalitis 85–6,
    (fig.) 86, 95, *(fig.) 96*, 287, 308–9
Refractory SE, stage of 201
Renal failure
    myoclonic SE in coma *(table) 99*
    tonic–clonic SE *(table) 55*, 60–1, 179,
        (table) 180
Respiratory acidosis, tonic–clonic SE
    58
Respiratory depression, and sedative
    drugs 195–6; *see also specific drugs*
Respiratory impairment and failure 54–8,
    (table) 55, 179, *(table) 180*; *see also*
    specific drugs
Resuscitation, and cardiorespiratory
    function, tonic-clonic SE 176
Rett syndrome, causing SE in mental
    retardation *(table) 73*
Rhabdomyolysis, and myoglobinuria,
    tonic–clonic SE *(table) 55*, 60,
    (table) 188
Rolandic epilepsy, benign childhood
    epilepsy syndromes 48, 306
Russian spring–summer tick-borne
    encephalitis 85, 95

Sakikku 1, *(fig.) 3*, 17
Salivation and hypersection, in SE 54,
    (table) 55, 61, *(table) 180*
Salpêtrière, Paris 2, 4, 19
Sandhoff disease, cause of childhood
    myoclonic SE 46
Santa Monica conference (1980) 16–17
Secondary generalised epilepsy, *see*
    Lennox–Gastaut syndrome
Sedatives
    barbiturate/nonbarbiturate 286
    and risk of respiratory depression
        195–6
SEEG (stereoencephalography) 87,
    127–9, 134

Serotonin, neurotransmitter in SE
    (table) 172
Severe myoclonic epilepsy in infants, *see*
    Myoclonic epilepsies
Sieveking, E. H. 4, 19
Situational related nonconvulsive
    generalised SE 137
Skin changes, in tonic–clonic SE 61
Sialidosis
    childhood myoclonic SE 46
    progressive myoclonic epilepsy 110
Simple partial SE
    convulsive 84–98
    defined 111
    frequency *(table) 32*
    nonconvulsive 110–16, *(figs.) 112*,
        114, 115
    prolonged aura 114
    see also Epilepsia partialis continua;
        Nonconvulsive simple partial SE
Slow wave sleep, electrical SE during, *see*
    Electrical status during slow wave
    sleep (ESES)
Small for dates, infant and SE in mental
    retardation *(table) 73*
Sodium valproate
    disseminated intravascular coagulation
        in SE 60
    in SE 286
Sodium valproate-induced hepatic failure
    in tonic–clonic SE 61
Somatoinhibitory SE 110
Sommer region, *see* Hippocampus
Somnulence, absence SE 80
SPECT scanning
    complex partial SE 129
    epilepsia partialis continua 97
Speech disturbance
    absence SE 80
    acquired epileptic aphasia 52
    benign rolandic epilepsy 48
    complex partial SE 123, *(fig.) 126*
    de novo absence SE of late onset 136
    electrical status during slow wave sleep
        (ESES) 50
    minor motor SE 107
    myoclonic–astatic epilepsy 48
    nonconvulsive simple partial SE 136
Spike and wave stupor, *see* Absence SE